"*The Teaching Transgender Toolkit is a first of i for any educator looking to help youth serving professionals, families, and communities be more trans sensitive and inclusive. These empathy building and skills-based tools are a great way to help your audiences support transgender communities better.*"
– Leslie M. Kantor, PhD, MPH, Vice President, Education, Planned Parenthood Federation of America

"*This is a most impressive work! It is thorough, well-informed, thoughtful, current and expert. The authors not only give us rich background information about transgender lives and experiences, they also provide a Toolkit that allows us to train others, shift the culture and transform the world. Resources don't get much better than this!*"
– Marcia Quackenbush, MS, MFT, MCHES, Senior Editor and Health Education Specialist, ETR

"*At last there is a comprehensive resource to inform, guide, and inspire educators, administrators, and other professionals in their efforts to be trans-inclusive and affirming. The Teaching Transgender Toolkit is a remarkable collection of lessons that will create positive and much needed change in the world. A copy should be in every school, medical office, social service agency, and home.*"
– Al Vernacchio, M.S.Ed., Sexuality Educator, Author of For Goodness Sex: Changing the Way We Talk to Teens about Sexuality, Values, and Health.

"*FANTASTIC Resource! Every educator in every setting should have The Transgender Toolkit as a resource, whether or not there is formal teaching specifically on transgender issues. I learned so much just reviewing it.*"
– Konnie McCaffree, PhD, Sexuality Education Consultant

"*This is a necessary toolkit for all sexuality educators. In this single publication, you will find a comprehensive guide to facilitating culturally competent transgender affirming education for a wide variety of audiences. This is a must own for all educators who wish to become more competent in raising awareness regarding transgender-related issues across multiple settings.*"
– Stephanie C. Chando, MSW, LSW, MEd, University of Pennsylvania Health System

> "This toolkit provides valuable lessons for those who desire to create spaces and provide resources which all people deserve. It is clear, respectful, and easy to use. This is a must have toolkit at all Universities and should be required for all Student Affairs professionals."

– Elizabeth Amaya-Fernandez, MPH, Senior Program Coordinator of Community Outreach; Center for Alcohol Studies, Rutgers University

> "The breadth, depth and scope of The Teaching Transgender Toolkit will have a profound impact on the delivery of compassionate, highly effective trans-inclusive sex education and healthcare. Long overdue, this user-friendly manual needs to be in the hands of every educator, therapist, and healthcare provider. As I read this manual, I kept a running tally of all the places I could use it; all the providers who will benefit. I'm most thankful for the way it is thoughtfully organized and can be used by organizations just beginning their process towards creating more inclusive environments and for those ready for intensive, advanced work."

– Lisa Schulze, M.Ed, CSE, Training and Education Coordinator, The Adolescent Health Project, Women's Fund of Omaha

> "This amazing, thorough, creative book should be in the hands of every educator, every family, and every school/health care provider in the nation. It is a life-saving manual that is exactly what we need."

– Mary Jo Podgurski, RNC, EdD

© Planned Parenthood of the Southern Finger Lakes 2015

First Printing, 2015.
Second Edition.

Published by Planned Parenthood of the Southern Finger Lakes
620 West Seneca Street
Ithaca NY 14850
www.teachingtransgender.org

All rights reserved. Only handouts may be reproduced for training participants, otherwise, no part of this publication may be reprinted or utilized in any form or by electronic, mechanical, or other means, now known or hereafter invented, or in any information storage or retrieval system, without permission, in writing, from the publisher.

Printed in the United States of America.

ISBN: 978-0-9966783-0-8

THE TEACHING *transgender* TOOLKIT

A FACILITATOR'S GUIDE TO INCREASING KNOWLEDGE, DECREASING PREJUDICE & BUILDING SKILLS

By
Eli R. Green, PhD, CSE
Luca Maurer, MS, CSE, CFLE

Table of *contents*

Introduction by Authors — i
Authors' Bios — ii
About Out for Health & Planned Parenthood of the Southern Finger Lakes — iii
Our Pedagogical Framework — iv
How To Use This Toolkit — v
Lessons at a Glance — xi
Our Lesson Plan Structure — xv

FOUNDATIONS & BEST PRACTICES FOR FACILITATORS — 1
Introduction By Dr. Elizabeth Schroeder — 2
Facilitator Self-Assessment — 3
Navigating Transgender Terminology (For Facilitators) — 5
Tips For Teaching Transgender Terminology — 10
The SIEO Model — 12
Understanding Transgender People's Experiences — 14
Understanding Intersecting Identities & Oppressions — 20
Handling Frequently Asked Questions — 23
Common Participant Reactions & Challenges — 31
Handling Inappropriate Language & Offensive Questions — 34
Handling Self-Disclosure — 36
Guidance On Transgender Documentaries — 38
Guidance On Transgender Guest Speakers & Panels — 42
Creating Supportive Learning Environments — 43
Adaptations For Accessibility — 46
Leading Effective Discussions — 50
Miscellaneous Bits & Pieces — 51
Glossary of Terms (For Participants) — 53

GETTING STARTED: OPENING ACTIVITIES — 59
1. Snapshots: Assessing Participants' Pre-Existing Knowledge — 60
2. Find Someone Who . . . — 62
3. Thinking About Gender Messages — 65

TRANSGENDER "101" — 69
Introduction By Jennifer Finney Boylan — 70
4. Wait. . . What?! Understanding Transgender Terminology — 71
5. Imagining Transgender — 76
6. Are You A Boy Or A Girl? Transgender In Childhood — 81

7. What Does Non-Binary Mean? Understanding And Supporting People
   Who Have Non-Binary Gender Identities — 85
8. Myth Or Fact: Stats & Stereotypes — 90
9. Coming Out: Always & Again — 96
10. Thanks for Sharing: Responses To Coming Out — 100
11. Everybody's Gotta Go: The Importance of Restroom Access — 112

UNDERSTANDING & ADDRESSING ANTI-TRANSGENDER PREJUDICE — 117
Introduction By Jaymie Campbell, MA, MEd — 118
12. A Thousand Cuts: Understanding Anti-Transgender Microaggressions — 119
13. At The Crux: Intersecting Identities — 125
14. Check Your Privilege: Understanding & Building Awareness — 130
15. In Solidarity With: Allies As Agents Of Social Change — 137

K-12 PROFESSIONALS — 145
Introduction By Dr. Emily Greytak — 146
16. Gender Messages In Children's Books — 148
17. Kids In The Hall: Transgender Kids In School — 153
18. Supportive Services: Creating Safe Havens Of Affirmation In Schools — 158

COLLEGE & UNIVERSITY PROFESSIONALS — 163
Introduction By Nancy Jean Tubbs — 164
19. Residence Life: Working Towards Safe & Affirming Residence Halls — 166
20. Safe And Inclusive Teams: Lessons For Athletics Staff In Higher Ed — 176
21. Creating Transgender-Affirming College Health Centers — 185

MEDICAL & MENTAL HEALTH PROFESSIONALS — 191
Introduction By Dr. Jennifer Hastings — 192
22. What To Do When The Phone Rings: Welcoming Transgender Clients — 193
23. The View From Here: Accessing Medical Care From A Transgender Perspective — 198
24. It's Not Always About Transition — 206
25. Providing Transgender Affirming Therapy: Applying Pre-Existing Clinical Strengths — 215

SERVICE PROVIDING & NON PROFIT SETTINGS — 219
Introduction By Rhodes Perry, MPA — 220
26. Context Is Everything: The Journey To Accessing Services — 222
27. How Inclusive & Affirming Are We? — 229

MAKING MEANING: CLOSING ACTIVITIES — 239
28. Impact & Reflection Circle — 240
29. Navigating Next Steps — 242
30. Reflection Sheet — 244

Works Cited — 247
Resources & Recommended Reading — 251
Contributor Bios — 263
Editorial Review Board — 266
Acknowledgements — 267

Introduction by Authors

DEAR FACILITATORS:

We are so excited that this book has found its way into your hands! While we have been writing the book for the past two years, our work here is based on our more than 35 years of combined experience leading thousands of transgender-related trainings. Individually, we have led these trainings in a wide variety of settings, including: K–12 schools, colleges/universities, domestic violence shelters, feminist organizations, mental health spaces, drug/alcohol recovery centers, LGBTQ centers, church basements, community groups, foster and congregate care settings, community health centers, doctors' offices, STI/HIV prevention organizations, sports teams, and more. Along the way, we created and honed our favorite "go to" lesson plans for each of these audiences. We have taken these lesson plans, critiqued, tested and re-evaluated them, and ultimately woven them together to create this guide.

As we write this, it is truly a revolutionary time for transgender people. As the June 9, 2014 cover of *Time* magazine declared, we are at a tipping point at which transgender people's existence, lives and rights are being acknowledged and affirmed in unprecedented ways. While the increasingly positive media coverage of transgender celebrities, such as Laverne Cox, Caitlyn Jenner, Janet Mock, Jazz Jennings and Chaz Bono are strong and encouraging indicators of a cultural shift towards greater acceptance of transgender people, there is still so much work to be done—particularly to benefit those who are further marginalized because of intersecting identities, especially transgender people of color. Transgender people continue all too frequently to face discrimination, prejudice and violence. These experiences have influenced our own lives as transgender individuals, and have had a profound impact on our friends, loved ones, and communities.

As individuals, our careers center on creating the world we wish to see: one in which all people—regardless of biological sex, gender identity, gender expression or sexual orientation—are safe, respected, and affirmed. Research and our own experiences as facilitators tell us that, when implemented effectively, education is a powerful tool for reducing prejudice and instigating social change. As with any type of education, this work can be both fulfilling and challenging. One of the consistent challenges we see has been the lack of tools for supporting those who wish to do this work. In writing this book, we seek to provide high-quality tools and support for those who wish to lead transgender-related professional development and community-based trainings.

As authors, we are incredibly proud of this work, and we understand that it is imperfect. In particular, we understand that as individuals, authors, and professionals we benefit significantly from racial, economic, and other systematic privileges, and that these privileges influence our work. While writing this book, we have continually challenged and held ourselves accountable to acknowledge, own, and be cognizant of how our privilege has influenced this work and will continue to do so. We see this toolkit as a starting point and encourage others to contribute to the evolution of this work by further building, adapting, and refining the lessons it seeks to impart.

—Eli R. Green & Luca Maurer

Authors' Bios

Eli R. Green, PhD is a nationally renowned educator and scholar, specializing in transgender education and inclusion. Dr. Green is an Assistant Professor in the Center for Human Sexuality Studies at Widener University, and is the founder of the Transgender Training Institute. In his award-winning research he has investigated the effectiveness of teaching transgender-related topics in undergraduate courses, particularly in relation to reducing prejudice towards transgender and gender non-conforming people. His ongoing research continues to evaluate the effectiveness of transgender-related trainings in community-based settings. In his role as an independent trainer and consultant, Dr. Green works extensively to support non-profits, direct service providers, medical providers, and educational professionals in expanding their LGBQ and transgender-related cultural competency. This work has included developing and facilitating multiple LGBQ- and transgender-specific curricula, teaching train-the-trainer courses, and providing ongoing technical assistance, coaching and mentorship to current educators and trainers. Dr. Green holds a PhD in Human Sexuality Studies from Widener University, and Master's Degrees in Human Sexuality Education (Widener University) and Applied Women's Studies (Claremont Graduate University). Dr. Green is a Certified Sexuality Educator (CSE) through the American Association of Sexuality Educators, Counselors and Therapists (AASECT). More about Dr. Green's work can be found at *www.EliRGreenPhD.com* and *www.TransgenderTrainingInstitute.com*.

Luca Maurer, MS is the founding director of The Center for Lesbian, Gay, Bisexual & Transgender (LGBT) Education, Outreach, and Services at Ithaca College. In this role, Maurer fosters the academic success and personal growth of LGBTQ and allied students, and offers college-wide services to enhance the campus community's understanding and appreciation of LGBTQ people and themes. Under Maurer's leadership, Ithaca College was named one of the 25 best campuses in the nation for LGBTQ students, and one of the top 10 transgender-friendly colleges and universities nationwide. Maurer has taught college courses on issues of health and sexuality at the graduate and undergraduate levels. Maurer also serves as a consultant and trainer on a variety of themes, including disability, LGBTQ topics, global health, diversity, inclusion, and intersectionality and has spoken throughout the country and internationally on these issues. The American Association of Sexuality Educators, Counselors and Therapists has designated Maurer a Certified Sexuality Educator (CSE) and Certified Sexuality Counselor (CSC). Maurer has served as Senior Advisory Editorial Board member of the *American Journal of Sexuality Education*, and as a member of the Editorial Board of *The Prevention Researcher*, a multidisciplinary journal focusing on successful adolescent development and at-risk youth. Maurer is also a Certified Family Life Educator (CFLE) through the National Council on Family Relations. Co-editor of *Doing Gender Diversity: Readings in Theory and Real-World Experience* published by Westview Press in 2009, Maurer's written work on sexual orientation, gender identity, disability issues, and HIV/AIDS has appeared in a variety of publications. More about Maurer's work can be found at *www.LucaMaurer.com*.

About...
Out for Health & Planned Parenthood of the Southern Finger Lakes

Beginning in 2008 Planned Parenthood of the Southern Finger Lakes (PPSFL) was awarded grant funding from the New York State Department of Health LGBT Health and Human Services Unit to support and enhance its regional LGBT Health and Wellness project, Out for Health.

The Program

Out for Health provides outreach, education, and information to LGBT people, their healthcare providers, and the community at large about the importance of inclusive, welcoming, and respectful care for LGBT people. We provide social and support groups and programs for youth and adults in rural communities, transgender hormone therapy and preventive healthcare services, advocacy, policy guidance, and training for schools, community groups, care providers, and businesses about being LGBT-inclusive and -affirming. We are proud to have been the first Planned Parenthood affiliate in New York State to offer transgender hormone therapy and preventive care services. The program was honored with an Achievement Award in 2014 from the Gay and Lesbian Medical Association (GLMA) in recognition of contributions to the LGBT community for exemplary commitment to improving the quality of health services for transgender people in upstate New York.

Connecting the dots.

Planned Parenthood is a proud member of the Causes in Common Coalition, an organizing initiative that brings together activists in the LGBT Liberation and Reproductive Justice Movements to work against common opponents and toward the shared goal of equal rights.

Our Pedagogical Framework *and Approach*

While this work has been influenced and informed by many pedagogical approaches, our foundational framework is based on Mezirow's (1991) Transformative Learning Theory and Bloom's (1956) Taxonomy of Educational Objectives.

Transformative Learning Theory:

Transformative Learning Theory proposes that learning is most effective when participants critically engage with their own perspectives, beliefs and values during the learning process. A key element of this process is helping participants "unlearn" previously acquired inaccurate information that has shaped their perspectives. Transformative learning also requires that participants engage emotionally with the content, particularly as it relates to changing a person's attitudes and reducing their prejudice toward other groups. Transformative learning builds on the idea that for learning to create meaningful change for participants, facilitators must engage both the cognitive (information and knowledge) and affective (feelings and values) domains of their learners.

Knowledge, Attitudes and Skills:

When applying Transformative Learning Theory to cultural competency trainings, we find it helpful to utilize Bloom's approach, which entails distinguishing between knowledge, attitudes, and skills. (For our purposes, we define skills as techniques of application that help participants determine how they will integrate what they have learned into their personal and professional lives.) We have designed our lessons specifically to engage one or more of these domains and have noted them on the first page of each lesson using the visual key above.

How to Use This Toolkit

Building Solid (Training) Foundations

We have designed this book to serve as a toolkit for people who wish to facilitate transgender-related trainings. Our goal is to create a guide that is accessible to people with a wide range of training and expertise as educators and transgender content experts. While we do not expect you to read this entire guide from cover to cover, we do recommend reading through the Foundations for Facilitators section.

The introductory section of *The Teaching Transgender Toolkit* provides facilitators with specific knowledge and tools that they can apply across all of the lessons included in this book. We begin with **Foundations & Best Practices for Facilitators**, which provides information about our core assumptions, language choices, and the transgender-related themes we have prioritized throughout this work so that facilitators can better understand our approach. We have created the **Facilitator Self-Assessment** as a tool that educators can use to assess their transgender-related topical strengths and areas in which they need to grow. Understanding that using common language is one of the core pieces of an essential training, we have included guides for facilitators (**Navigating Transgender Terminology** and **Tips for Teaching Transgender Terminology**) and handouts for participants (**Glossary of Terms**) to ensure that everyone is familiar with the terms used throughout the book and trainings. We have also included several pieces that provide a foundation for teaching transgender-related content, including **The SIEO Model, Understanding Transgender People's Experiences, Understanding Intersecting Identities & Oppressions**, and **Handling Frequently Asked Questions,** to help ensure that facilitators have strong foundational knowledge of key topics, language, challenges, and controversies that will potentially emerge in any transgender-related training. The **Common Participant Reactions & Challenges, Handling Self-Disclosure, Handling Inappropriate Language & Offensive Questions**, and **Miscellaneous Bits & Pieces** sections provide detailed guidance on navigating the unique complexities of facilitating transgender-related trainings. The sections on **Creating Supportive Learning Environments, Leading Effective Discussions, Adaptations for Accessibility, Guidance on Transgender Documentaries**, and **Guidance on Transgender Guest Speakers & Panels** will be particularly useful for facilitators who are newer to leading trainings, have limited formal training in pedagogical approaches, or are looking for additional guidance on how to optimize educational methods within a transgender-related context. In combination, these sections will help ensure that facilitators are very well prepared to implement successful transgender-related trainings.

Choose Your Own (Training) Adventure

We have presented our 30 lesson plans in a "choose your own adventure" style. Specifically, we have designed "standalone" lessons that also work particularly well when combined with others to create a longer training. To that end, we have provided icebreakers, foundational/101 lessons that expand knowledge, affective-based lessons that explore values, attitudes and beliefs, skill-building lessons that help participants understand how to be transgender-affirming, and closing activities, all of which can be combined to create extended trainings. Collectively, these lessons help participants increase their foundational knowledge of transgender-related topics (including "unlearning" misguided or false information), assess and improve their attitudes toward transgender people, and build skills that will help them to be personally and professionally affirming of transgender people and their loved ones.

Tailored for Target Audiences

Since there are so many distinct audiences who need transgender-related trainings and each audience is best served by a tailored approach, we have written many of our 30 lessons with specific groups in mind. In addition to our more general **Transgender 101** and **Understanding and Addressing Anti-Transgender Prejudice** sections, we have also created separate sections for **K-12 Professionals, College & University Professionals, Medical & Mental Health Professionals,** and **Social Services & Non-Profit Settings.** Each section is introduced by a noted expert in the topical area that helps to frame the content. Those who write our introductory pieces are our colleagues, our mentors, our mensches. They have shared their varied reflections—by turns professional, poignant, historical, and humorous—and the ways in which they have played integral roles in engaging others in learning about transgender themes and transgender lives. Although they work in a variety of settings, a common thread is their commitment to furthering understanding and affecting lives positively. Their perspectives remind us all of the ways in which teaching and learning of transgender content is not merely important but *essential* to social change. More information about each of these authors is available in the **Contributor Bios** section on page 263.

Facilitator Preparation

The **Foundations & Best Practices for Facilitators** section provides extensive guidance and support to help facilitators lead effective trainings, but it is also important that facilitators seek additional information and support. The **Resources & Recommended Reading** section of this book (page 251) provides resources with which to build and expand transgender-related knowledge for facilitators and participants alike.

Some communities may also have transgender organizations, LGBTQ community centers, or educator networks that offer additional ideas, information, and support.

Selection of Lessons and Activities

As with all training materials, each activity needs to be carefully evaluated by the facilitator for its appropriateness for use in a particular community, with a particular group of participants, at a particular time. Since each lesson is designed for a unique audience, not all activities will be appropriate for all groups. When selecting lessons, consider the cognitive and affective information that will need to be processed during the lesson, and remember that participants will be able to process only limited amounts of information in a certain timeframe before becoming overwhelmed or confused. Similarly, it is important to consider the potential emotional investment required by participants, as some lessons are designed to evoke strong affective responses. For facilitators who wish to focus on skills-building, lessons should build knowledge and evaluate attitudes prior to focusing on skills.

When arranging a training for a new audience or first establishing a relationship with an organization to provide trainings, another important consideration is a group's level of pre-existing transgender-related knowledge. It is not uncommon for groups to overestimate their knowledge of or comfort with transgender-related topics. It is also common for there to be multiple levels of knowledge or comfort within a group—one or two participants may have advanced knowledge, while others may have heard the term "transgender" only in passing. Most participants will likely fall somewhere in the middle or towards the lower end of this spectrum of knowledge and comfort. Some groups do, however, truly have advanced knowledge. It is important to ask careful questions in advance of the training about how prior knowledge was established. This will help to determine whether a group is over-reporting its knowledge, or is truly advanced:

- Has your group been trained before? By whom? When did the training occur?
- In what ways does your group currently engage with transgender people?
- What steps has your group taken to increase transgender cultural competency?

Regardless of whether a group has advanced knowledge, it is still very important to include foundational pieces or steps—particularly related to terminology. In our experience, when reviewing terminology we find that even advanced groups quickly find that they are using outdated, inaccurate or conflicting terms. At the very least, we encourage facilitators to explain which terms will be used during a training session and how they are to be defined for the purposes of the training. This will help to reduce confusion and conflation.

Other important considerations when selecting lessons:

- The goals and objectives of the participants/group/inviting agency
- Your goals and objectives as a facilitator
- The background of the participants/group
- The training setting and how the information will be applied

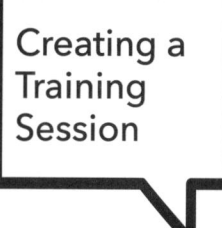

Creating a Training Session

When selecting lessons to combine, we strongly recommend that the training session begin with an opening activity and terminology. Ideally, all training sessions will also include an affective lesson (see those labeled with a ☺) to help participants evaluate their own attitudes and values related to transgender people. Including these pieces prior to addressing applications will help to ensure that any skills-based messages are based on a solid foundation of understanding and awareness. Closing activities will give participants the opportunity to reflect on what they have learned and think specifically about how they will be able to apply what they have learned once they leave the training.

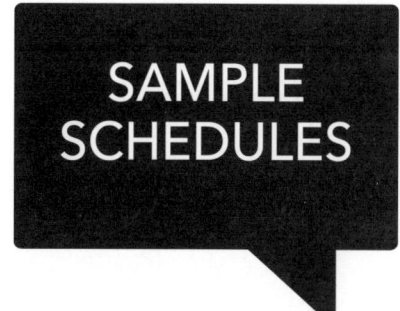

SAMPLE SCHEDULES

These are some sample schedules for half-day, full-day and series trainings, based on the target audience, amount of time available, and the goal of creating a training that incorporates knowledge, attitudes and skills. Each schedule refers to specific lessons in the book by number.

UNDERSTANDING TRANSGENDER FOR COLLEGE STUDENTS (As a part of a semester long course):

1. Lesson 3: Thinking About Gender Messages
2. Lesson 4: Wait, What?! Understanding Transgender Terminology
3. Lesson 9: Coming Out: Always & Again
4. Lesson 12: A Thousand Cuts: Understanding Anti-Transgender Microaggressions
5. Recommended Add-in: Panel First Person Experiences or Documentaries

TRANSGENDER 101 FOR FRIENDS & FAMILY OF A TRANSGENDER OR GENDER NON-CONFORMING CHILD (Half Day)

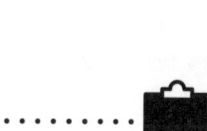

1. Lesson 1: Snapshots: Assessing Participants' Pre-Existing Knowledge
2. Lesson 4: Wait, What?! Understanding Transgender Terminology
3. Lesson 6: Are You a Boy or a Girl? Transgender in Childhood
4. Lesson 10: Thanks for Sharing: Responses to Coming Out
5. Lesson 16: Gender Messages in Children's Books
6. Lesson 28: Impact & Reflection Circle

TRAINING FOR SOCIAL AWARENESS & CHANGE (Full Day):

1. Lesson 2: Find Someone Who . . .
2. Lesson 4: Wait, What?! Understanding Transgender Terminology
3. Lesson 7: What Does Non-Binary Mean? Understanding And Supporting People Who Have Non-Binary Gender Identities
4. Lesson 9: Coming Out: Always & Again
5. Lesson 13: At the Crux: Intersecting Identities
6. Lesson 14: Check Your Privilege: Understanding & Building Awareness
7. Lesson 15: In Solidarity With: Allies As Agents of Social Change
8. Lesson 28: Impact & Reflection Circle

TRANSGENDER 101 FOR SOCIAL SERVICE STAFF (Full Day):

1. Lesson 1: Snapshots: Assessing Participants' Pre-Existing Knowledge
2. Lesson 4: Wait, What?! Understanding Transgender Terminology
3. Lesson 5: Imagining Transgender
4. Lesson 10: Thanks for Sharing: Responses to Coming Out
5. Lesson 26: Context is Everything: The Journey to Accessing Services
6. Lesson 27: How Inclusive & Affirming Are We? Inclusion Audit for Social Service Providers
7. Lesson 29: Navigating Next Steps

PROVIDING TRANS-AFFIRMING SERVICES FOR MENTAL HEALTH PROVIDERS (Full Day):

1. Lesson 3: Thinking About Gender Messages
2. Lesson 4: Wait, What?! Understanding Transgender Terminology
3. Lesson 14: Check Your Privilege: Understanding & Building Awareness
4. Recommended Add-in: Panel First Person Experiences or Documentaries
5. Lesson 22: What To Do When the Phone Rings: Welcoming Transgender Clients
6. Lesson 25: Providing Transgender-Affirming Therapy: Applying Pre-Existing Clinical Strengths
7. Lesson 28: Impact & Reflection Circle

PROVIDING TRANS-AFFIRMING SERVICES FOR MEDICAL PROVIDERS (Half Day):

1. Lesson 1: Snap Shots: Assessing Participants Pre-Existing Knowledge
2. Lesson 4: Wait, What?! Understanding Transgender Terminology
3. Lesson 23: The View from Here: Accessing Medical Care from a Transgender Perspective or, Lesson 24: It's Not Always About Transition, or, Lesson 21: Creating Transgender-Affirming College Health Centers
4. Lesson 22: What To Do When the Phone Rings: Welcoming Transgender Clients
5. Lesson 29: Navigating Next Steps

PROFESSIONAL DEVELOPMENT TRAINING FOR MIDDLE SCHOOL TEACHERS (Half Day):

1. Lesson 3: Thinking About Gender Messages
2. Lesson 4: Wait, What?! Understanding Transgender Terminology
3. Lesson 6: Are You a Boy or a Girl? Transgender in Childhood
4. Lesson 17: Kids in the Hall: Transgender Kids in School
5. Lesson 29: Navigating Next Steps

PROFESSIONAL DEVELOPMENT TRAINING FOR SCHOOL COUNSELORS & SUPPORT PROFESSIONALS (Half Day):

1. Lesson 3: Thinking About Gender Messages
2. Lesson 4: Wait, What?! Understanding Transgender Terminology
3. Lesson 17: Kids in the Hall: Transgender Kids in School
4. Lesson 18: Supportive Services: Creating Safe Havens of Affirmation In Schools
5. Lesson 29: Navigating Next Steps

TRAINING FOR RAs & RESIDENCE LIFE STAFF (Half Day):

1. Lesson 2: Find Someone Who . . .
2. Lesson 4: Wait, What?! Understanding Transgender Terminology
3. Lesson 8: Myth or Fact: Stats & Stereotypes
4. Lesson 19: Residence Life: Working Towards Safe & Affirming Residence Halls
5. Lesson 11: Everybody's Gotta Go: The Importance of Restroom Access
6. Lesson 30: Reflection Sheet

TRAINING FOR ATHLETIC DEPARTMENT STAFF (Half Day):

1. Lesson 1: Snapshots: Assessing Participants' Pre-Existing Knowledge
2. Lesson 4: Wait, What?! Understanding Transgender Terminology
3. Lesson 8: Myth or Fact: Stats & Stereotypes
4. Lesson 20: Safe And Inclusive Teams: Lessons For Athletics Staff In Higher Ed
5. Lesson 29: Navigating Next Steps

Training Duration

In addition to carefully selecting lessons for audience and content, it is also very important to be strategic about managing the duration of the training. Whenever possible and feasible, we recommend asking for a minimum of 3 hours training time, longer if you are trying to help build skills. Sometimes this is met with resistance, and facilitators may feel pressured to conduct shorter trainings. Common reasons for requests for shorter training times include low training budgets, scheduling conflicts, concerns that the facilitator will feel uncomfortable with or burdened by longer training times, or the assumption that participants already have sufficient foundational knowledge (or the converse, that there is not that much to learn about transgender people).

While some groups may not be able to allocate the extra time, many groups respond favorably once they understand that shorter trainings are less effective. It may be useful to cite the related best practices (Green, 2009) and emerging research that demonstrates that longer training times are more effective (Green, 2014). Specifically, when trying to reduce participants' level of anti-transgender prejudice, training for less than 2 hours has been shown to be completely ineffective (e.g., at the end of such trainings, participants' levels of prejudice remained unchanged and were the same as those of people who never had the training). Trainings that last 3-4 hours are ideal for reducing participants' anti-transgender prejudice. (Note that the 3-4 hours of training can be spread over multiple sessions, although that may present additional logistical challenges). At the time of publication, no studies had evaluated how much time it takes for participants to successfully acquire related cultural competence skills, but based on what we know about education and pedagogy, we can safely assume that it will take more training time than 2 hours.

If a group cannot accommodate a longer training time or hold multiple trainings to reach the target time, it is essential that you very carefully assess whether or not to move forward with a shorter training time. Even the most talented, experienced and skilled facilitators cannot make participants learn faster or absorb more information than can be cognitively or emotionally processed during a specific timeframe. Whether we are eager to reach new audiences or assume that 1 or 2 hours of training is better than none, it is important to note that trainings can actually increase participants' confusion or prejudice (Green, 2014). It is very strongly recommended that facilitators who conduct short trainings focus exclusively on sharing concrete and concise pieces of factual information rather than building empathy or skills. Likewise, it is important to manage the expectations of the group and clearly explain that shorter training times will allow for only very basic sessions.

Additional Resources

In addition to this book, we have also provided additional facilitator resources at our website **www.TeachingTransgender.com**. We will also be periodically adding new resources and recommended readings to the website, and use our Facebook/Twitter accounts to share current events articles related to transgender, non-binary and gender non-conforming people and communities.

Where noted in the lessons, we have provided supplemental printable materials to help reduce your advanced preparation time. These supplemental materials are available at: **www.TeachingTransgender.com/printables** and can be accessed with the password: **TTTprep15**

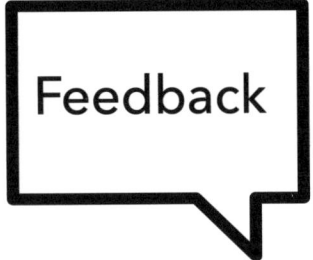

Do you wish to provide feedback about our content or lessons? We would love to hear it! Head to **www.TeachingTransgender.com** to send us a message.

Lessons at a glance

Knowledge	Attitudes	Skills

1. **Snapshots: Assessing Participants' Pre-Existing Knowledge**
   This quick warm-up activity helps participants think about their current knowledge and questions and provides the facilitator with a quick "snapshot" picture of participants' pre-existing knowledge.

2. **Find Someone Who . . .**
   This icebreaker helps build a positive learning environment by helping participants get to know each other, while introducing some transgender-related concepts.

3. **Thinking About Gender Messages**
   This fun warm-up activity helps participants think about how and what they learned about gender while they were growing up.

4. **Wait, What?! Understanding Transgender Terminology**
   This foundational activity helps participants learn the basics of transgender-related terminology through an interactive worksheet and guided discussion, which helps to clarify common misunderstandings and confusion related to transgender people, experiences and terminologies.

5. **Imagining Transgender** ☺
   This affective activity asks participants to imagine what it would be like to be either a transgender child or a transgender adult, and consider what daily life might be like as a transgender person.

6. **Are You A Boy Or A Girl? Transgender in Childhood** 💡 ☺
   With video clips of transgender children and guided discussion, this lesson helps participants understand the experiences of transgender children and establishes a framework for understanding what it means to affirm a transgender child's identity.

7. **What Does Non-Binary Mean? Understanding And Supporting People Who Have Non-Binary Gender Identities**
With a brief lecture, video clips, and a brainstorming activity, this lesson provides participants with an intermediate-level understanding of the concept of non-binary gender identities, the identities and experiences of people with non-binary identities, and the challenges that people with non-binary identities may face.

8. **Myth Or Fact: Stats & Stereotypes**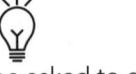
During this lesson, participants will be asked to consider whether common statements made about transgender people are myths or facts, while the facilitator helps to explain and clarify each of these statements based on current research.

9. **Coming Out: Always & Again**
By considering how they might handle having to come out as transgender in a dozen common situations, participants will gain a better understanding of how often and under what circumstances transgender people have to consider coming out.

10. **Thanks For Sharing: Responses To Coming Out**
Using quotes from popular media, this lesson establishes a framework for understanding the range of responses that transgender people receive when coming out—from outright rejection to complete affirmation—with a focus on cultivating affirming responses.

11. **Everybody's Gotta Go: The Importance Of Restroom Access**
Since restrooms are a frequently cited concern for both transgender people and allies trying to create safer spaces, this lesson explores challenges of restroom access from the perspective of transgender and gender non-conforming people and examines the implications of not having access to safe restrooms.

12. **A Thousand Cuts: Understanding Anti-Transgender Microaggressions**
This powerful activity asks participants to experience what it is like to have your gender questioned or commented on in a range of settings. This empathy-building activity is combined with information about microaggressions and how they affect the daily lives of transgender and gender non-conforming people.

13. **At The Crux: Intersecting Identities**
By guiding participants through an activity that reflects on prejudice at systematic, organizational and individual levels, this lesson underscores understanding intersectionality as a critical component of understanding transgender and gender non-conforming peoples' experiences of prejudice and discrimination.

14. **Check Your Privilege: Understanding & Building Awareness**
Using multiple teaching methods to raise awareness and increase skills, this lesson encourages participants to examine cisgender privilege and specific strategies for leveraging cisgender privilege to serve as better allies and advocates for transgender and gender non-conforming people.

15. **In Solidarity With: Allies As Agents Of Social Change**
Based on the premise that allies have an essential role in contributing to a world that is affirming of transgender and gender non-conforming people, this lesson provides participants with helpful information, strategies and scenarios for practicing the essential skills of being better allies.

16. **Gender Messages In Children's Books**
Designed for those who have small children or work with them professionally, this lesson helps participants examine the hidden gender messages in children's books, and contrasts these with books that are affirming of children who are transgender or gender non-conforming.

17. **Kids In The Hall: Transgender Kids In School**
    With reference to current research documenting the experiences of transgender and gender non-conforming youth in schools, this lesson increases awareness of the challenges that transgender and gender non-conforming middle and high school students face and explores strategies for creating affirming schools.

18. **Supportive Services: Creating Safe Havens Of Affirmation in Schools**
    Building on pre-existing skills used to support cisgender students, this lesson uses case studies to help participants explore how they can best support students who are transgender, non-binary, or gender non-conforming.

19. **Residence Life: Working Towards Safe & Affirming Residence Halls**
    Through the use of vignettes and guided discussion, this lesson helps Resident Assistants and professional Residence Life staff consider the unique needs of transgender college students and strategize about how to create safe and affirming residence halls.

20. **Safe And Inclusive Teams: Lessons For Athletics Staff In Higher Ed**
    Using case examples, this lesson provides an opportunity for athletics and recreation professionals to critically examine their current policies and practices and determine steps for creating athletics programs that are safe and affirming for transgender, non-binary, and gender non-conforming students.

21. **Creating Transgender-Affirming College Health Centers**
    By conducting a participant-led "Health Center Check-up," this lesson provides participants with the opportunity to compare their current policies and practices with the best practices for providing general and transgender-specific affirming student health care.

22. **What To Do When The Phone Rings: Welcoming Transgender Clients**
    Using a guided brainstorm activity, this lesson asks medical and mental health practitioners (both direct and indirect staff) to assess their services from a transgender person's perspective, and then provides specific strategies for implementing policies and practices that are transgender-affirming.

23. **The View From Here: Accessing Medical Care from A Transgender Perspective**
    With documentary film, real-life case examples, and guided discussion, participants will explore the challenges of accessing medical care while transgender, particularly as it relates to discrimination and bias in medical settings.

24. **It's Not Always About Transition**
    This lesson helps participants identify best practices for working with transgender people in medical settings, especially transgender people who are seeking routine, preventative and general health care, and provides community-informed strategies for working with transgender, non-binary and gender non-conforming patients.

25. **Providing Transgender Affirming Therapy: Applying Pre-Existing Clinical Strengths**
    This lesson helps mental health practitioners and therapists connect their pre-existing professional strengths with transgender-affirming best practices by exploring and evaluating culturally competent and affirming approaches to working with clients as they navigate the unique challenges of being transgender, non-binary or gender non-conforming.

26. **Context Is Everything: The Journey to Accessing Services**
    With a detailed case example, this lesson provides social service staff—from the reception desk staff to direct service providers—with an increased understanding of the specific barriers that transgender people may have to navigate while seeking supportive services.

27. **How Inclusive & Affirming Are We? Inclusion Audit For Service Providers**
    By leading participants through guided imagery while exploring their physical spaces and overall organizational values, this lesson encourages participants to view their office or organization through the perspective of a transgender person accessing services, and to implement changes to make their space affirming.

28. **Impact & Reflection Circle**
    This large-group closing activity asks participants to consider what they have learned during the training and share how what they have learned has affected them personally or professionally.

29. **Navigating Next Steps**
    This small-group closing activity asks participants to identify, consider, and share the personal or professional action steps that they will implement to become better allies and advocates for transgender, non-binary and gender non-conforming people.

30. **Reflection Sheet**
    This individual closing activity provides participants with the opportunity to reflect on what they have learned during the training and the related action steps they will take in their personal or professional lives as a result of this training.

Our Lesson Plan *structure*

Type of Lesson: At the start of each lesson, we have included a symbol to indicate whether the lesson primarily addresses knowledge, attitudes, or skills.

Knowledge   Attitudes   Skills

Overview & Rationale: A brief explanation of what the lesson includes and why it is important.

Audience: A description of the intended audience for each lesson, including target group and size.

Objectives: The specific knowledge, attitudes, and skills that participants should acquire from the lesson, in measurable terms.

Background Knowledge for Facilitators: Key content essential for facilitators to be familiar with before implementing the lesson. (See our **Facilitator Self-Assessment** on page 3 and **Resources & Recommended Reading** on page 251 for specific recommended references and resources for each topic).

Time: Estimated time for implementation. The actual time needed will depend on the facilitator, the group, participants' prior knowledge and experience, and the degree of participants' participation.

Materials: Items needed for the lesson, plus related handouts and facilitator resources. Common materials include copies of handouts, easel paper, markers, masking tape and index cards.

Preparation: Advanced steps needed to make sure the lesson is ready for implementation.

Procedure: A step-by-step guide to teaching the lesson.

Tips for Facilitators: Guidance for facilitators to consider using while leading the specific lessons. These tips are based on our experiences with testing and refining these lessons across diverse audiences and types of participants.

Evaluation Questions: Questions to help determine whether the facilitators have successfully met the learning objectives for the lesson. Evaluation questions are provided within each lesson, so that facilitators can select and compile the questions that are relevant to the specific lessons conducted and particular facilitator goals. (Please note that these evaluation questions are intended to help assess whether the training objectives have been successfully met, and are not intended as statistical measures.) These questions can be combined from each of the lessons used into one post-training evaluation survey.

Facilitator's Guide: These guides provide facilitators with answers and talking points that correspond to activities that include significant reporting back or group discussion components.

Handouts: These are photocopy-ready materials that will need to be duplicated for participants' reference or use during activities.

FOUNDATIONS & BEST PRACTICES
for Facilitators

WHY Foundations & Best Practices Are Essential

By Elizabeth Schroeder, EdD, MSW
Sexuality Education & Training Expert

• • •

Several unfortunate fallacies complicate workshop facilitation: first, that it is easy; second, that anyone can do it; and third, that all you need to do is impart information and you've succeeded. These fallacies are likely associated with inexperience and misunderstanding what it means to facilitate a program as opposed to giving a one-directional presentation. And when it comes to training on such a nuanced, sensitive and complex topic as gender, professionals need to approach the topic and process with particular intentionality and care.

True facilitation demonstrates an understanding and respect for the fact that much of what takes place during a training or workshop is not written in a book or lesson plan. Material presented will confuse, inspire, anger or provoke other reactions that must be processed within the group environment to help reduce resistance to hearing and internalizing the information. This requires that facilitators be flexible, patient and assertive in balancing the trade-off between creating a space in which all ranges of reactions—positive or negative—can be expressed and ensuring that participants leave with the factual information they need.

There is no better way to feel empowered as a facilitator than to be well-informed and well-prepared—which is where this toolkit comes in. The top questions training participants ask regarding gender identity are very basic: What are the correct terms to use with someone who identifies as transgender or gender non-conforming, and how do I—whether as a cisgender or transgender person myself—interact with this client, patient or student in ways that are respectful and focus on their needs? The terminology and tools provided in the foundations section will help you provide your training participants with the information and skills they need. When preparing to facilitate a training, be sure to read and refer back to the best practices found in the foundations section to help ensure that your training runs smoothly and produces the best possible results.

It is also important to ask yourself the same questions that you will pose to workshop participants in connection to any training presented in this toolkit, and to be honest about your strengths and comfort zones, and where you still struggle, whether in terms of content and skills or feelings relating to the content. Such self-reflection will enable you to identify what additional training or support you may need before facilitating a workshop on working with transgender individuals.

CONGRATULATIONS! In using the toolkit, you are joining in a much-needed effort to build comfort and understanding that will promote social justice and equality for people of all genders.

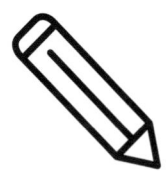

FACILITATOR SELF-ASSESSMENT

Should I lead a transgender training?

This is a great first question that all facilitators should ask themselves! Not all facilitators should facilitate all trainings—it's important to know our strengths and areas in which we need growth, particularly when facilitating sensitive topics. While you don't need advanced degrees in transgender studies or decades of experience as a facilitator to lead an effective transgender training, it is important that you have strong foundational knowledge of the topics you will be presenting. There will naturally be topics you are better prepared to facilitate or more comfortable facilitating, and that is okay. To help you identify your areas of growth, we have created this "Facilitator Self-Assessment," complete with recommended resources to help you expand your personal and professional knowledge base.

If a training participant were to ask you a question about any of the following topics, how comfortable and confident are you that you could provide a correct, detailed answer?

> Select a number from 1 (not at all) to 5 (completely).

General Knowledge/Transgender 101

1. Differences between sexual orientation and gender identity/expression ① ② ③ ④ ⑤
2. Avoiding disrespectful and offensive transgender-related language ① ② ③ ④ ⑤
3. Variations in preferred and affirming transgender-related language ① ② ③ ④ ⑤
4. A variety of individual first-person stories of transgender identity ① ② ③ ④ ⑤
5. The process of coming out as transgender, or as having a non-binary gender identity ① ② ③ ④ ⑤
6. Explaining non-binary and fluid gender identities and expressions ① ② ③ ④ ⑤
7. Common reactions from parents, children, and extended family ① ② ③ ④ ⑤
8. Common reactions from friends, peers, and social networks ① ② ③ ④ ⑤
9. Narratives of transgender people who have been affirmed and are happy ① ② ③ ④ ⑤
10. Navigating social transition, including name and pronoun changes ① ② ③ ④ ⑤
11. Navigating changing name and gender markers on identity documents ① ② ③ ④ ⑤
12. Transgender people in history and literature ① ② ③ ④ ⑤
13. Representations of transgender people in the media (positive & negative) ① ② ③ ④ ⑤
14. Positive role models within the transgender and ally communities ① ② ③ ④ ⑤
15. Navigating ongoing disclosure (visibility/stealth) ① ② ③ ④ ⑤

Sexuality and Relationships

16. Navigating dating and partner disclosure ① ② ③ ④ ⑤
17. Transgender people's sexual behaviors, expression, pleasure and satisfaction ① ② ③ ④ ⑤
18. Navigating safer sex as a transgender person (contraception and STI prevention) ① ② ③ ④ ⑤

19. Prevalence and rates of intimate partner violence and sexual assault ① ② ③ ④ ⑤
20. Making decisions about fertility, conception, pregnancy, and/or parenting ① ② ③ ④ ⑤

Navigating the World While Transgender & Related Legal Protections

21. The unique challenges of transgender youth in foster care or juvenile justice ① ② ③ ④ ⑤
22. The unique challenges transgender people face when aging ① ② ③ ④ ⑤
23. The unique challenges transgender people face on sports teams ① ② ③ ④ ⑤
24. The unique challenges transgender people face with police and prisons ① ② ③ ④ ⑤
25. The impact of discrimination on transgender individuals and communities ① ② ③ ④ ⑤
26. Common microaggressions transgender people experience ① ② ③ ④ ⑤
27. Experiences of bullying, harassment and violence in schools ① ② ③ ④ ⑤
28. Intersections of transgender identity with race, class, age, ability ① ② ③ ④ ⑤
29. Current organizational and public policy related to the needs of transgender people ① ② ③ ④ ⑤
30. Local, state and national laws regarding transgender-inclusive non-discrimination protections ① ② ③ ④ ⑤

Navigating Medical Transition

31. The current WPATH Standards of Care and medical best practices ① ② ③ ④ ⑤
32. Accessing pubertal suppression for transgender youth ① ② ③ ④ ⑤
33. Making decisions about transition-related medical care ① ② ③ ④ ⑤
34. Medical interventions and options (surgical/hormonal) ① ② ③ ④ ⑤
35. Degrees of satisfaction with (or regret for) various types of medical transition ① ② ③ ④ ⑤
36. Challenges with accessing preventive, routine, and emergency medical care ① ② ③ ④ ⑤
37. Challenges with insurance companies, particularly around transgender care exclusions ① ② ③ ④ ⑤

Being An Affirming Ally and Advocate

38. Strategies for being supportive of someone who is coming out as transgender ① ② ③ ④ ⑤
39. How to be an effective transgender ally or advocate ① ② ③ ④ ⑤
40. How to provide affirming, culturally competent services to transgender people ① ② ③ ④ ⑤
41. Examples of fully transgender-affirming organizations and companies ① ② ③ ④ ⑤

For any question or section for which you rated yourself at a 3 or below, you can use the Resources & Recommended Reading located on page 251 of this book to help build your knowledge about that specific aspect of transgender experience prior to training on that topic.

As you prepare for your trainings, you may find it useful to review these questions and draft possible explanations and answers for each one. This will help you track your knowledge base, and can be useful as a quick reference during the training.

NAVIGATING
TRANSGENDER TERMINOLOGY

. . .

Transgender terminology is challenging, even for the experts. Teaching it adds another level of complexity! There are many terms, and each has a complex history and meaning that has evolved over time. They will be defined differently by everyone you ask, and terms that some find offensive seem affirming to others. Our participants often find the nuances and complexities (not to mention the sheer number of terms) to be confusing and overwhelming. At the same time, accurate terminology is also central to being culturally competent around transgender issues.

During the time we have spent writing this book, the language used within transgender communities has changed. Similarly, our own views on best and preferred terms have evolved—and will continue to do so well after this book is in your hands. All of these factors create a unique challenge for us as authors as we provide you with our preferred terms and rationales for using them. Generally speaking:
- Transgender terminology is complex and evolves relatively quickly (especially online)
- Commonly used words mean different things to different people
- What is considered most affirming (or offensive) will vary by audience and location

Accordingly, we are providing our own definitions and rationale for the terms that we use throughout this book. We have taken exceptional care to be strategic about the terms we have chosen and do our best to explain why we have done so. Consider this section a reference for you as a facilitator. We have provided a separate alphabetical handout on page 53 that can be copied for participants.

Terms we use frequently:

Affirming:
The unequivocal support for an individual person's gender identity or expression, regardless of the biological sex they were assigned at birth; systematic support that ensures that transgender people and communities are fully represented, included, valued and honored.

Gender Identity:
A person's deep-seated, internal sense of who they are as a gendered being—specifically, the gender with which they identify themselves. All people have a gender identity.

Biological Sex:
A person's combination of genitals, chromosomes and hormones, usually categorized as "male" or "female" based on visual inspection of genitals via ultrasound or at birth, supported by the assumption that a person's gender identity will be congruent with their sex assignment. Everyone has a biological sex.

Sex Assigned at Birth:
The decision made about a person's sex based on the visual appearance of the genitals at birth. The sex someone is labeled at birth.

Transgender:
An adjective used to describe a person whose gender identity is incongruent with (or does not "match") the biological sex they were assigned at birth. We have chosen to use "transgender" as an umbrella term to refer to the full range and diversity of identities within transgender communities because it is currently the most widely used and recognized term.

Cisgender: (pronounced /sis-gender/)
An adjective used to describe a person whose gender identity is congruent with (or "matches") the biological sex they were assigned at birth. (Some people abbreviate this as "cis").

Gender Expression:
A person's outward gender presentation, usually comprised of personal style, clothing, hairstyle, makeup, jewelry, vocal inflection and body language. Gender expression is typically categorized as masculine or feminine, less commonly as androgynous. All people express a gender. Gender expression can be congruent with a person's gender identity, but it can also be incongruent if a person does not feel safe or supported, or does not have the resources needed to engage in gender expression that authentically reflects their gender identity.

Gender Conforming:
A person whose gender expression is perceived as being consistent with cultural norms expected for that gender. According to these norms, boys/men are or should be masculine, and girls/women are or should be feminine. Not all cisgender people are gender conforming and not all transgender people are gender non-conforming. (For example, a transgender woman may have a very feminine gender expression).

Gender Non-Conforming:
A person whose gender expression is perceived as being inconsistent with cultural norms expected for that gender. Specifically, boys/men are not masculine enough or are feminine, while girls/women are not feminine enough or are masculine. Not all transgender people are gender non-conforming, and not all gender non-conforming people identify as transgender. Cisgender people may also be gender non-conforming. Gender non-conformity is often inaccurately confused with sexual orientation.

Gender Neutral:
A term that describes something (sometimes a space, such as a bathroom, or an item, such as a piece of clothing) that is not segregated by sex/gender. Some language can also be gender neutral.

Coming Out:
The process through which a transgender person acknowledges and explains their gender identity to themselves and others.

Social Transition:
A transgender person's process of a creating a life that is congruent with their gender identity, which often includes asking others to use a name, pronoun, or gender that is more congruent with their gender identity. It may also involve a person changing their gender expression to match their gender identity

Affirming Pronouns:
Refers to the most respectful and accurate pronouns for a person, as defined by that person. This is also sometimes referred to as "preferred gender pronouns," although this phrasing is increasingly outdated. To ascertain someone's affirming pronouns, ask: "What are your pronouns?"

Sexual Orientation:
A person's feelings of attraction (emotional, psychological, physical, and/or sexual) towards other people. A person may be attracted to people of the same sex, to those of a different sex, people of the same and different sexes, or to people regardless of sex or gender. And some people do not experience primary sexual attraction, and may identify as asexual. Sexual orientation is about attraction to other people (external), while *gender identity* is a deep-seated sense of *self* (internal). All people have a sexual orientation that is separate from their biological sex, gender identity and gender expression.

Some terms that are generally used in a medical or mental health context:

Gender Dysphoria (GD):
The formal diagnosis in the American Psychiatric Association's *Diagnostic and Statistical Manual, Fifth Edition (DSM 5),* used by psychologists and physicians to indicate that a person meets the diagnostic criteria to engage in medical transition. In other words, the medical diagnosis for being transgender. Formerly known as *Gender Identity Disorder (GID)*. The inclusion of Gender Dysphoria as a diagnosis in the DSM 5 is controversial in transgender communities because it implies that being transgender is a mental illness rather than a valid identity. On the other hand, since a formal diagnosis is generally required in order to receive or provide treatment in the US, it does provide access to medical care for some people who wouldn't ordinarily be eligible to receive it.

Medical Transition:
A long-term series of medical interventions that utilizes hormonal treatments and/or surgical interventions to change a person's body to be more congruent with their gender identity. Medical transition is the approved medical treatment for *Gender Dysphoria*.

Pubertal Suppression:
A low-risk medical process that "pauses" the hormonal changes that activate puberty in pre-pubertal adolescents. The result is a purposeful delay of the development of secondary sex characteristics (e.g. breast growth, testicular enlargement, facial hair, body fat redistribution, voice changes, etc.). Suppression allows more time to make decisions about hormonal interventions and can prevent the increased dysphoria that often accompanies puberty for transgender youth.

WPATH:
The World Professional Association for Transgender Health (WPATH) is the international group of medical, mental health and educational professionals who publish the *Standards of Care (SOC) for the Health of Transsexual, Transgender, and Gender Non-Conforming People*. A primary function of the SOC is to provide guidance for medical and mental

health professionals in supporting access to medical transition and pubertal suppression as a means of reducing Gender Dysphoria.

Some terms we use to explain prejudice toward transgender people:

(Anti-Transgender) Prejudice:
Negative attitudes, beliefs, or reactions to transgender people. Examples of anti-transgender prejudice include: believing that transgender people are mentally disturbed, being uncomfortable sharing space with a transgender person, or thinking that transgender people should not be allowed to use public bathrooms. We use "anti-transgender prejudice" in this book instead of the more common "transphobia" because "phobia" implies a fear of transgender people, while prejudice refers to a broader range of negative attitudes toward and biased beliefs about transgender people.

(Anti-Transgender) Discrimination:
Any of a broad range of actions taken to deny transgender people access to situations/places or to inflict harm upon transgender people. Examples of discrimination include: not hiring a transgender person, threatening a gender non-conforming person's physical safety, denying a transgender person access to services, or reporting someone for using the "wrong" bathroom.

Microaggressions:
Small, individual acts of hostility or derision toward transgender or gender non-conforming people, which can sometimes be unintentional. Examples of microaggressions include: use of non-affirming name or pronouns, derogatory language, asking inappropriate or offensive questions, and exhibiting looks that reveal distaste or confusion. (See page 119 for more detailed information and examples of microaggressions).

Systematic Anti-Transgender Prejudice:
A system that denies the existence of or devalues the worth of transgender people and cannot be tied to the discriminatory actions of any one individual. Examples of systematic prejudice include: not being able to access affirming identity documents (such as a birth certificate, driver's license or passport), lack of federal or state laws that prohibit discrimination against transgender people, and lack of gender-neutral bathrooms.

Some other terms we use less frequently:

(Transgender) Ally:
A cisgender person who supports, affirms, is in solidarity with, or advocates for transgender people. The word "ally" is contentious in some circles, in which case "advocate" or the phrase "in solidarity with" is used instead.

Gender Binary:
The idea that gender is strictly an either/or option of male/men/masculine or female/woman/feminine based on sex assigned at birth, rather than a continuum or spectrum of gender identities and expressions. The gender binary is often considered to be limiting and problematic for all people, and especially for those who do not fit neatly into the either/or categories.

Gender Marker:
The marker (male or female) that appears on a person's identity documents (e.g., birth certificate, driver's license, passport, travel or work visas, green cards, etc.). The gender marker on a transgender person's identity documents will be their sex assigned at birth until they undergo a legal and logistical process to change it, where possible.

Intersex or Disorder of Sex Development (DSD):
A category that describes a person with a genetic, genital, reproductive or hormonal configuration that results in a body that often cannot be easily categorized as male or female. Intersex is frequently confused with transgender, but the two are completely distinct and generally unconnected. Participants may be more familiar with the term *hermaphrodite,* which is considered outdated and offensive.

LGBTQ:
An acronym commonly used to refer to Lesbian, Gay, Bisexual, Transgender, Queer and/or Questioning individuals and communities. LGBTQ is often erroneously used as a synonym for "non-heterosexual," which incorrectly implies that transgender is a *sexual orientation.*

Questioning:
A person who is exploring or questioning their gender identity or expression. Some may later identify as *transgender* or *gender non-conforming,* while others may not. Can also refer to someone who is questioning their sexual orientation.

Trans:
This is sometimes used as an abbreviation for "transgender."

Transgender men and boys:
People who identify as male, but were assigned female at birth. This is preferred because other language, such as *FTM* or *female-to-male,* puts more emphasis on biological sex rather than affirming gender identity. Also sometimes referred to as transmen.

Transgender women and girls:
People who identify as female, but were assigned male at birth. This is preferred because other language, such as *MTF* or *male-to-female,* puts more emphasis on biological sex rather than affirming gender identity. Also sometimes referred to as transwomen.

Some terms used to describe non-binary gender identities:

Non-Binary:
A continuum or spectrum of gender identities and expressions, often based on the rejection of the gender binary's assumption that gender is strictly an either/or option of male/men/masculine or female/woman/feminine based on sex assigned at birth.

Agender:
A person who does not identify as having a gender identity that can be categorized as male or female, and sometimes indicates identifying as not having a gender identity.

Bigender:
A person who experiences gender identity as two genders at the same time, or whose gender identity may vary between two genders. These may be masculine and feminine, or could also include non-binary identities.

Genderfluid:
A person whose gender identity or expression shifts between masculine and feminine, or moves across this spectrum.

Genderqueer:
A person whose gender identity is neither male nor female, is between or beyond genders, or is some combination of genders.

Pangender:
A person who identifies as all genders.

Two Spirit:
A term used by Native and Indigenous Peoples to indicate that they embody both a masculine and a feminine spirit. Is sometimes also used to describe Native Peoples of diverse sexual orientations, and has nuanced meanings in various indigenous sub-cultures.

Some terms we don't use (and why):

Preferred Gender Pronouns/Pronoun Preference:
Refers to the most affirming pronoun for a person, as defined by that person. We avoid using the term "preferred" because it implies that it is optional or a choice. We use the phrase "affirming pronouns" instead. These are sometimes also called "chosen pronouns." The most common pronouns are female (she/her/hers) and male (he/him/his). Gender-neutral pronouns include "they/them/theirs" or "ze/hir/hirs."

Transexual/Transsexual:
This is one of the most enduring transgender-related terms, and has evolved significantly over the years. Most commonly, "transsexual" is an older term used to refer to a transgender person who has had hormonal or surgical interventions to change their bodies to be more aligned with their gender identity than the sex that they were assigned at birth. This term has generally fallen out of favor in the United States because it over-emphasizes a person's medical transition rather than affirming their gender identity. Since historically it was a medical term, some people feel it is unnecessarily pathologizing. However, some transgender people in the US and in other countries use the term "transsexual" as an affirming identity label. In such situations, it is not considered derogatory. Unless a person refers to their own identity or reports another person's self-identification as transsexual, "transgender" is generally the best term to use.

Trans*:
Trans* is a relatively new term that seeks to represent the diversity of non-cisgender gender identities, particularly non-binary ones, within transgender communities. Some of these identities include: bigender, genderfluid, gender non-conforming, genderqueer, non-binary, agender, genderless, non-gendered, third gender, crossdresser and two-spirit identified people. While we fully support the goal of decreasing the marginalization of non-binary gender identities, we have chosen not to use trans* for two primary reasons. First, it is a relatively new term, and it is unclear how popular this term will become or how

long it will remain current. Second, we find it most useful with participants who already have a strong understanding of transgender identities, experiences and communities. Some people purposefully use trans* as the term they feel best describes their gender identity. Others shun it, for a variety of reasons. Since our target audience for this book is facilitators working with participants who are seeking foundational knowledge and skills, we have elected to use "transgender" as our primary term, and provide additional ideas and resources that facilitators can use to include and represent non-binary gender identities.

Terms we recommend avoiding:

The following terms are generally considered to be outdated, offensive or derogatory when discussing people who are, or are perceived to be, transgender or gender non-conforming. And as noted above, usage and preferred terms can vary by audience and community. This is not an exhaustive list.

- Tranny, or Trannie
- Hermaphrodite
- Transvestite
- Transgendered
- Transgendering
- Transgenders
- It
- She-Male, or He-She
- "The Surgery"
- Pre-Op, or Post-Op
- Deviant
- Fooling, or Deceiving
- "Real" sex
- Sex Change

Instead of saying this:	Say this:
"Real" sex, "real" gender, genital sex	Sex assigned at birth
A transgender	Transgender person, or, Person who is transgender
Transgenders	Transgender people, or, People who are transgender
Transgendered	Transgender
FTM, used to be a woman, born a female	Transgender man, or, Transman
MTF, used to be a man, born a male	Transgender woman, or, Transwoman
Sex Change, The Surgery, Transgendering, pre-operative, post-operative	Medical Transition
Hermaphrodite	Intersex person or Person who is intersex
Sexual preference, homosexual	Sexual orientation

REMEMBER

It is very likely that these terms and definitions will continue to evolve over time.
Check out **www.teachingtransgender.com** for updated references and resources.

TIPS
FOR TEACHING TRANSGENDER TERMINOLOGY
...

As we noted in the last section, transgender terminologies are by their very nature complex, nuanced, and can be confusing, particularly for people who are learning them for the first time. Here are some facilitator tips and tools you can use to navigate these complexities while you are teaching:

Always explain how you define the terms you use. Your participants may not have heard the terms before, or they may have alternative understandings of what the terms mean. Explaining how and why you use each term will help to reduce confusion. Often, part of the learning process is unlearning false or inaccurate information that participants have acquired previously—including terminology and language. Modeling being kind and patient in addressing instances in which participants use non-preferred terms can be particularly important as people navigate new terminology. Assume a desire to learn, and correct language missteps quickly, and then move on.

Be alert for conflations of gender identity and sexual orientation. It's still common for participants to confuse the two ideas, so it is important to emphasize that all people have both a gender identity and a sexual orientation that are separate parts of their identities. As a facilitator, be sure you are clear on each of these concepts, and invite regular feedback from participants to determine that they understand the difference. Repeat the definitions of these two concepts when facilitating, and use the handouts provided in this guide as additional resources.

Speak slowly. It sounds very basic, but don't underestimate the need to speak slowly while explaining definitions. It's similar to learning a new foreign language—our participants' brains need more time to put the words and definitions together and create meaning for them. When we speak too quickly, especially at the start of a session, we lose our participants. It will also be helpful to validate participants' confusion as they navigate this new language.

Repeat your definitions as you facilitate. Repetition throughout the session helps your participants absorb the meanings of terms and reduces confusion. For example, you might repeat the definition of transgender as "a person whose gender identity is incongruent with the sex they were assigned at birth" several times throughout the training. Even when leading longer trainings, it can be helpful to restate the definitions later in the session, because it helps build participants' confidence that they are "getting it."

Provide handouts with the terms and definitions. Depending on their individual learning style, not all participants will be able to process complex auditory information. Many participants find it useful and reassuring to know that they have a handout with the information written out that they can reference throughout the training. Guide participants' attention to terms on the handout to help keep them focused. (See page 53 for the participant **Glossary of Terms** handout.)

Ask participants to explain or clarify the terms they use. Participants will come to a session with their own terms and definitions—some of which may be outdated, offensive or inaccurate. If you are unsure how a person is using a term, ask them to clarify: "When you use the term ____, are you referring to a person whose gender identity is incongruent with the sex they were assigned at birth, or are you talking about a transgender person who has specifically undergone medical treatment?" This will help clarify things for that participant, but will also role-model using respectful, accurate terminology for the other participants.

Honor the nuances and complexities. While leading sessions on terminology, we are often trying to distill complex topics into clear and concise bits of information. This is a necessary part of teaching and learning, but can also result in oversimplification. This might sometimes play out with particularly astute participants making connections between pieces of information you provide and asking for further clarification. For example, a participant may reflect back: "If we are affirming a person's gender identity, and they identify as a man, then why would we call them a transgender man instead of just a man?" or, "Why is it called a person's 'pronoun preference' if we want to avoid talking about gender identity as a choice or a preference?" These are great questions that indicate that participants are applying what they are learning! Congratulate them on making the connections and explain your rationale.

Recognize Context. It is important to note that common and preferred language will vary (sometimes greatly) across contexts. For example: a term that is used frequently in Brooklyn may be used rarely, if at all, in Oklahoma; a term that is affirming to older transgender people may be considered outdated by younger transgender people; a term that is prevalent within a certain ethnic or cultural group may be considered offensive to others.

Be open to hearing other preferred language. While a majority of participants will not have advanced knowledge of transgender terminology, there are participants who do. They may be transgender themselves, or have friends or loved ones who are, and have strong opinions about what language is most affirming (or offensive). They may ask pointed questions about why you are using specific terms instead of others, or ask for the rationale behind a specific phrase. Be prepared to explain your language choices in a non-defensive way, provide clarifying information, provide an opportunity for the participant to explain their perspective, and validate that there are many perspectives on what language is most affirming (or offensive).

Use Gender-Neutral Language. Gender is everywhere—even in our language. As a facilitator, it is important that you role-model using gender-neutral language whenever possible, and when it makes sense to do so. Gender-neutral terms do not imply everyone is cisgender, or assume that the sex that someone was assigned at birth is accurate.

- Use language such as "partners" "parents" "children" "siblings" instead of . . .
- Use person-centered language such as "a person's penis" or a "person's vulva" instead of . . .
- Use the singular they ("they/them/theirs"), rather than assuming or presuming pronouns
- Use neutral terms such as "folks" and "everyone" instead of gendered groupings such as "ladies and gentlemen," "boys and girls" and "guys"

THE **SIEO** MODEL

One of the fundamental challenges that participants have when learning about transgender identities for the first time is figuring out how this information fits in with what they already know about the world. The SIEO Model (Green, 2013) is one way of helping participants situate and organize new information about transgender identities and assists participants in understanding the difference between sex assigned at birth, gender identity, gender expression and sexual orientation.

Biological Sex	Gender Identity	Gender Expression	Sexual Orientation
Female	(Cisgender) Woman	Feminine	Heterosexual
Male	(Transgender) Woman	Masculine	Lesbian
Intersex / Disorder of Sex Development	(Cisgender) Man	Androgynous	Gay
	(Transgender) Man	Aggressive	Bisexual
	Non-Binary	Femme Queen	Queer
	Genderqueer	Butch	Asexual
	Pangender	Femme	Same Gender Loving
	Agender	Drag King/Queen	+++
	+++	+++	

+++This is not an exhaustive list of labels, and there are many other identity labels that are used and are not reflected here. Check the **Glossary of Terms** and **Navigating Transgender Terminology** for guidance on and examples of other terms.

Biological Sex: A person's combination of chromosomes, gonads, and hormones. Most of the time, these combinations will result in typically male or female configurations, but some births may be considered to be intersex, meaning that the child's combination of chromosomes, gonads or hormones present in a way that is not strictly male or female. A person's biological sex is then recorded on a person's identity documents, and becomes their sex assigned at birth.

Gender Identity: A person's internal, psychological sense of who they are as a gendered being. A person who is cisgender has a gender identity that is congruent with or matches the sex that they were assigned at birth. A person who is transgender has a gender identity that is incongruent with or does not match the sex that they were assigned at birth. A transgender man is a person who identifies as a man but was assigned female at birth. A transgender woman is a person who identifies as a woman but was assigned male at birth. For transgender people who have non-binary gender identities, such as genderqueer or pangender, their gender identity does not fit neatly into either the man or woman category, but is incongruent with the sex that they were assigned at birth. "Cisgender" and "transgender" are both adjectives that provide additional information about a person's identity.

Gender Expression: How a person communicates gender identity to others, i.e., through gender cues such as hair length, facial hair, make-up, attire, etc. A person's gender expression is the most visible part of the person's gender. Some people express their gender in a feminine or femme way, while others express their gender in a masculine or butch way. Some people express androgyny, which is generally considered an equal mix of masculinity and femininity. Most people fall somewhere on the spectrum of masculine to feminine, expressing both masculine and feminine qualities or characteristics at the same time. People whose gender differs from what is traditionally expected based on their sex assignment at birth are referred to as gender non-conforming. Drag performers (drag queens and kings) take on specific gender expressions when performing.

Sexual Orientation: Reflecting those to whom a person is emotionally, physically, sexually and/or psychologically attracted. All people have a sexual orientation that is entirely separate from their gender. Sexual orientation is about other people—those with whom one wishes to engage in relationships, including sexual relationships. Common sexual orientations include heterosexual, lesbian, gay, bisexual, queer, and asexual, and there are many other labels that people use to describe their sexual orientations.

Talking Points:

- Every person has a biological sex/sex assigned at birth and a gender identity. Most people's sex assigned at birth matches their gender identity (cisgender). A person whose gender identity is incongruent with their sex assigned at birth is transgender.

- When using gendered language, it is always best to use the language that affirms someone's gender identity. For example, instead of referring to someone as having been assigned male at birth, we would instead use transgender woman, because that affirms her gender identity.

- Every person has a gender expression. Some people's gender expressions are consistent with traditional gender norms of femininity and masculinity, while other people's are inconsistent with such gender norms, and can be described as gender non-conforming. Gender non-conforming people (especially those who are visibly transgender) face more persistent and intense discrimination and violence.

- Every person also has a sexual orientation that is separate from their own gender identity and expression. While many people assume that someone who is gender non-conforming is not heterosexual, not all people who are gender non-conforming are lesbian, gay, bisexual or queer. Heterosexual people can be gender non-conforming, and LGBQ people can be gender conforming.

- When using labels for sexual orientation, it is generally best to use the language that affirms someone's gender identity (not the sex they were assigned at birth). For example, the sexual orientation of a transgender woman who is exclusively attracted to women is best characterized as lesbian. Likewise, the sexual orientation of a transgender man who is attracted to women is best described as heterosexual. Most importantly, mirror the language that people use to describe their own identities.

- A person's sexual orientation is not determined by their partner's sex assigned at birth (or by the status of their partner's medical transition). For example, if a cisgender man exclusively dates women and is in a relationship with a transgender woman, he is heterosexual.

UNDERSTANDING TRANSGENDER PEOPLE'S EXPERIENCES

...

In this book we emphasize several key themes regarding the lives and experiences of transgender people. Whether you will be facilitating just one lesson or using the book to create a day-long (or longer) series of presentations, the following points will help you guide rich, authentic discussions. They will also help participants keep the most important points in mind as they strive to understand the experiences of transgender people. Since intersectionality—especially but not limited to the staggering and pervasive effects of individual, structural and institutional racism—is particularly critical in understanding transgender people's identities and experiences, we have designated a separate section for this topic, starting on page 20.

15 KEY THEMES

1. Being transgender is only one aspect of a person's experience
2. Coming out and navigating being transgender is a life-long process
3. Affirming names and pronouns are essential
4. Choices concerning social and medical transitions are highly personal
5. Social and medical transitions require a lot of intense personal change and growth
6. Gender is complex and multi-faceted—everyone's identity is unique
7. Some transgender people have non-binary gender identities
8. Experiences of affirmation or rejection by families of origin have a profound impact
9. Dating and relationships can be harder to navigate
10. Sexuality, sexual expression and sexual behavior are also harder to navigate
11. Creating families (fertility, conception and parenting) presents unique challenges.
12. Bathrooms, locker rooms, and other gender-segregated spaces create barriers
13. There is limited information about transgender aging
14. There are hierarchies within transgender communities, particularly related to medical transition and passing
15. "LGBQ" communities are not always supportive of transgender people

1. Being transgender is only one aspect of a person's experience

Transgender people, like cisgender people, are multidimensional. Their gender identity is only one aspect of their lives. It's important not to reduce transgender people to their gender identity alone. Being transgender may not be the central theme of a transgender person's life or the most important part of their experience. For some, it is more a part of their past history than something they think about in daily life.

Tip for Facilitators: Participants may be tempted to reduce a transgender person to their gender identity. They may focus single-mindedly on that one aspect rather than seeing the whole person. Facilitators can help participants put this into perspective by reminding them about all the parts that make up every person's experience, and how it might feel if others thought of them in terms of only one of those things.

2. Coming out and navigating being transgender is a life-long process

Transgender people have to make decisions about how, whether, and when to come out throughout their lives. There is no single "coming out" conversation, announcement, or event. Instead, there are many. These may include coming out to oneself, family, friends, coworkers, teachers and peers, medical providers, and others. Sometimes transgender people can plan and prepare for coming out conversations in advance, which often happens when deciding to come out to a friend or family member. At other times, an unexpected situation or opportunity might make one feel forced to come out, such as when applying for a job or a loan or explaining name discrepancies on financial, school, or identity documents. In some cases an emergency or medical event necessitates disclosing one's transgender status. Transgender people may experience concern or anxiety about navigating these situations. They can be unsettling, unexpected, ill-timed, and even dangerous. For some, this may influence their comfort in dealing with new people or situations.

Tip for Facilitators: Participants may expect coming out to be a one-time thing. Facilitators can help participants think about all the ways in which a transgender person might have to come out over the life course, or sometimes even within a single day.

3. Affirming names and pronouns are essential

Referring to people using their chosen name and pronouns conveys basic respect. Not doing so—either purposefully or accidentally—is generally perceived as disrespectful and hurtful. It denies that person their humanity. In some instances it can be dangerous because it can reveal someone's transgender identity in a world in which discrimination and violence is severe, pervasive, and persistent.

Tip for Facilitators: Participants may insist they should be able to know a transgender person's previous name. They may also think it is all right to tell other people a transgender person's previous name. Or, they may balk at using pronouns with which they are unfamiliar or "slip" and use the wrong pronouns on purpose. Facilitators can help participants think about how deeply important each person's name and pronouns are to them, and what it might feel like if someone refused to call them what they wanted to be called.

4. Choices concerning social and medical transitions are highly personal

Not all transgender people are able to or want to medically or socially transition. Transition is often (inaccurately) considered to be the center and focus of a transgender person's life. Many people assume that being transgender is primarily about medical transition, rather than being about people being their authentic selves. Those who cannot or do not want to transition are often expected or pressured to explain this to others. These decisions are often complicated and are always highly personal. There are many factors that go into an individual's decision to transition socially. These can include comfort with being out, the importance of being affirmed by others, having sufficient emotional or physical energy, whether loved ones (including families of origin and chosen families) will be affirming and supportive, level of personal autonomy, and local cultural climate. These may also include job security or the ability to navigate potential rejection, prejudice and discrimination. Medical transition involves many factors, which can include age, overall health status, access to affirming providers, comfort with medical interventions, types of interventions that are available, the anticipated quality of the results, healing time, access to physical and emotional support, potential side effects, and of course, financial resources.

Tip for Facilitators: Participants may be very curious or focused on medical or social transition details. Or they may not "believe" someone is transgender unless they have medically transitioned. Facilitators can assist here by noting how not all transgender people want to transition, or are able to transition, and by reminding participants of the wide range of gender identities and expressions that humans exhibit.

5. Social and medical transitions require a lot of intense personal change and growth

For people who decide to transition socially and/or medically, transition is a process. It can bring with it significant self-reflection, personal change, challenge and growth. It is intensely personal, and yet much of it is negotiated in public. That is, it takes place surrounded by others who can easily observe these changes. A person's name, pronouns, speech, movement, dress, hairstyle—all of these may be changing. Transition can mean many challenges and opportunities, both expected and unexpected. During social or medical transitions, these changes may occupy a central role in a person's life. It takes time to process and understand these changes.

Tip for Facilitators: Participants may think the transition process is self-centered or selfish. Facilitators can help participants think about how transition is unique to each person who experiences it yet must be played out for all in the transgender person's life to see on an everyday basis.

6. Gender is complex and multi-faceted—everyone's identity is unique

Gender is both individual and cultural. Every person has their own experiences of gender and their own unique identities. These are multi-faceted and sometimes complex. For most people, gender identity is congruent with biological sex—they are cisgender. For other people, gender identity is incongruent with biological sex—they are transgender. Some transgender people have more complex identities and relationships with their bodies. They sometimes fall outside of the gender binary—the expectation that everyone identifies simply as a man/male or woman/female. Which is to say, not all transgender people identify as men or women, or even as transgender. Many words are used to describe non-binary gender identities, including: genderqueer, non-gender, agender, and pangender. Which labels are most affirming will vary from person to person. And sometimes people will decide to use the term "transgender" to describe their identity or experience because it is more easily understood by others, even though their identities are non-binary.

Tip for Facilitators: Participants may feel confused or uncomfortable with the wide variety of words people use to describe gender. Facilitators can help participants think about the power and importance of language, especially when it comes to describing oneself.

7. Some transgender people have non-binary gender identities.

Not all people experience their gender identity as being "opposite" to the sex they were assigned at birth. Some identify as having non-binary gender identities. That is, they do not experience their gender identity as fitting into the assumption that gender is strictly an either/or option of male/men/masculine or female/woman/feminine based on sex assigned at birth. There is a wide diversity of non-cisgender gender identities that are non-binary within transgender communities. Some of these identities include: bigender, genderfluid, gender non-conforming, genderqueer, non-binary, agender, genderless, non-gendered, third gender, crossdresser and two-spirit identified people. (See the **Navigating Transgender Terminology section** on page 5 for more information about each of these terms). Most people have long believed that both sex and gender are fixed, binary concepts. On this view, a person is one or the other—not both, neither, or something else entirely. The idea that some people may experience their gender along a continuum or outside of this framework altogether can be challenging for many people to grasp, or to respect. For this reason, people who have non-binary gender identities may experience marginalization and discrimination from both cisgender people and transgender people whose identities are closer to being binary.

Tip for Facilitators: Participants may struggle with understanding non-binary identities because they have always been (formally or informally) taught that gender is a binary and you must be one or the other. Facilitators can help participants think about all of the ways in which gender can fall along a spectrum. Participants are likely able to recognize the various ranges of gender expression as a spectrum, and facilitators can help participants build on this foundation and extend it to biological sex and Disorders of Sex Development, and then to gender identity and non-binary identities.

8. Experiences of affirmation or rejection by families of origin have a profound impact

Research shows that LGBT youth and young adults who experience rejection by their parents have poorer mental and physical health. Those who have parents that are accepting fare far better. Feeling supported and valued by loved ones is very important. Such support promotes emotional well-being and resilience. And, having a strong support network helps to reduce the pain of a world that can be discriminatory and harsh.

Tip for Facilitators: Participants may be tempted to think of a transgender person as if they exist in a vacuum. They may not consider their relationships—whether positive or strained—with loved ones. Or, they may wonder why transgender youth or young adults experience such profound health disparities. Facilitators can help participants think about all the people in a transgender person's life. This may include family or origin, chosen family, close friends, co-workers, peers—and the impact those people can have in supporting or rejecting the transgender person.

9. Dating and relationships can be harder to navigate

Making decisions about dating and relationships can be difficult and stressful for everyone. People negotiating these situations must choose to share vulnerability. And they may share pieces of their history that are otherwise private or difficult. Navigating how and when to disclose one's gender identity adds yet another dimension to the already complicated dance of dating and relationships. In a world where there is still much myth and misinformation about transgender people, this can become even more layered and potentially highly charged.

Tip for Facilitators: Participants may have unrealistic ideas about transgender people and relationships. They may have strong opinions about how soon a transgender person should tell a potential date they are transgender. Facilitators can help participants think about how cisgender people have to navigate dating, and consider commonalities and differences between cisgender and transgender peoples.

10. Sexuality, sexual expression and sexual behavior are also harder to navigate

Expectations about men and women, and about bodies and behavior, can be tightly wrapped up in many people's experiences of sexuality. Transgender people may have to make decisions about disclosing details of their gender identity as well as details about their bodies. All this is in addition to having to counter myths, stereotypes, or fear in potential partners. And, many people confuse gender identity with sexual orientation, or lack information about transgender people. There are also sometimes unique physical challenges. For instance, there may be a lack of safer sex materials that work with transgender people's genitals. Or, experiences of gender dysphoria may influence how a person physically or emotionally engages in sexual behavior.

Tip for Facilitators: Participants may have very specific questions about how transgender people have sex or what their genitals look like. Facilitators can help participants think about how these can be very personal questions for anyone. They can provide resources to help participants learn this information from credible sources. They can also encourage participants to consider situations in which such questions might be appropriate (for instance in a medical situation where this information is necessary, or when negotiating sexual activity with a partner), or are considered inappropriate (most other situations).

11. Creating families (fertility, conception and parenting) presents unique challenges.

People who come out as transgender after becoming parents must make decisions about if, when, and how to come out to their children. These decisions may be further complicated by issues of legality, partner support, and degree of acceptance by an extended family. People who come out as transgender and want to become parents will have to make decisions about how they will become parents. Some aspects of medical transition may change how or whether a transgender person can become pregnant or make someone pregnant, now or in the future. In some cases, transgender people may not have the financial means to preserve their eggs or sperm for later use. Or, they may not be able to anticipate a future desire to become a parent.

Tip for Facilitators: Participants may assume transgender people cannot become parents using their own eggs or sperm. Or, they may be confused about how or whether it is possible for transgender people to become parents. Facilitators can help participants think about how transgender people can build or add to their families—which may not differ much from how cisgender people do. Facilitators can also refer participants to resources on fertility and transgender people.

12. Bathrooms, locker rooms, and other gender-segregated spaces create barriers

It can be difficult for transgender people to access safe, private restrooms and changing facilities. Non-private and gender-segregated spaces cause significant barriers that can prevent transgender people from fully participating in society. Transgender people often experience threats, harassment, or even violence if someone thinks they may be in the "wrong" restroom. Transgender people may restrict their fluid intake and diets based entirely on access to safe restrooms and changing spaces. Having to constantly manage health and personal safety can have short-term and long-term health consequences. It can also affect a transgender person's ability to succeed at work or school, to travel, or to interact in their community.

Tip for Facilitators: Participants may not understand how sex-segregated restrooms impact transgender people. Or they may have misinformation about restroom safety. Facilitators can help participants think about the impact that the lack of a restroom might have on a person's everyday life. They can also provide resources to counter myth and misinformation.

13. There is limited information about transgender aging

Our knowledge regarding how to support transgender youth and young adults is quickly increasing. But our knowledge and understanding of the unique needs of transgender people while aging is not as well understood. Minority stress, violence, and lack of access to affirming health care can contribute to shorter lifespans for transgender people than their cisgender counterparts. As the cultural climate continues to become more affirming, transgender people will live longer lives. Research continues to explore how various aspects of medical transition, particularly surgical, will hold up over time and what special care might be required. There is very limited research on this topic, and the information available is often anecdotal. There is also a need to work toward transgender cultural competence in retirement centers, long-term care facilities, and other aging-specific settings, so that transgender people have access to affirming aging and end-of-life care.

Tip for Facilitators: Participants may be familiar with issues that affect transgender young people but not consider the needs of aging transgender people. Facilitators can help participants think about how aging issues affect transgender people in ways that are similar to and different from the effects of aging on their cisgender peers.

14. There are hierarchies within transgender communities, particularly related to medical transition and passing

There is no one "transgender experience," or even a single united "transgender community." There are many transgender communities and sub-communities. Transgender people are not immune to internalized homophobia or transphobia. These prejudices sometimes play out in transgender communities to create hierarchies that further marginalize some transgender individuals or groups. Often, people within transgender communities who have had access to medical transitions have "passing" privilege. That is, they are not "visibly" transgender. They have gender expressions that conform to cultural norms for their gender, or are considered conventionally attractive, and have greater privileges within transgender communities. Transgender people who cannot or do not desire to medically transition, or have non-binary gender identities, are sometimes marginalized within transgender communities. So are gender non-conforming people, or those who do not have passing privilege. Moreover, transgender people who are marginalized in the greater culture because of age, ability, ethnicity, political affiliation, race, religion, sexual orientation, or socioeconomic status will also have to deal with all those issues within transgender communities, often finding themselves further marginalized within an already highly marginalized community.

Tip for Facilitators: Participants may imagine a single transgender experience, and transgender community. They may not be aware of how intersecting oppressions can further marginalize people within transgender communities. And they may not have considered the role of "passing privilege." Facilitators can help participants think about the diversity of experiences within transgender communities. They can also encourage participants to consider the impact of hierarchies within transgender communities.

15. "LGBQ" communities and individuals are not always supportive of transgender people

As in heterosexual and cisgender communities, some lesbian, gay, and bisexual people are still learning about gender identity and transgender people as well. LGBQ people take in the same misinformation, myths, fear, or sensationalism of transgender people and experiences that is common in mass media. It can be just as difficult for LGBQ cisgender people to understand what it means to be transgender as it can be for heterosexual cisgender people. Transgender people may feel stuck between a heterosexual cisgender society that does not fully understand their experiences and LGBQ communities that should but also do not. Historically, some large national organizations that focus on social justice related to sexual orientation have distanced themselves from transgender people, or have refused to support initiatives that include transgender people. While more of these organizations are changing to be more inclusive of transgender people, these changes are slow in coming, and sometimes occur "in name only."

Tip for Facilitators: Participants may assume that all LGBQ cisgender people embrace transgender people. And they may believe that all transgender people socialize only with cisgender LGBQ people. Facilitators can help participants think about how all cisgender people are exposed to anti-transgender prejudice, myth, and misinformation. And they can help participants think about how that might affect transgender people, cisgender LGBQ people, and cisgender heterosexual people.

UNDERSTANDING INTERSECTING IDENTITIES & OPPRESSIONS

...

All people have experiences of gender, orientation, race, ethnicity, class, religion, ability and age that are intersecting and complex. To truly contribute to social change, transgender education must pay particular attention to how intersecting identities and oppressions affect the lives of transgender people. Just as each cisgender person constitutes a unique constellation of experiences and background with differing degrees of societal privilege or ease, so each transgender person must navigate society through the lens of not only gender identity but also race, class, and other elements of identity that can combine in interesting and complicated ways.

This section provides some examples illustrating how multiple identities may uniquely affect transgender people. When facilitating any of the lessons in this book, it's important to think about how participants can be equipped with a basic understanding of what oppression is, and how multiple oppressions may interact with transgender people's experiences and access to public and private goods in the world. It is important for facilitators to think seriously about how these intersections can be highlighted during lessons and make a consistent effort to include corresponding themes.

ABLEISM:

Prejudice against people who are perceived as physically, mentally, or intellectually atypical. Questions illustrating how being transgender intersects with ableism:

- Will medical providers doubt my gender identity because I have also been diagnosed with Bipolar Disorder?
- Once I find one of the few affirming medical and mental health providers in my area, how accessible is the public transportation I need to use to get to their office?
- Due to my chronic illness, will my body physically be able to handle hormonal or surgical interventions?
- As a transgender person with Down Syndrome, how will my intellectual abilities affect how people validate my gender identity?
- What are the American Sign Language signs for transgender-related terms, and will people understand them?

AGEISM & ADULTISM:

Prejudice against older people, and prejudice against young people. Questions illustrating how being transgender intersects with ageism and adultism:

- Will people believe me because I am a child?
- Will malpractice laws prevent me from undergoing surgical interventions before I turn 18?
- If I am a minor in foster care, will my foster parents respect and affirm my identity?
- How will being older affect my capacity to transition medically?
- If I develop age-related dementia, how will the people in my life affirm my gender?
- Will I be able to find a long-term care facility that will respect and affirm my identity?

CITIZENSHIP:

Rights and privileges afforded to being a documented citizen, or lack thereof if one is undocumented or not a citizen. Question illustrating how being transgender intersects with citizenship:

- Does my country of origin or country of immigration allow me to change my identity documents, (e.g. passport, driver's license)?
- As a genderqueer person, how will I navigate not being able to have identity documents that validate my gender identity?

- Can I return to my country of origin if I have medically transitioned?
- Is it illegal for me to be transgender in my country of origin? To visit certain countries?
- If I am undocumented, how will I have access to affirming identity documents?
- Do I have to delay social or medical transition in order to obtain citizenship?
- If I am detained for deportation due to lack of documentation, with which sex will I be housed and will I be safe from violence from peers and guards?
- What will the impact be of my not being able to change my name or gender markers once I have applied to become a US citizen?
- Since the US does not have legal protections for transgender people, will I be unable to seek or receive asylum from my own country based on persecution there due to my gender identity?

CLASSISM:

Lack of access to social and economic power based on socioeconomic status. Question illustrating how being transgender intersects with class:

- Will I be able to use sexual and reproductive services (e.g., egg harvesting, freezing sperm, fertility)?
- Can my family afford pubertal suppression drugs?
- How will I pay for medical transition, if my insurance doesn't cover it?
- Can I afford to buy a gender-affirming wardrobe?
- Will my access to jobs be restricted because of my gender identity or expression?
- How will I be able to find the information I need online if I can't afford Internet access?

ETHNICITY & CULTURAL HERITAGE:

One's ethnic and cultural backgrounds and experiences. Questions illustrating how being transgender intersects with ethnicity and cultural heritage:

- Does my cultural background acknowledge that transgender and genderqueer people exist?
- How will I respond to the lack of gender-neutral words and affirming terms in my native language?
- How will I navigate the traditional dress and roles of my culture?
- Is gender non-conformity forbidden by law or custom?

HETEROSEXISM:

The assumption that all people are, or should be, heterosexual and that heterosexual people must be gender conforming (based on sex assigned at birth). Questions illustrating how being transgender intersects with heterosexism:

- Will people assume that, because I am transgender, I must be attracted to the opposite sex?
- Might my marriage or custody of my children be subjected to heightened scrutiny because I am a transgender person?
- If people know that I am a transgender woman, will my heterosexual male partner be subjected to gay bashing?

RACISM:

Prejudice based on one's racial background or perceived racial background. Questions illustrating how being transgender intersects with race:

- How will being targeted by the police as a transgender or genderqueer person of color affect my safety?
- Since people of color are more likely to be targeted as potential shoplifters, will I be able to shop for affirming clothing without additional scrutiny or harassment?
- How will historical stereotypes of Native Americans influence how people perceive my gender identity?
- How will I be able to succeed in school, given that gender non-conforming students face high rates of bullying, and teachers are less likely to intervene on behalf of students of color?
- If I experience rejection from my family, friends or community because I am transgender, who will I turn to so that I can process and cope with the racism that I experience as a person of color?

RELIGION:

One's faith, agnosticism or atheism. Questions illustrating how being transgender intersects with religion:

- Does my religion condemn transgender people?
- Does my faith tradition require that men and women be separated during worship or life?
- Will I have to choose between affirming my gender and my faith?

- How will I handle my faith's requirements to cover my head (e.g. hijab, yarmulke, wigs, apostolnik) or sit in a certain part of a worship space?
- Does my religion prohibit me from modifying my body?
- Will I be allowed to be a faith leader? Will my faith leaders support me?
- Will I be allowed to participate in the traditions and rites of passage that are gendered?

SEXISM:

The ways in which people are treated differently based on whether they are perceived as men or women. Questions illustrating how sexism intersects with being transgender:

- Will my income change after I medically transition because of the pay disparities between men and women?
- As a transgender man, how will I handle other men's sexist comments or treatment of women?
- As a transgender woman, will I experience heightened scrutiny about whether my fashion choices are considered to be "trying too hard" or "too sexual"?
- As a transgender woman, will people within the LGBQ communities expect me to be "femme"? Will people invalidate my gender identity if I want to express masculinity?
- As a gay transgender man, will other gay men reject me because I don't have traditional male genitals?
- As a genderqueer person, how will other people's discomfort with my non-binary identity impact me?

These are not exhaustive lists, because the intersections between transgender identity and all other aspects of identity are incredibly complex and truly limitless. While in-depth discussions of these intersections may fall outside of the scope of a specific training (and are outside the scope of the Toolkit), it is a moral imperative to remind participants that these intersections exist and must be considered in order to understand all transgender people's experiences in the world. One strategy for doing so is to contextualize the information being presented.

For example, when discussing the high rates of bullying that transgender and gender non-conforming children face while in school, facilitators can include statements such as:

> *Based on what we know about intersecting oppressions, we know that our transgender students of color or low socioeconomic status will have even higher negative outcomes because they are also experiencing the negative impacts of racism and classism."*

Or, when discussing how transgender people must navigate multiple barriers to coming out, the facilitator could say something like:

> *We know that transgender people face many barriers when it comes to employment. For some transgender people who were born in countries that do not allow them to change their identity documents, they may face additional obstacles. Potential employers will be alerted to their transgender status immediately, or perhaps not even understand that the person applying is the same person to whom the identity documents were issued."*

Similarly, when covering how transgender or genderqueer people may have a difficult time accessing medical transition services they want and need, a facilitator can explain:

> *Being able to access transgender care is not simply about locating knowledgeable, affirming care providers and having the financial resources or health insurance coverage to do so. It also includes having the physical access to do so: for example, finding public transportation and healthcare offices that are designed so that entrances, exam rooms, and equipment are fully accessible to people who have physical disabilities. It also means having cultural and linguistic access to communicate with and understand care providers: for instance, providers who are able to speak the languages of their patients, have interpreters available in other languages and American Sign Language, and have written materials available in multiple languages, and for patients with low English language literacy."*

It's important for facilitators to consider and incorporate these themes in all sessions, so that participants can understand the impact of multiple oppressions and how they affect transgender people's experiences.

HANDLING FREQUENTLY ASKED QUESTIONS

...

In every lesson, there are common questions and themes that are asked of all trainers. Some of the most frequently asked questions (FAQs) and the themes are listed below, with answers and talking points provided for each starting on page 24.

General FAQs

1. What causes someone to be transgender?
2. How common is it to be transgender?
3. When does someone know they are transgender?
4. Is transgender a mental illness?
5. Do transgender people have "both" parts? Are they intersex?
6. What is the difference between transgender and transsexual?
7. What is the difference between transgender and being in drag?

Medical Transition FAQs

8. How does medical transition work?
9. What causes someone to want to medically transition?
10. What does a person have to do to obtain "clearance" to medically transition?
11. Is medical transition covered by health insurance?
12. What if the person changes their mind after they medically transition?
13. Is it safe to medically transition? What are the risks?
14. Why would someone mutilate their body?
15. Why would a transgender person not want to medically transition?
16. How long does medical transition take?
17. When does someone become the other gender?

Sexuality & Reproduction FAQs

18. If a person is transgender, then what is their sexual orientation?
19. What is the sexual orientation of a cisgender man attracted to transgender women?
20. Can transgender people have children?
21. How do transgender people have sex? Can they reach orgasm?
22. What do transgender people's genitals look like?

Intentions & Deception FAQs

23. Why are transgender people trying to trick or confuse people about who they are?
24. Why don't transgender people want to share their names or details about their histories?
25. Why do transgender people hide that they are transgender from sexual partners?

Legal FAQs

26. Are there legal protections for transgender people? What are they?
27. When can someone legally change their name?
28. When can someone legally change the gender marker on their identity documents?
29. Can transgender people legally get married?
30. How do marriage equality laws affect transgender people?

Answering Frequently Asked Questions

These questions can be challenging to answer, but are often essential to participants' comfort and learning. We have provided general explanations and talking points for each of the questions. Overall, when responding to questions, we recommend the following strategies:

- Correct stereotypes, misinformation and insensitive language
- Validate and appreciate the person's desire to learn and ask questions
- Provide examples that normalize and affirm transgender people
- Address the potential underlying intentions or assumptions of the questions being asked
- Work to increase empathy by helping participants to think about what it would be like if they were transgender

What Should I Do If I Don't Know an Answer to a Question?

There are always situations in which even the most advanced and expert trainers are stumped by a participant's question. If you are asked a question and you are not sure of the answer, resist the urge to make your "best guess." Instead, admit that you are not sure and that you will research it and report back. Then be sure to follow up and provide the information later.

General FAQs

1. What causes someone to be transgender?

While there are many theories purporting to explain what causes transgender identity, there is no known definitive answer—and it is likely that there is no one cause that explains every transgender person's identity or experience (American Psychological Association, 2014). Often when we are looking for what causes someone to be transgender, it is because we see being transgender as a problem that we should be able to prevent or fix. This implies that there is something wrong with people who are transgender. Rather than trying to determine potential causes, it is essential if we are to support transgender people that we focus on reducing the extensive prejudice they experience. That is what causes a majority of the harm and negative outcomes experienced by transgender people.

2. How common is it to be transgender?

For a variety of reasons, we don't have reliable numbers indicating how many transgender people exist. To obtain a truly accurate statistic we would have to include a question on the census and we would have to make sure that transgender people were able to answer honestly without fear of repercussion. Without such data, all current numbers are "best guesses," which can vary based on how questions are asked, how transgender is defined, where the data are collected, who is surveyed, and how safe they feel so they can answer honestly. The Williams Institute (Gates, 2011) estimates that about .3% of US adults (about 700,000 people) are transgender. Other surveys estimate that as many as 1% or more are transgender. These are increasingly considered low estimates, and new studies are under way.

3. When does someone know they are transgender?

There is no single age when people know that they are transgender or come out as transgender (American Psychological Association, 2014). Some transgender people know from a very young age and communicate their gender identity when they are 2 or 3 years old. Some transgender youth have a better sense of their gender identity around the time of puberty (9-10 years old), or later in adolescent and teen years. Other transgender people come out later in life, around the time of a significant change (going to college, the passing of a close relative, etc.). Some people come out much later in life or towards the end of life. The one constant is that transgender people come out only when they are ready to do so, and when they either feel safe enough to do so, or feel that they can no longer continue living without being who they know they are.

4. Is transgender a mental illness?

No. Gender Dysphoria is a diagnosis in the American Psychiatric Association's *Diagnostic and Statistical Manual, Fifth Edition (DSM 5)*, used by psychologists and physicians to indicate that a person meets the diagnostic criteria to engage in *medical transition*. In other words, this is the medical diagnosis for being transgender. It was formerly known as *Gender Identity Disorder (GID)*. The inclusion of Gender Dysphoria as a diagnosis in the DSM 5 is controversial within transgender communities because it implies that being transgender is a mental illness rather than a valid identity. Such a diagnosis should not mean, though, that one's gender identity is itself as a disorder. The disorder is a function of incongruity between one's gender identity and sex assignment at birth. On the other hand, since a formal diagnosis is generally required in order to receive or provide healthcare treatment in the US, it does provide some people with access to medical care they wouldn't ordinarily be able to receive. Many people have complicated feelings about this diagnosis. It can bring on stigma associated with having a mental health diagnosis, but it can also provide access to care. Some transgender people may experience mental health challenges such as depression, anxiety, or other issues. But these are not a result of being a transgender person. They can be the result of the significant stress, stigma and discrimination transgender people may experience by living in a society in which transgender people are still not fully accepted or understood (World Professional Association for Transgender Health, 2012).

5. Do transgender people have "both" parts? Are they intersex?

No. "Hermaphrodite" is an outdated and offensive term that refers to people who have what is known as a Disorder of Sex Development (also and more commonly known as being intersex). People who are intersex have a combination of chromosomes, genitals and hormones that cannot easily be categorized as male or female. This is completely separate and different from being transgender (Intersex Society of North America, 2008)—which is when a person's gender identity is incongruent with the sex they were assigned at birth. Some intersex people may also be transgender, but a majority of people who are transgender do not have intersex conditions.

6. What is the difference between transgender and transsexual?

"Transgender" and "transsexual" are both related to incongruity between a person's experience of having a gender identity and their sex assigned at birth. "Transgender" is an umbrella term used to refer to the whole range of people whose sex assigned at birth is an incomplete or inaccurate description of their gender. "Transsexual" is an older term (GLAAD, 2014) that was historically used to indicate that a transgender person had had some form of medical transition (e.g., hormonal or surgical interventions). While still used by some, "transsexual" is used less today because not everyone desires or is able to access medical transition. Since historically it was a medical term, some people feel it is unnecessarily pathologizing. Unless a person is referring to their own identity or reporting another person's self-identification as transsexual, "transgender" is generally the best term to use.

7. What is the difference between being transgender and being in drag?

A person who is transgender experiences incongruity between their gender identity and the sex they were assigned at birth. This disconnect is felt on a deep-seated level. A person who performs drag chooses to express a different gender for the sake of fun of performance—not because of a having a gender identity that is incongruent with the sex they were assigned at birth (McClouskey, 2015). Most people who perform drag (drag queens/drag kings) generally do not identify as transgender.

Medical Transition FAQs

8. How does medical transition work?

Some transgender people choose hormonal or surgical interventions (or both) to help their bodies become more physically congruent with their gender identities. Medical transition can be a long-term process and may differ greatly from person to person. Not all transgender people want to medically transition and a person should not be judged by whether or not they have a desire to, are able to, or how they choose to medically transition. There are many different options and procedures potentially involved and each transgender person who desires to medically transition will make decisions about which combinations of interventions are best for them (Center of Excellence for Transgender Health, 2011). While many transgender people do wish to medically transition, not all are able to due to health or life circumstances (such as cost, location, lack of logistical or family support, etc.). It can be very difficult for transgender people to access the information, financial resources, and documentation required for medical transition health services.

9. What causes someone to want to medically transition?

Transgender people choose to transition for a variety of reasons. Having ones' body be incongruent with one's inner sense of gender can be very stressful emotionally and physically, and transitioning (socially or medically) can help address this disconnection and support one's sense of well-being and wholeness (WPATH, 2012). For some, medical transition reduces the intense dysphoria associated with having a gender identity that is incongruent with sex assigned at birth. For others, it can help them feel more authentic in their own bodies, and help them lead more authentic lives. Some people are also motivated to transition so that their gender identity is acknowledged and respected by other people.

10. What does a person have to do to get "clearance" to medically transition?

The most commonly referenced standards are those provided by the World Professional Association for Transgender Health (WPATH). The best practices are framed within the idea that medical transition is a beneficial option for transgender people that can enable them to live physically, psychologically and emotionally healthier lives. To support the process, the WPATH Standards of Care recommend that a transgender person work with a culturally competent and transgender-affirming mental health professional to make an informed and supported decision to transition medically. Some medical providers require a letter of support from a person's therapist before providing hormonal or surgical interventions (World Professional Association for Transgender Health, 2012). Alternatively, some medical providers use an "informed consent" model for hormonal interventions (Reisner, et al, 2015). The provider will screen the transgender person for any mental or physical health risks, review all the possible risks and benefits of hormonal interventions for that particular person, and then the transgender person decides whether to accept the risks and benefits by signifying their consent to be treated. In order to access surgical interventions, surgeons will generally require one letter from a mental health provider and one letter from a medical provider.

11. Is medical transition covered by health insurance?

Not usually. While there are a few insurance plans that cover medical transition, plans that cover all possible options for medical transition—or even most options—are few and far between (Lambda Legal, n.d.). These plans are typically available only to people who work for large companies that are staunchly LGBTQ supportive, or in a small handful of states that require that transgender health care be included in health insurance plans. It is much more common that people who have health insurance will have plans that have outright transgender exclusions, where any procedures related to medical transition, or to any transgender-related health care at all (for instance counseling), are specifically excluded from coverage. Since most hormonal and surgical interventions are not covered by health insurance, part of the process for many transgender people contemplating medical transition is figuring out if or how they can finance it with their own personal financial resources. Even when medical transition is partially or fully covered by medical insurance, there are very few providers, particularly surgeons, so people will generally have to pay out of pocket for out-of-network care charges as well as travel expenses (including airfare, extended hotel stays, follow-up visits, etc.) to travel to where the providers are located. Cost is persistently a barrier making it difficult for transgender people to access medical transition.

12. What if a person changes their mind after they medically transition?

While there are people who change their minds, this is very rare (Smith, et al, 2005). Several studies have found that most of people who undergo medical transition report improved quality of life, greater comfort with their bodies, reduced depression and anxiety, and overall increased satisfaction with their lives. Sometimes well-meaning cisgender people worry about this because they are trying to use their own perspective to understand transgender people, and it would seem very unsettling to them if they were to suddenly find themselves in a different gender one day (and they would very likely want to change back!). This is different from being transgender because having a gender identity that is different from one's sex assigned at birth does not happen suddenly. Saving money for accessing medical transition can take a long time, so by the time a person is able to transition medically, they have had ample time to be confident in their decisions.

13. Is it safe to medically transition? What are the risks?

Yes. Medical transition is considered the appropriate medical treatment for people who are transgender and wish to transition (WPATH, 2012). There are significant risks associated with *denying* transgender people access to medical transition. While all hormonal and surgical interventions have inherent risks, medical transition is generally considered safe. Whenever possible, individual transgender people should consult with an affirming medical provider to discuss the risks and benefits that are specific to their own health and access ongoing routine health screenings. In fact, transgender people who have access to affirming healthcare providers and who are interested in and able to have hormones prescribed often access routine health monitoring (blood pressure, cholesterol, other basic blood tests and physical exams) more regularly, and they are in better health than the rest of the population.

14. Why would someone mutilate their body?

For a person whose body is incongruent with their gender identity and is a source of significant dysphoria, medical transition is the *opposite* of mutilation. Medical transition can help create a body that is more comfortable and authentic for a person, which improves their sense of well-being and wholeness (WPATH, 2012). Similarly, cisgender people use hormones and surgeries to increase their comfort and satisfaction with their bodies for a variety of reasons—yet, cisgender people do not need to "prove" themselves to a mental health or medical provider prior to accessing such interventions.

15. Why would a transgender person *not* want medically transition?

Some transgender people don't medically transition simply because they cannot afford to due to financial constraints, geographic access, or because of other constraints or aspects of their lives. Others choose not to because they do not feel it is necessary in order for them to live authentic lives (Grant, et al, 2011). Still others may have concerns because of continued discrimination against transgender people—they may want to transition, but fear the risks of living in a society that is still not very accepting.

16. How long does medical transition take?

Every person's process is unique and will happen differently, based on the interventions chosen and pre-existing factors such as genetics. There are some good online medical resources that estimate how long hormones take to achieve certain masculinizing or feminizing body changes such as hair growth, breast development, skin and muscle changes, voice change, genital changes, etc. (WPATH, 2012), but most effects of hormonal interventions build over years. Surgical interventions may provide more immediate changes, but many surgical interventions involve multiple stages that are conducted over time. For both hormonal and surgical interventions, cost will be a significant factor, and lack of funds often delay or extend the process. Likewise, lack of accessible and affirming medical providers often extend the process due to inconsistent access to care.

17. When does someone become the other gender? (Legally, logistically?)

There is no one point at which a person becomes "the other gender." Every person's transition is unique, and only that person will be able to determine when they are satisfied with the progression of their transition. The state or country in which a person was born or in which they reside while they are transitioning (or after) will have a significant impact on how and when a person is able to legally change the gender marker (M/F, see more information in the Navigating Transgender Terminology section) on their identity documents. Each state and country has its own requirements for when—or if—a person is allowed to change the gender marker on their identity documents (Lambda Legal, n.d.).

Sexuality & Reproduction **FAQs**

18. If a person is transgender, then what is their sexual orientation?

Like cisgender people, transgender people can have any sexual orientation (American Psychological Association, 2014). Sexual orientation is about those to whom a person is romantically, emotionally, psychologically, physically, or sexually attracted. Labels related to sexual orientation are generally based on a person's gender identity and the genders of the people to whom they are attracted. For example if a transgender man is exclusively attracted to other men, he is likely to label himself as gay. If a transgender woman is exclusively attracted to other women, she is likely to label herself as a lesbian. If a transgender man is attracted exclusively to women, or if a transgender woman is attracted exclusively to men, then they are likely to label themselves heterosexual. If a person is attracted to both men and women, or all genders, they may label themselves as bisexual or queer.

19. What is the sexual orientation of a cisgender man who is attracted to transgender women?

People often question the sexual orientation of people who are attracted to transgender people—particularly male partners of transgender people who identify as straight. The same guidelines that apply to labeling transgender people's sexual orientation apply to cisgender people's orientation. If a cisgender man is attracted to a transgender woman, then he is attracted to a woman, and is therefore heterosexual because the transgender woman's sex assigned at birth is irrelevant. If a cisgender man is attracted to men, he is likely to label himself as gay. If a cisgender woman is attracted to women, she is likely to label herself as a lesbian. If a cisgender person is attracted to people of another gender, then they are likely to label themselves as heterosexual. These principles are true regardless of the sex that someone was assigned at birth (American Psychological Association, 2014).

20. Can transgender people have children?

Yes. Like cisgender people, transgender people can build families in many ways. Some transgender-related hormonal or surgical interventions may temporarily or permanently remove a person's ability to produce sperm or release eggs. In these cases, while they may not be able to reproduce using their own eggs or sperm, then can still create families in other ways such as through partnership, foster parenting or adoption. Still other transgender people have the resources to have their eggs or sperm saved before undergoing any interventions that might affect their fertility (Center of Excellence for Transgender Health, 2015). This allows them to keep their options open for future family-building through assisted reproductive technologies.

21. How do transgender people have sex?

Human beings have a whole range of sexual behaviors from which to choose, and there is no one way that transgender people have sex. Transgender people have sex in all the ways cisgender people have sex; which is to say that different people use different parts of their bodies in different ways to bring themselves or other people pleasure (Scarleteen, 2014). Some people may use sex toys or prostheses, while others do not. Medical transition will often impact how a person experiences their body, and may increase their comfort with their body and how they experience pleasure.

22. What do transgender people's genitals look like?

People often fixate on transgender peoples' genitals and ask intensely personal and invasive questions about transgender peoples' bodies and surgical status in particular (Oh, 2015). While it is natural to be curious, these questions are rarely appropriate, and should be asked only when it is medically necessary or if they are engaging in consensual sexual activity with a transgender person. One good guideline is to consider whether or not it would be appropriate to ask a cisgender person about their genitals in the same situation—if not, it is not appropriate to ask a transgender person. Depending on a person's decisions regarding medical transition, their genitals may look similar or dissimilar to cisgender people's genitals. It's important to remember that not all transgender people have financial or logistical access to the hormonal or surgical interventions that they would like, and as a result, may have significant dysphoria about their genitals or about other parts of their bodies. It's also important to remember that not all transgender people want to access hormonal or surgical interventions. Similar to cisgender people, all transgender people are individuals and have a unique experience of their own gender and comfort or discomfort with their bodies. Many transgender people experience little or no significant dysphoria about their genitals.

Intentions & Deception **FAQs**

23. Why are transgender people trying to trick or confuse people about who they are?

They aren't. Being transgender is not about trying to fool or deceive other people about the sex that someone was assigned at birth—it is about a person's living an authentic life that reflects their gender identity (Valenti, 2014). Stories of deception are generally myths that come from popular media portrayals of transgender people, particularly transgender women, as being the punch line in a joke or the plot twist in a story line. Sometimes, a person may *feel* tricked or deceived because they did not know a person was transgender, and feel surprised that their assumptions were incorrect. They may place blame on the transgender person for this. This incorrectly assumes that transgender people are always easily identified as such because they are visibly transgender, or that other people always have a right to know about someone's gendered history.

24. Why don't transgender people want to share their names or details about their histories?

Like cisgender people, transgender people usually want to get to know someone before they discuss personal details of their lives or their past—particularly ones that can be highly emotionally charged, embarrassing, or simply private (GLAAD, 2015). Discrimination and violence against transgender people is also rampant, and so disclosing information that reveals their transgender status is something that a transgender person may consider very carefully before deciding to share it with others. Transgender people are much more than just their gender identity, but it can be hard to be appreciated for all facets of one's personality when others know they're transgender.

25. Why do transgender people hide that they are transgender from sexual partners?

There are many reasons a transgender person would not immediately disclose their transgender identity to a potential romantic or sexual partner. Like cisgender people, transgender people usually want to get to know someone before they discuss deeply personal or intimate details of their lives—particularly because they want a potential partner to get to know them for who they are now rather than for their gendered history. Discrimination and violence against transgender people are also significant concerns, especially in dating and romantic situations, and so transgender people have to make very careful decisions about when to disclose (Stotzer, 2009).

Legal FAQs

26. Are there legal protections for transgender people? What are they?

As this book goes to press, there is no federal law protecting people from discrimination based on gender identity or expression. Only a few states, cities and towns have nondiscrimination laws that offer such protections (Movement Advancement Project, 2015). Only 19 states and Washington DC offer non-discrimination protections for transgender people. See www.lgbtmap.org/equality-maps/non_discrimination_laws for the most current information on statewide nondiscrimination laws. Some individual schools and workplaces have site-specific non-discrimination policies that include transgender people. For example, President Obama enacted a policy that all federal employees are protected from discrimination based on gender identity or expression, and Title IX requires that all transgender people be free from discrimination in schools that receive Title IX funding. Regardless of the available legal protections, it is important to note that laws against discrimination don't specifically *prevent* discrimination; they provide recourse for people who experience discrimination. For example, the James Byrd and Matthew Shepard Hate Crimes legislation increases the severity of punishment for those who are found guilty of having committed a hate crime against a transgender or gender non-conforming person because of their gender identity or expression.

27. When can someone legally change their name?

Name change processes differ from state to state. Theoretically, anyone can change their name by following proper procedures. In some jurisdictions this is a matter of filing required paperwork and supporting documentation, while in others it may involve a court appearance, fingerprinting, a background check, and more. Changing a first name can often be more complicated than changing a last name—particularly if that name change represents a change in gender (Lambda Legal, n..d.). The costs of legally changing a name varies by location, and by the types of documents on which the name is to be changed. Other expenses, such as the cost of certified copies of court orders and fees to update driver's licenses, passports, and other identity documents, contribute to the overall cost.

28. When can someone legally change the gender marker on their identity documents?

Changing the gender marker on a person's identity documents is generally an extensive, expensive and complicated process, the specifics of which will depend largely on where they live, where they were born, and the type of document on which the change is to be recorded, such as an official government identification card, a driver's license, a birth certificate, a passport or some other identity document (Lambda Legal, n.d.). For each of these documents there are specific processes, rules to follow, and fees, and each requires specific information or physician/therapist/hospital records for gender change requests. Thus a transgender person has to decide which documents to change (depending on which they are allowed to change, based on specific requirements, their transition status and the documentation they can provide), and then decide how they will allot their time and money. Transgender people must also make difficult decisions about whether and how to do this, as it will immediately "out" them to the staff and offices to which they submit the new documents. It could be extremely uncomfortable or scary for a transgender person living in a small town where everyone "knows" everyone else to apply for such a changes on their identity documents. In short, the process of securing identity documents with correct gender markers can be time consuming, expensive, harrowing and frustrating. On the other hand, successfully obtaining an identity document with the correct gender can also be a very validating experience and a cause for celebration.

29. Can transgender people legally get married?

Yes. Due to U.S. Supreme Court decision Obergefell v. Hodges in 2015, transgender people may legally marry whomever they wish in the U.S. Before this decision, each state could decide whether to allow same-sex marriage, and the right of transgender people to marry was subject to a patchwork of regulations and policies (Lamda Legal, n.d.), many related to states' attempting to "prevent" same-sex marriages. Nor, during this time, was the right of transgender people to marry someone of another sex firmly established. In some states, if a transgender person had undergone surgical transition, they could marry someone of another sex. In other states, there were cases where this was contested, or simply not allowed at all. In some countries, transgender people may marry whomever they wish, while in other countries there are regulations that may prevent transgender people from marrying.

30. How do marriage equality laws affect transgender people?

The Obergefell v. Hodges Supreme Court decision of 2015 extended marriage equality nationwide, giving same-sex couples the freedom to marry in all 50 states. Thus transgender people in the U.S. should be able to legally marry, regardless of another person's sex or the gender marker shown on their identity documents (Marriage Equality and Transgender People, 2015). For people living in U.S. territories, or those wishing to hold their weddings there, whether same-sex couples can marry is still being established. Before June 2015, the right of transgender people to marry someone of any sex was not firmly established. There have also been legal cases in which issues of divorce, inheritance, or child custody have been contested by non-supportive spouses or family members when the other person in a marriage is a transgender person. In places with marriage equality laws, transgender people may marry whether or not they have transitioned or obtained identity documents with their correct gender marker. Yet, due to myths, misinformation, or anti-transgender prejudice, questions and challenges regarding the right of transgender people to marry may persist. It is imperative that transgender people who are married, or who are considering marriage, protect their rights. Legal documents including wills and healthcare proxies are recommended in case a marriage is contested by healthcare providers, courts, family members, or others. Organizations including Lambda Legal and the National Center for Transgender Equality provide resources on this still-evolving issue.

COMMON PARTICIPANT
REACTIONS & CHALLENGES

Based on our extensive experience facilitating trainings, we have identified 20 common reactions or challenges from participants who are learning about transgender-related topics. Familiarizing yourself with these common reactions will help you better tailor your responses to meet the needs of each group. Since most participants have limited information about or experiences with transgender people, their participation in the training may be the first time they have considered how they feel about transgender people. Participants' backgrounds, openness, and desire to learn will affect how they engage with the content, with their fellow participants, and with you as a facilitator. Many of these reactions will present themselves during a training session, and sometimes participants will exhibit multiple reactions at the same time. Some reactions may visibly surface during the training, but many of the participants' individual reactions and processes will remain invisible to you as a facilitator. Knowing the patterns that apply to how participants commonly react will help you better "read" the room and adjust the facilitation accordingly.

Understanding these reactions can also be particularly useful when you encounter training situations in which participants are resistant, hostile, or openly prejudiced. These participants may be unlikely to change their views, values or perspectives during the training, although change may occur later. With such participants, it may be most effective (and the best use of your energy as a facilitator) to focus on the "moveable middle"—specifically helping folks who are ambivalent to recognize the prejudiced responses of their peers and apply it by becoming more affirming, providing opportunities for those who are already affirming to practice and demonstrate their support.

Although some participants' thoughts and feelings will remain invisible to facilitators, it's common for a majority of participants in a group—the moveable middle we've just mentioned—to express middle-of-the-road responses, with fewer at the poles of outright hostility or overt affirmation. A major part of your role as a facilitator is to highlight positive reactions, focus on moving the middle and create/maintain a group dynamic that uses positive peer pressure to encourage all participants to become transgender-affirming.

POSITIVE OR AFFIRMING

1. Excitement to learn. Participants may be excited they finally have an opportunity to explore transgender-related topics in a formal setting that creates a space for them to ask questions and receive expert, concrete information.

2. Lifting the veil. Participants may be surprised that there is so much to learn about transgender people, and so much that they didn't know or hadn't previously considered.

3. Having empathy. Participants may have heartfelt and empathetic responses that often lead to a desire to change personal behaviors or cultural values to be more transgender-affirming.

4. Desire to advocate or be an ally. Participants may have a desire to, and seek guidance about, how they can be better advocates for or allies of transgender people and communities.

5. Self-disclosure of relevance to personal life. Participants may feel safe enough or comfortable enough to reveal (privately or in the group) that they have loved ones who are transgender, or that they themselves have questioned or struggled with gender identity.

6. Validation and affirmation. Participants may exerience a sense of relief that their own identities, experiences and attractions are being validated and affirmed. This can be particularly powerful if this is the first time a participant has experienced this. Some participants may also express relief that they were able to let their guard down because the space was validating and affirming.

RESPONDING TO Positive or Affirming Participants: Responding to participants who share positive or affirming reactions can be straightforward. Re-state or summarize the themes they raise for clarity, and in order to reinforce, validate, and model for other participants. For instance, "What I hear you saying is that you're pretty enthusiastic to be here today in a place where everyone can share their ideas and questions, and get the most up-to-date and accurate information." Or, "Sounds like you want to be the best advocate for the needs of transgender people that you can be."

MIDDLE OF THE ROAD / AMBIVALENT

7. Overwhelmed & confused. Participants may feel very overwhelmed and confused by the amount of new information being presented. Learning new terminology while unlearning false information and stereotypes can often elicit this reaction. This is a common learner reaction, particularly for those who have minimal previous knowledge.

8. The wheels are turning. Participants may process information at a slower pace than is presented during the training and may need more time to formulate their questions or thoughts. These participants may be particularly likely to ask "101" and foundational questions after you have moved past the "101" portion of the training.

9. Biological determinism. Participants may have a hard time separating gender identity from sex assigned at birth, particularly as it relates to affirming gender identity. This is generally rooted in the overwhelming cultural belief that biological sex and gender identity are universally congruent. A common response is that biology is more important than gender identity and that sex assigned at birth is not something that can or should change. This often presents as consistently referencing the sex that a person was assigned at birth as the defining or determining factor in their gender.

10. Conflating orientation and identity. Participants may have a hard time separating gender identity from sexual orientation. Some participants may falsely believe that transgender *is* a sexual orientation because the T is included in LGBTQ. Other participants have a hard time basing sexual orientation labels on gender identity (as opposed to inaccurately basing labels on sex assigned at birth).

11. Lack of experience, contact, or application. Participants may have a hard time integrating objective information about transgender people, particularly if they have minimal contact or experience with them. This may be particularly true for people who believe that they do not or will not have contact with transgender people, professionally or socially.

12. Unsure how to integrate knowledge into their worldview/experiences. Participants may see that the culture is largely hostile toward transgender people, but are unsure of their role in that, and/or are unsure of how this information applies to them. This may include some degree of embarrassment or wariness about appearing ignorant.

13. Incongruence with media messages. Participants' previous knowledge may be based on inaccurate, false, or hostile stereotypes about transgender people, which may be exacerbated by inaccurate terminology used in the media.

14. Discomfort at paradigm shifting. Participants may feel that understanding transgender people's identities and experiences of gender requires them to change their fundamental understanding of gender as a biologically based binary.

15. Desire to distance oneself from anti-transgender prejudice. Participants may not feel comfortable affirming transgender people, but do not wish to seem overtly prejudiced or hostile. They may feel internal or social pressure to avoid appearing prejudiced.

16. Denial of Difference. Participants may adopt an "I treat everyone the same" perspective, as a way of avoiding dealing with their own biases/prejudices. In doing so, they excuse themselves from contributing to social change because they feel that they are not a part of the problem (often because they are not physically harming or directly interacting with transgender people).

RESPONDING TO Ambivalent Participants: These moveable middle participants have the greatest potential for personal growth and learning potential. Responding to participants who share ambivalent reactions is about supporting and encouraging participants to explore ideas that are confusing or challenging to them. How the facilitator responds to such reactions should allow them to be learning tools for other participants. As they watch how the facilitator handles middle-of-the-road responses, they may feel better equipped to act similarly when others in their lives share similar reactions. "These are a lot of new terms and new ideas. It can feel overwhelming. Let's go back to that last idea again to give everyone another chance to consider it one more time," or "That's a question many people ask, so let's take a few moments to talk that through" are examples of responses facilitators can offer in support of ambivalent participants while encouraging then to continue to incorporate new or complex ideas into their knowledge base and experience.

NEGATIVE OR HOSTILE

17. Lack of empathy. Participants may feel that having a transgender identity is a choice, and that any challenges, discrimination or hostility that transgender people experience is a result of their choice. This is often rooted in a lack of willingness or ability to empathize with transgender people. A related reaction is empathy for those who are "tricked," such as cis women in bathrooms with transgender women or a person dating someone who later discloses they are transgender.

18. Moral or religious opposition. Participants may have strong religious beliefs, or faith leaders who believe there's a moral imperative against affirming transgender people. This may be supported by specific biblical passages or rhetoric from faith leaders. Another reaction of this type is expressed in the phrase "love the sin, hate the sinner." (Note: not all religions or faith-based persons reject transgender people).

19. Hostility or disgust. Participants may have a strong personal reaction of revulsion or disgust, particularly at the idea that transgender people should be validated and affirmed. This is sometimes rooted in a belief that transgender people are mentally ill, or a misguided belief that transgender people maliciously deceive others about the sex they were assigned at birth to trick or hurt others.

20. Defensive response. Participants may have a strong affective response without indicating clearly why, and it may present in a way that appears irrational or overly defensive. This may be rooted in a negative personal experience with a specific transgender person, based on false information and stereotypes, or feeling generally resistant to changing their own values and attitudes.

RESPONDING TO Negative & Hostile Participants: Responses to participants who have negative or hostile reactions should focus on minimizing harm. These reactions can undermine the learning environment, arouse anger or confusion among participants, or cause participants or the facilitator to feel unsafe. They can also, in hostile cases, contribute to derailing or sidetracking the session, especially if the facilitator or participants insist on engaging or arguing with the negative or hostile speaker. There may be educational moments, but participants who share this type of reaction often shut down and refuse to learn. Facilitators should be prepared to set firm boundaries and time limits on these situations, and to correct misinformation quickly and clearly. For example: "It sounds like you have complicated feelings on this, which is common. But it is not okay to use derogatory language when referring to transgender people (or anyone in the room)." "I think it's time to move on, we've spent some time on this and I want to make sure there's still time for others' questions or comments."

HANDLING INAPPROPRIATE LANGUAGE & OFFENSIVE QUESTIONS

Reframing Offensive Language Without Shaming or Shutting Down

One of the most common facilitator challenges that presents during a transgender-related training occurs when a participant uses language that is outdated, offensive, or derogatory. On the one hand, we want to make sure that participants understand that their language choices are not respectful or affirming and may be hurtful. On the other hand, we need to assume that participants are using the best language they have at that moment, and we want them to feel comfortable enough to participate so that they can learn. We also need to role-model how to call someone out on when their language is not respectful or affirming. It can be a lot to manage in the moment.

Proactive Planning: In such cases a facilitator can address such challenges with language at the beginning of the session and validate that participants may be nervous to ask questions out of fear of being offensive. For example, a facilitator might say:

> *Before we get started today, I want to acknowledge that you are all here to learn and that one barrier to learning is being nervous about using 'incorrect' language. I understand that you may be unsure about what that language might be, so I want to give you permission to use the language that you have during our discussions. If you use a term that is outdated or offensive, I will share that information and then I will model the affirming language instead. What I will try to do is repeat back what you have said, using the affirming language instead."*

Often participants will be visibly relieved that you have validated this concern, provided assurance that you won't shame them, and that you will provide them with more affirming options.

> *In the Moment:* When a participant does use an inappropriate term, quickly but gently address the issue by noting, *"That was a word that was used in the past but today we use the word _____ instead,"* or *"Although we may still hear that word sometimes from our peers or in the media, it's considered very disrespectful."*

Correcting Non-Affirming Labels and Pronouns

During the learning process some participants will struggle with using affirming language and pronouns when discussing transgender people. Many participants will focus on the sex someone was assigned at birth because they think of sex assigned at birth as permanent and unchanging. This often results in using non-affirming pronouns or gender markers. For example, during a discussion about transgender people's access to changing their identity documents, a participant may struggle with getting past a transgender woman's history of having been assigned male at birth, and they may incorrectly refer to her as a transgender man and "he," or also incorrectly referring to a transgender man as a woman or "she". It can be very hard for participants to stop thinking about the sex someone was assigned at birth. This does not necessarily indicate that a participant is *unwilling* to be affirming, but it does indicate how hard it can be to shift from assuming the finality of the sex assigned at birth to affirming a person's seemingly incongruent gender identity. If a participant is struggling or clearly taking care with the words they are using, this is usually a great indicator that the participant is trying to shift their thinking.

It is important to be patient with participants as they practice their new skill of using affirming language and validate their efforts to do so. Participants may find it useful when the facilitator provides them with prompts or corrections as they are testing out the new language. For example, when a participant uses the label "transgender woman," it can be useful for the facilitator to say *"Okay, just to clarify, we are talking about someone whose gender identity is that of a woman."* Or, if someone speaks about a transgender man using female pronouns, the facilitator can gently remind the participant to use "he" instead by saying *"Because we are talking about someone who identifies as a man, to affirm his gender identity we will use male pronouns."*

Responding to Inappropriate Questions or Remarks

Another common challenge facilitators have to navigate when leading transgender-related trainings is responding to questions that are intensely personal, biased, or outright offensive. In the section **Handling Self-Disclosure** on page 36, we have named some of the assumptions and questions that emerge during trainings, but this is not an exhaustive list. The appropriate response will depend on the person involved, context and the questions/statements. As a facilitator it is important to consider where the participant is coming from and what is motivating their reaction. (See **Common Participant Reactions & Challenges** on page 31.) Whenever possible, tailor your response to the motivation.

Other strategies include:

- Offering your own personal affective response (e.g. "I am struggling a bit with responding because it is really hard for me to hear you talk about transgender people that way"),
- Asking other participants to respond (e.g., "what do other folks think about this?"),
- Redirect the conversation (e.g., "that is a topic that takes us off track, so I am wondering: can we move forward with focusing on ____ instead?").

HANDLING SELF-DISCLOSURE

. . .

Facilitating transgender content can be personally and professionally challenging. Participants can and do make assumptions about who you are, your history, and why you care. Regardless of your gender identity or history, it is important that facilitators think proactively about whether you will come out, why you will come out, and how you will come out.

Coming Out As Transgender

There are many pros and cons to consider when coming out as transgender as a facilitator in a training. For example, research has shown that people experience a sharp decrease in prejudice after meeting someone who is transgender, and sharing your identity or story can be validating. On the other hand, coming out can be emotionally draining, triggering, or a risk to personal safety. It is also important to note that not all transgender people have the luxury of deciding whether or not to come out. People who are "visibly" transgender may not have the privilege of deciding whether or not to disclose, having to focus more on *how to come out or manage participants' impressions. Whether you decide to discuss your personal identity or not, it is likely that some participants will be preoccupied by figuring out or processing your identity.*

There is no "correct" answer to the question whether or not a facilitator should come out as transgender or discuss their personal identity during a training but it is important to be deliberate about how you approach it. Every facilitator needs to make a decision for themselves, based on the training setting, type of participants, personal comfort, emotional availability and energy. It is not always necessary to come out, nor is it necessary to come out every time you facilitate. Each situation will be different and can be handled accordingly.

There are also many ways to come out:

- Including your identity as a part of your introduction to participants
- Coming out and telling your detailed personal story
- Coming out but declining to tell your detailed personal story
- Referencing your identity or experiences as one example during a training
- Naming your identity in response to questions about experiences of being transgender
- Mentioning your identity in passing without elaborating or providing details
- Coming out only if directly asked about your identity
- Coming out when someone is being particularly affirming and you want to acknowledge that
- Coming out to shut down someone who is challenging, derogatory or hostile

When deciding whether to come out as transgender, take some time to consider why you are doing so, how it contributes to your goals as an educator, and how you want to approach it. Here are some questions to consider:

- Will I disclose being transgender? Why?
- How will I respond if people assume I am transgender?
- How will I respond if people assume I am cisgender?
- How will I respond if people ask me if I am transgender?
- How will I respond if people ask me personal questions about my history or genitals?
- Will I talk about my personal experiences? If so, how much will I reveal and why?
- How will I balance representing my own experience with that of representing other people's experiences within the transgender communities?
- How will I handle the emotional impact of hearing potentially ignorant, prejudiced or hurtful statements about transgender people?

Coming Out As Cisgender

As in coming out as transgender, there are pros and cons to consider when deciding whether or not to come out as cisgender. For example, participants may feel more comfortable asking questions of a cisgender person because they are less concerned with offending the facilitator, and being a strong ally or advocate for transgender people can serve as excellent role modeling. On the other hand, participants may question your expertise or may feel more comfortable voicing prejudiced opinions. Whether or not you decide to discuss your personal identity, it is likely that some participants will be preoccupied by figuring out if you are transgender. Again, there is no "correct" answer to the question whether or not you should come out as cisgender, but it is important to be deliberate about it.

When making decisions about whether to come out as cisgender, take some time to consider why you are doing so, how it contributes to your goals as an educator, and how you want to approach it. Here are some questions to consider:

- Will I disclose being cisgender? Why?
- How will I respond if people assume I am transgender?
- How will I respond if people assume I am cisgender?
- How will I respond if people ask if I am transgender?
- How will I respond if people ask me personal questions about my history or genitals?
- How will I respond if people question my expertise because I am not transgender?
- How will I handle the emotional impact of hearing potentially ignorant, prejudiced or hurtful statements about transgender people?

If you have a transgender loved one:

If there is a transgender person in your family or life, you will have some additional questions you will need to consider when making decisions about whether or not to disclose:

- Will I disclose that I have a loved one who is transgender? Why?
- Do I have that person's permission to disclose (with or without identifying information)?
- How will I talk about their personal experiences? How much will I reveal and why?
- How will I balance representing that person's experiences (or my own experiences of them) with representing other people's experiences within transgender communities?
- How will I handle the emotional impact of hearing potentially ignorant, prejudiced or hurtful statements about transgender people?

GUIDANCE ON TRANSGENDER **DOCUMENTARIES**

...

Documentary movies can be useful in helping participants make connections between the information being presented during a training and transgender people's lived experiences. Participants often find informational pieces to be abstract until they are able to apply it to someone's narrative. Documentaries can help, particularly when the movies are strategically selected and the related discussions are carefully facilitated. Here we provide some general guidelines to help you navigate using documentaries as a part of your teaching.

General tips:

- Selecting nonfiction documentaries over fictional drama is strongly recommended. Fictional films are often highly sensationalized, can be very complex to facilitate, and usually have many other components (the specific actors, costumes and make-up, complicated or unusual plotlines that are not true to life) that can distract from the main transgender themes you wish to cover.

- Be sure to select and screen any movie ahead of time. This enables you to determine its appropriateness for the group, and also to facilitate discussion that connects general transgender themes with the specifics of the particular movie selected.

- Every movie has a point of view. Some seek to portray transgender people as accurately and realistically as possible. But others may veer into sensationalizing transgender people, focusing too much on medical issues, endorsing a "trapped in the wrong body" idea, discouraging a whole-person perspective, promoting only a gender binary view, appropriating cultures, or falling into other potential pitfalls that may hinder learning. For more advanced groups, the facilitator may want to discuss this aspect further, and ask the group to share their thoughts on bigger-picture ideas such as the motivation or aims of the filmmaker for making such a movie, commenting on the effectiveness of the movie in portraying those ideas, and related topics.

- Be sure to note that the movie portrays the story of only one (or several, depending on the movie) transgender people. Transgender people and transgender communities are diverse, and such a movie is typically meant to provide a glimpse into the world of just one (or a few) transgender people. Although some common themes may affect transgender people and non-transgender people differently, it is important not to generalize and apply this one movie to the lives and experiences of all transgender people and communities.

- Use caution when selecting and presenting movies posted on YouTube or other user-generated movie-streaming sites. There can be both great advantage and significant challenges when attempting to use these in educational settings. While the movies are easily available for free, provide access to personal stories that otherwise are not represented, and may be closed-captioned, they generally represent only one person's experience and can also include inaccurate information, which may not be easily discerned by the average viewer.

Selecting Movies:

Questions for consideration when selecting the most appropriate movies for your audience and goals:

- What is your goal for using a movie—for example, do you want participants to develop more empathy for transgender people, more fully understand the experiences of transgender youth, learn more about healthcare barriers for transgender people?

- Which documentaries represent a diversity of gender experiences—for example, those that illustrate a range of gender identities and expressions?

- Which documentaries represent the range of transgender people's experiences in the world, and include positive portrayals of transgender people living full, authentic and happy lives?

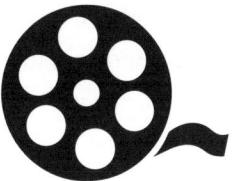
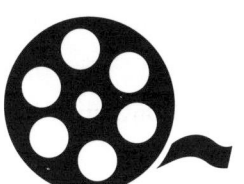
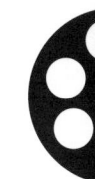

- In what ways can the movie(s) selected, and a facilitated discussion, be as inclusive as possible with regard to race, class, ability, age, and other dimensions of diversity?
- From whom/what voices/experiences will my audience learn most? What will be most relatable, meaningful, and positive for your audience? For example, traditional college-age students might relate best to movies that feature traditional college-age people. Consider selecting movies based on characteristics you would expect to see in members of your audience.
- If providing an online educational experience, which movies are available online for your participants?

Other considerations:

- Cost to obtain movie
- Ease in obtaining/access to movie—for instance, consider borrowing from friends or colleagues, requesting through your local or campus library, online and streaming sources, and other methods
- Length of movie
- Depending on your setting/venue, do you need to secure public performance rights for the movie?

Resources for locating movies and films:

- University or public libraries
- Campus- or community-based LGBT Centers
- YouTube has many possibilities. Be sure to consult the general tips, below, when selecting possible movies
- Netflix and other online and streaming sources
- LGBTQ-specific movie distributors, for example Frameline, Wolfe Video, and others
- Several transgender- and LGBTQ-specific national and regional organizations, such as Out and Equal, Massachusetts Transgender Political Coalition, and Transgender People Speak, have created their own movies on selected themes

Documentaries

There are many high-quality documentaries that focus on transgender issues. But sources and availability can change quickly, as can prices. Some may be found online at no cost, others through libraries, and a number are occasionally available through subscription-based streaming services. Many can be purchased through companies that specialize in films or entertainment or educational media, or directly from filmmakers or distributors. Occasionally a local community-based LGBT Center or a university may have titles for loan as well. Searching the name of the movie you're seeking online and through local library databases is likely the quickest and simplest way to find out about availability. Depending on the setting and audience, facilitators may also need to make sure they have the appropriate license for their screening purposes.

On the following pages you will find a list of transgender-related documentaries, generally released in the past ten years, along with some information about the themes they address. Not all documentaries will be suitable for all audiences or learning goals/objectives.

Thematic Key:

Movie Title:	Title of movie, year movie was made
Length (mins):	Duration of movie in minutes
Trans Women:	Movie includes portrayals, themes, and experiences of transgender women
Trans Men:	Movie includes portrayals, themes and experiences of transgender men
Gender NonCon:	Movie includes portrayals, themes and experiences of gender non-conforming people
USA Specific:	Movie is based on portrayals, themes and experiences of transgender people in the US
Race/Ethnicity:	Movie addresses race/ethnicity or intersectionality as a specific theme
Youth:	Movie includes portrayals, themes and experiences of transgender children or adolescents
Faith:	Movie includes portrayals, themes and experiences of religion, spirituality or faith
Ability:	Movie includes themes pertaining to ability, disability
Family:	Movie includes themes pertaining to family, family relationships, family acceptance/rejection
Relationships:	Movie includes themes pertaining to relationships in transgender people's lives
Medical:	Movie includes themes pertaining to medical issues, medical transition, health, and healthcare
Discrimination:	Movie includes themes pertaining to transgender people's experiences of anti-transgender discrimination and prejudice
Historical:	Movie includes portrayals and themes pertaining to the history of transgender people, historical background information about transgender people and movements

Note: This is not an exhaustive list, and the thematic key is meant to serve as only a guide for helping to select a potential film. Check out the resources page of www.teachingtransgender.com for additional film options.

MOVIE TITLE	Length (mins)	Trans Women	Trans Men	Gender NonCon.	USA-specific	Race/Ethnicity	Youth	Faith	Ability	Family	Relationships	Medical Transition	Discrimination	Historical
100% Woman (2004)	60	✔								✔		✔		
Austin Unbound (2011)	44		✔	✔				✔						
Becoming Me – In The Life (2012)	28	✔	✔	✔	✔		✔			✔	✔			
Becoming Me – The Gender Within (2009)	41	✔	✔	✔	✔			✔	✔		✔	✔	✔	
Boy I Am (2006)	72		✔			✔				✔	✔			
Call Me Malcolm (2005)	90		✔		✔			✔						
Cruel & Unusual (2006)	64	✔			✔					✔		✔		
Diagnosing Difference (2009)	64	✔	✔	✔	✔							✔		
Everyone Matters (2009)	10	✔	✔	✔	✔	✔						✔		
FREE CeCe (expected in 2016)		✔		✔	✔							✔		
Girl Inside (2007)	70	✔								✔	✔			
Georgie Girl (2001)	70	✔				✔								✔
Growing Up Trans PBS Frontline (2015)	84	✔	✔	✔	✔		✔			✔	✔			
How Do I Look (2006)	81	✔		✔	✔	✔	✔			✔				✔

MOVIE TITLE

Movie Title	Length (mins)	Trans Women	Trans Men	Gender NonCon.	USA-specific	Race/Ethnicity	Youth	Faith	Ability	Family	Relationships	Medical Transition	Discrimination	Historical
I Am: Transgender People Speak (Series)	1-7	✔	✔	✔	✔	✔		✔	✔		✔			
I'm Just Anneke (2010)	14		✔		✔					✔				
I am Jazz (2012)	45	✔			✔		✔			✔				
In The Turn (2014)	113	✔			✔		✔			✔				
I Stand Corrected (2011)	86				✔									
Just Call Me Kade (2002)	26		✔		✔		✔			✔				
Kuma Hina (2014)	75				✔									
No Dumb Questions (2004)	24	✔			✔					✔				
No Dumb Questions 5 Years Later (2008)	8	✔			✔					✔				
On The Male Side of Middle (2011)	12		✔				✔			✔	✔			
Paris Is Burning (1990)	71			✔	✔	✔								✔
Passing Ellenville (expected in 2015)		✔	✔		✔		✔	✔		✔	✔	✔		
Pay It No Mind: The Life & Times of Marsha P Johnson (2012)	55	✔			✔	✔								✔
Prodigal Sons (2009)	86	✔			✔				✔	✔	✔			
Queer and Pleasant Danger (2014)	72	✔			✔					✔		✔		
Red Without Blue (2006)	74	✔			✔					✔				
Riot Acts: Flaunting Gender Deviance in Music Performance (2009)	72	✔	✔	✔	✔									
Screaming Queens: The Riot at Compton's Cafeteria (2005)	57	✔		✔	✔	✔								✔
She's a Boy I Knew (2007)	70	✔								✔				
Southern Comfort (2001)	90	✔	✔		✔						✔	✔	✔		✔
Still Black: Portrait of Black Transmen (2008)	67		✔		✔	✔				✔	✔		✔		
Straightlaced (2009)	67			✔	✔		✔			✔	✔		✔		
The Believers (2006)	80	✔	✔	✔	✔		✔								
Three to Infinity: Beyond Two Genders (2015)	84		✔		✔	✔	✔			✔	✔	✔			
TRANS The Movie (2012)	104	✔	✔	✔	✔		✔			✔	✔	✔			
Transcending Gender: Portraits from the Community (2010)	39	✔	✔	✔						✔	✔	✔			
Transforming Gender (2015)	45	✔	✔			✔				✔	✔	✔			
TRANSforming Healthcare (2011)	17	✔	✔	✔	✔						✔	✔	✔		
Transgeneration Series (2005) *60-90 minutes	90*	✔	✔		✔	✔	✔		✔	✔	✔	✔			
TransMormon (2014)	14	✔			✔			✔	✔		✔				
Transparent (2005) (Documentary, not the fictional tv series)	61		✔		✔					✔	✔	✔			
Two Spirits (2009)	65	✔		✔	✔	✔	✔			✔	✔		✔		
Zanderology (2014)	41		✔		✔					✔	✔	✔			

GUIDANCE ON TRANSGENDER GUEST SPEAKERS & PANELS

Having guest speakers who are transgender is a not a new activity, but when well facilitated, it remains one of the most effective ways to reduce participants' prejudice toward transgender people and help them make personal connections to the materials. By inviting transgender people to speak about their personal experiences, transgender identity becomes "real" for participants. Many participants experience profound empathy and appreciate the opportunity to ask questions in real time. As a facilitator, it is your role to identify the best speakers for the situation, manage the expectations of participants, and ensure the safety and security of your guest speakers.

Finding Guest Speakers

- Consider whether you would like to have someone come to your location and speak, or whether or not you will host a virtual session. If you are having someone speak in person, make sure that you take steps to protect your speakers' safety and privacy.

- Consider the identities that you would like to have represented in the session, paying particular attention to which types of guest speakers will be most relatable for your participants. When possible, be sure to include a variety of diverse identities and backgrounds. You may also wish to consider including partners, parents/family members, and/or transgender allies.

- Depending on your location, you may be able to reach out to local LGBTQ community groups, non-profit organizations and colleges/universities. If this is not an option, word of mouth or personal connections may be effective.

- Whenever possible, seek out recommendations and endorsements from trusted peers who have seen a person speak. This can help you assess the person's public speaking abilities, appropriateness, and potential for success.

- If you want to use students as guest speakers, there are a few additional factors to consider. It is important to help students think about their comfort when presenting to peers, their level of outness, their level of personal safety, and how much time has passed since their disclosure. Student panelists may require additional coaching due to the intense personal nature of guest speaking and panels.

- Prior to contacting potential speakers, investigate your honorarium budget and make sure you know what you will be able to offer and whether or not travel expenses can be reimbursed. While some people will donate their time to speak, it is inappropriate to automatically assume this. Guest speakers are providing time and expertise, which is important to respect and value. If you cannot provide honorariums, personalized thank you notes should be sent. Gift cards or other useful tokens are generally appreciated as well.

- Once you have identified a potential speaker, have a conversation with that person to make sure they are a good match for your particular needs—not all speakers are good matches for all sessions. Explain exactly what you hope participants will take away from the session, any concerns you might have, the amount of time requested, potential dates and an honorarium, and what the participants are expected to know prior to the session. You will want to ask what they are hoping to take away from the session as the speaker, what concerns or questions they might have, and if there are any questions or topics that are "off limits" for them.

Preparing the Audience

Once you have identified your speaker(s) and determined that they match up with your needs, your next step will be to help prepare your audience. It is generally a good idea to give your participants advance notice when a guest speaker will be present. This will give them time to formulate their questions. When announcing a guest speaker, think carefully about the amount of information to reveal about the speakers' identity and history, taking care to respect the guest speaker's wishes.

Prior to the guest speaker session, it may be useful to help your participants assess their current beliefs, stereotypes, and expectations with respect to transgender people, and to think critically about how the session will go. For example:

- As an audience member, what do you hope to learn from this session?
- Based on your current knowledge, what are your expectations about what this person will have to say about their experience?
- What do you think might be some of the reasons this person engages in guest speaking about transgender identity?
- If you were the guest speaker, what concerns might you have about this session?
- If you were the guest speaker, what would you want participants to take away from the session?

It is very important to establish ground rules with participants prior to such a presentation. If your guest speaker has stated that they are not comfortable answering certain types of questions (such as: the name they were given at birth, or their genital status) make sure that this is clear to your participants in advance. Also, remind participants that the speaker can always "pass" on questions that they are not comfortable answering.

It may be useful to provide the opportunity for participants to write some of their initial questions on index cards in advance of the session. This gives participants the opportunity to ask for your support in articulating their questions, choosing their language, and determining whether or not their questions are respectful. During the session, having these pre-written questions can help participants overcome nervousness and provides a starting point for the Q&A part of the session.

Participants are likely to have many questions, but may not understand whether their questions are invasive, invalidating, or intrusive. As the facilitator, you should ask participants in advance to consider how it might feel to be asked intensely personal questions by strangers. Stress to the participants that, while the guests are coming to the sessions to answer questions, that doesn't mean that all questions are fair game.

Suggested Prepared Questions

Sometimes, even a talkative group will become quiet and feel shy about asking questions. Preparing questions in advance of the session provides an opportunity for facilitators to role-model respectful language, ensures that the information most relevant to your audience is covered, and can help to balance out the types of questions that are asked. Using these questions at the start of the session also gives the speaker and participants the opportunity to become comfortable with each other, and can help avert awkward silences while participants formulate questions.

When preparing your own questions for the session, it is best to start off with general questions and progress to more specific questions. It is also useful to predetermine a "summary" question that will be asked as the last question of the session.

Some sample *general questions* might include:

- How would you explain "transgender" to someone who had never heard the term?
- What are some of the biggest challenges that transgender people face?
- What is the relationship between the LGB and transgender communities?

Some sample *specific questions* might include:

- At what point did you have a sense that you might be transgender?
- When you were coming out as transgender, how did the people in your life receive the information?
- How has being transgender affected your intimate relationships?
- How has being transgender affected your social life?
- How do you identify your sexual orientation?
- How did your family react to your coming out?
- How has being transgender affected your choices related to parenting?
- How has being transgender affected your professional life and career?
- What role does religion play in your life?
- For you, what has been the best part about being transgender?
- For you, what has been the most challenging part about being transgender?
- Have you personally experienced discrimination or prejudice because of your identity?
- What has informed your personal decisions concerning medical transition?

Some *summary questions* might include:

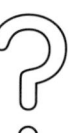

- What would you tell someone who is struggling with their gender/gender identity?
- How can the people in this room offer the most support to transgender communities?
- What is one thing you would want everyone here to take away from this session?

CREATING SUPPORTIVE LEARNING ENVIRONMENTS

...

A supportive group atmosphere and a supportive non-judgmental facilitator are essential to effective education about transgender issues and themes. Participants may be nervous, cautious, or even suspicious as they address this complex and sensitive topic, which may sometimes require a serious examination of their own ideas, values and behaviors. Try to create a safe, non-threatening environment in which people can talk openly and honestly. The goal is to provide experiences that strengthen people's motivations and capacities to take responsibility for their own learning, behavior, and increase their cultural competence around themes of gender identity and gender expression. A few basic interaction guidelines for facilitators include:

1. Create a physically comfortable learning environment

To the extent possible, try to ensure that the room is private and comfortable. If you can, arrange chairs or desks in a circle or semi-circle so that participants can look at each other while talking. Discourage interruptions that may be distracting (make sure that participants can leave the room without disturbing others) or violate privacy (close doors and avoid allowing non-participants to walk through the space). Take care to make sure that the space and the setup are accessible to those with different types of physical ability.

2. Explain logistics

At the start of a training session, participants may be focused on logistical issues—such as when breaks will occur, whether food will be provided, and whether they will be allowed to leave early. It can be particularly useful to address these logistics at the beginning of the session so that participants can direct their full attention to the training materials. When planning for breaks, keep in mind that breaks can help participants maintain their focus and keep their energy up, and they provide some unstructured processing time. It can be useful to include a buffer of an extra five minutes or so for participants to return to the space and get settled, so if you intend to allow a 15-minute break, you may wish to ask them to return in 10 minutes. It can also be helpful to remind participants that their returning on time will help keep the rest of the training on schedule so that they will be finished on time.

3. Create boundaries around technology and connectivity

Since many participants will have cell phones, tablets, or computers with them, it can be useful to clearly communicate your boundaries and comfort regarding participants' use of technology during the training time. Be clear about whether it is okay for participants to check their phones, use social media, or use their computers. Reminders to turn phones to silent or vibrate (and don't forget to check your own) can help to reduce embarrassing distractions during the training.

4. Encourage self-care

Since the materials presented in a training may be emotional, overwhelming or confusing for participants, it is important to encourage them to engage in self-care as needed. Letting participants know at the start of the training that they can leave the room if they need to use the bathroom or answer a phone call allows participants to take time for self-care without calling attention to themselves.

5. Carefully consider "ground rules"

As the facilitator, you will make strategic decisions about when and how to incorporate ground rules. Depending on the setting and type of participants, ground rules or group guidelines may help participants feel comfortable—particularly if they have previously participated in sessions in which they have been used successfully. For other participants, ground rules can feel like a distraction, a deterrent, or a setup. When planning your training, it can be helpful to ask in advance if ground rules are a cultural norm for the setting or participants. Consider the overall amount of time that you have available for the training, how much affective content and group discussion are included, and whether or not you will be able to successfully monitor these ground rules during the training. If you elect to use ground rules, consider your specific ground rules carefully and choose four or five that are most relevant to your training goals and that are achievable. For example, while "Be respectful" is often commonly listed as a well-intentioned ground rule, it puts the burden on the participants to know what is or is not respectful to transgender people, and they may truly not know that their questions or comments are offensive or disrespectful. If one of your goals as an educator is to help participants understand what language or questions are affirming (or non-affirming), it is unfair to expect participants to know this at the start of the training.

Some ground rules to consider:
- Try to Assume Good Will
- Use "I" Statements (instead of generalizing)
- One Person Speaks at a Time (limit side conversations)
- Move Forward, Move Back (be aware of how much you are talking)

ADAPTATIONS FOR ACCESSIBILITY

...

As a facilitator, your role is to provide opportunities for participants to learn more about transgender people and themes. Doing this most successfully means feeling confident and informed not only about the material you'll present but also about being able to meet the needs of the participants with whom you'll be working. One important element of meeting participants' needs is understanding how they may learn best, aspects that may prove to be unintended barriers, and what strategies you can use to ensure that everyone can fully participate and be included in the session you have planned. For this reason, a critical first step to accessibility is making sure that contact information for communicating accommodation needs is explicitly available, whether the facilitator is teaching their own independent session or they're part of a larger event.

There are many ways to modify or adapt the lessons in this book to best suit participants who have disabilities. Likewise, a variety of changes can be easily made to the lessons in this book to suit the needs of facilitators who have disabilities. A full exploration of this field is outside the scope of this book. However, there are many resources available online and through local libraries with information that can assist facilitators in learning more about the needs of people who have specific disabilities. Many communities also have a local education or advocacy group centered on the needs of people who have disabilities. Each of these sources can also supply helpful information about methods facilitators can use to minimize challenges and amplify the strengths that may be present for people who have various types of disabilities.

Here are some basic tips and tools for all facilitators to consider. This is not an extensive or complete list, but a jumping-off point for each reader to consider how their facilitation creates an accessible learning experience for participants. The most important consideration is that individuals who have disabilities are, first and foremost, individuals. Like people who do not currently have a disability, each person who has a disability has specific and unique skills and challenges.

Simply finding out that an individual has a disability does not automatically set out a prescribed set of adaptations for facilitators to use.

Knowing that someone has a disability in your session does not mean you should assume you know what will work best for them. For instance, knowing there will be a deaf person in your session tells you that someone in your session is deaf, but you will have to find out how best to address that specific *individual* person's needs. Some deaf people use sign language, or perhaps an interpreter; others use neither. Some use speech reading (sometimes referred to in the past as reading lips); others do not. Some deaf people use devices or technology that will require your active participation to enable it to do its job (like a Bluetooth or FM transmitter to be passed to each person when they speak); others use technology that requires little adaptation from the facilitator and participants (e.g., hearing aids or cochlear implants), while others use no assistive devices at all. Some have limited English literacy skills because their primary language is American Sign Language or because they were not able to fully access their education while in school due to institutional barriers; for others, written materials are the best source of information. As you can imagine, the most important element to providing inclusive sessions is finding out what best suits the participants in your session.

The more information the facilitator can obtain ahead of time to best serve the needs of the participants, the better. This will allow time to make modifications to the activities or the structure of the session(s), or both. If you'll be presenting to a group you work with regularly, you may already know about adaptations or accommodations that are in place to support each person's participation. If you'll be working with participants you do not know, you may learn that someone has a disability because they contact you to request accommodations in advance. And sometimes, you will not have any information about participants' needs before you are in front of the group, facilitating a session. In these situations, you may become aware of a participant who has disabilities only at that moment. Or, you may never become aware that they have a disability at all, if they do not tell you. In any of these cases, it is your job as the facilitator to best structure your session so that everyone may participate and benefit.

Also, remember that there are and will almost certainly be people who have disabilities who are participants in your sessions, whether you are aware of them or not. The lessons in this book were created with the intent of demonstrating and utilizing a variety of learning methods and modes. If while reading through the lessons you see an idea or activity in one lesson that you know will make it easier for participants who have disabilities to fully participate, feel free to use that in another lesson.

- Refresh your understanding of basic etiquette for interacting with people who have disabilities.
- Effective communication requires understanding and respect. If you are unsure, ask what you can do to facilitate in a manner that will best support everyone's needs.
- Your role as facilitator is to think through the session you will present, and consider what will be required for full inclusion of all participants.

Basic tips for making lessons inclusive

People who are deaf or hard of hearing:

- Make sure that movies or videos you plan to use are captioned.
- Have transcripts available for movies or videos you plan to show. If it's possible to also make these available before the session, it will give participants an opportunity to review and become familiar with the material before the session.
- To signal a transition in a session, for instance to ask participants engaged in small-group work to focus their attention back to the large group, consider a visual signal such as using the light switch to flash the room lights, or another signal.
- Know the etiquette for interacting with deaf people who have an interpreter in the session. And, consider Certified Deaf Interpreters whenever possible, because they bring linguistic and cultural competency that a hearing interpreter may not provide.
- If you are inviting a third party to facilitate communication (transcriptionist, interpreter, etc.) it's a best practice to provide notes to that person at least a day or so prior to the event. These should include specific terminology—for instance, differentiating gender from sex, and other terms with which they may not be familiar ("genderqueer," for example). Providing proper nouns and people's pronouns, if known, is also helpful. Although pronouns aren't particularly important in Deaf culture, in transgender deaf spaces they are, and pronouns are usually fingerspelled when the person is introduced.
- Encourage participants to move around the room as needed during the session, especially if facilitation and interaction take place not just at the front of the room but from other points as well.
- Seek out additional sources of information about deaf allyship, if you are still learning about this.

People who are blind or who have low vision:

- Use vocal cues—say hello to the person, provide instructions aloud to describe the activity.
- Make sure movies or videos you plan to use have video description. This is sometimes also called audio description.
- Have transcripts available for movies or videos you plan to show. They may be accessed by participants by using a variety of adaptive technology, or through Braille. If it's possible to also make these available before the session, it will give participants an opportunity to review and become familiar with the material before the session.
- For lessons that include printed material, such as scenarios for discussion or role playing or other handouts, have participants break into small groups and invite participants who wish to do so to read the materials aloud to the group. The facilitator may also read written materials aloud to the group, depending on the activity.
- Provide an auditory description of what is displayed or written in newsprint, PowerPoint slides, or chalkboards.
- Communicate with participants about what seating arrangement will work best for their needs. Take into account lighting and glare from windows and reflected on surfaces, on chalkboards, newsprint, or screens used for the session. Also consider whether seating participants nearest these, or to the side, will help maximize accessibility for participants whose visual fields are restricted.

- Encourage participants to move around the room as needed during the session, if facilitation and interaction takes place not just at the front of the room but at other points, too.
- Seek additional sources of information about being an ally to people who are blind or have low vision.

People who have physical mobility challenges:

- Invite participants to hold up signs or use other signals rather than having to move to another side of the room for activities that require participants to stand or move around of the room to signify "agree/disagree."
- Rather than moving the large group, or small groups, around the room to various stations for an activity, move the stations to them—rotate easel paper to each group of participants rather than rotating participants to each easel.
- Ask participants how they want to participate instead of assuming. Don't assume participants don't want to or can't perform physical activities, such as tossing a koosh ball in an icebreaker activity, or moving to another location in the room.
- Encourage participants to move around the room as needed during the session, or to stand rather than remaining seated, or vice versa, during activities.
- Seek additional sources of information about being an ally to people who have mobility challenges.

People who experience mental health challenges:

- Embrace opportunities to explore mental health issues, including the ways in which they disparately affect transgender people and some of the conditions that cause these disparities.
- Because Gender Dysphoria is still considered a mental health condition in the US, facilitating some of these lessons may provide unique opportunities for participants to consider issues such as the history and uses of diagnosis, treatment, stigma, ways in which medicalization may help or hinder individuals' development and needs, and other general mental health concepts.
- Be sure you are up to date on key concepts and ideas that are important to understanding mental health.

- Some participants (whether they have received a mental health diagnosis or not) may find some of the content of the lessons challenging or upsetting. Or it may arouse other unsettling or difficult feelings. Let participants know before starting the lesson that this may occur and that they have the right to pass on any activity, and let them know about local resources that are available to support them. Review the support materials in this book for additional information on creating safe, supportive learning environments for talking about such topics.
- Seek additional sources of information about being an ally to people who have mental health disabilities.

People who have learning disabilities:

- Utilize a variety of learning styles (auditory, visual, kinesthetic, experiential).
- Allow enough time for participants to engage in each element of the lesson.
- Be sure to provide transition time between activities.
- Provide materials and instructions in several formats (written, oral).
- If appropriate, provide some of the lesson information in advance for participants to review using assistive technology, or simply to have more time in advance to familiarize themselves with it.
- Encourage participants to move around the room as needed during the session, or to stand rather than remaining seated, during activities.
- Seek additional information about being an ally to people who have learning disabilities.

People who have intellectual disabilities:

The lessons in this book were not specifically designed for use with people who have intellectual disabilities, although a skillful facilitator will be able to draw from the lessons and support materials in this book to create learning opportunities suited for use with such audiences. People who have intellectual disabilities are just are curious and interested in transgender topics as everyone else. They hear about transgender topics through media and everyday conversations, may have transgender friends or relatives, or may be transgender themselves.

The most effective learning strategies for people who have intellectual disabilities include:

- Breaking information into small chunks
- Presenting small amounts of information that are repeated over time
- Presenting ideas in logical ways—specifics of biology are usually not as important as their practical applications
- Providing information in concrete ways
- Providing context—not just information, but how it fits into real life—making content relevant, ideally as the subject arises, taking advantage of "teachable moments"

Since creating and conducting optimal learning opportunities for people who have intellectual disabilities is a sub-specialty in itself, there are many excellent resources online from which to draw. The material in this book may provide the keys to outstanding, enriching educational presentations with people who have intellectual disabilities when used by a facilitator skilled in best practices and approaches for working with people who are a part of this community.

LEADING **EFFECTIVE** DISCUSSIONS

• • •

Giving participants the opportunity to talk about their perspectives and experiences is an essential component of helping participants create meaning and connect the topic to their own lives. Accordingly, many of the lessons included in this book contain a guided discussion component. In each lesson, we have provided discussion questions and key talking points for each. In addition, the following strategies will help ensure a smooth and productive group discussion:

- Make sure that you are driving the discussion—it's essential that you have a sense of where the conversation should go and the key points that need to be covered during the discussion. Framing comments and questions as a bridge to the next talking point can be particularly helpful when participants lead the conversation astray with questions or comments.

- When participants ask questions or make statements, repeat the questions or talking points to the group before answering or moving on. Many participants' voices do not carry, which can make it difficult for other participants to hear. Additionally, this gives you the chance to reframe a question or statement using the most affirming language.

- Alternate voices in conversations to make sure that many people have the opportunity to speak if they so desire. Some participants may take longer than others to gather their thoughts, and some participants may not feel comfortable speaking in large groups. If you find that one particular participant is dominating a discussion, there are a few strategies that can be useful. For example, *"Thanks for sharing, X. What are other people's perspectives on this?"* or *"I would love to hear more from the left side of the room. Any thoughts you would like to share?"*

- If you are unsure of the point a participant is trying to make or you are unsure why they are asking a particular question, it can be useful to ask for more information to help clarify. *"Can you tell me a bit more about the situation?"* or *"That's an interesting question. Why do you ask?"* can help clarify the point. You can also try: *"I want to make sure I understand your point/question. [Repeat back in own words.] Do I have that right?"*

- Silence or low participation in a discussion can indicate confusion about what is being asked, that participants are uncomfortable speaking in the large group, or that there is an unknown (to you) dynamic between participants. It can be useful to clarify whether everyone understands the question that is being asked by asking it in different words. If silence persists, it may be useful to divide people into smaller groups and have them discuss the issue at hand and report back. Alternatively, it may be worthwhile to take a short break or ask if there is anything that you can do to help people feel more comfortable participating. Generally speaking, groups of participants are uncomfortable with silence, and a participant will speak up to end the silence.

MISCELLANEOUS
BITS & PIECES
...

Should I role-model asking for pronouns?

For many years, it was considered best practice to ask participants to share their most affirming pronoun(s) while introducing themselves during a training. This can be a great tool for helping participants understand the experience of having to describe or validate their gender identity to others. That said, asking for a person's pronouns at the beginning of a training can also increase discomfort and confusion, and can sometimes result in microaggressions and other statements of prejudice. Asking for pronouns may also place a burden (including a safety risk) on any transgender people who may be in the audience. Facilitators should make decisions about this based on pre-existing knowledge of the group, the amount of time available for the session, and the group's potential for applying affirming pronouns in their personal or professional lives.

How much should I talk about medical transition?

It is common for participants to want to focus on medical transition, likely in large part because this is a persistent focus of media coverage about transgender people, and many are curious about how medical transition works. Generally speaking, conversations about the specifics of medical transition are largely unnecessary for most audiences (with medical providers being a notable exception). The key take-away point should always be that medical transition helps reduce the dysphoria that transgender people experience, and is a long-term process, not just one event (such as a surgery). For a great example of how to redirect conversations away from medical transition, see Laverne Cox's interview with Katie Couric: http://bit.ly/1cO9jFT.

What should I do if there are transgender people in my training?

It is generally wise to assume and act as if there are transgender people present in a group. Sometimes, there may be transgender people within the group who are not visible or do not wish to be out, and you may never know. At other times, there will be visibly transgender people within a group, or a person will out themselves as transgender during introductions. Having a person who is visibly or out as transgender often changes the dynamics of the training—for both the facilitator and the participants. Participants may feel less comfortable asking questions or speaking freely, or they may specifically ask the transgender person to explain their personal experience. From the facilitator perspective, when other participants know of transgender persons among them, this can increase self-consciousness and elicit a desire to "protect" or "win over" the transgender participants. There is no particular solution or strategy for these scenarios—but it is important to be aware of the dynamics that may occur.

How should I handle religious objections to transgender people?

Religions and faith groups have unique perspectives on transgender people—while conservative religions often reject transgender people, others adopt a "love the sinner, hate the sin" approach. There are also religions and faith groups that are completely affirming of and advocate for transgender people. Even within each of these faith traditions there will be considerable individual variance in how rejecting or affirming a person is, so it is important to avoid making assumptions. In instances in which a participant names their religion as a fundamental barrier to their acceptance and affirmation of transgender people, it is often best not to engage in "debates" with such an individual because it is very unlikely that anything you say will change their mind. Instead, continue to focus on the moveable middle. (See **Common Participant Reactions & Challenges** on page 31.) If you anticipate this as a challenge during a training, you may wish to have literature or referrals to national and local affirming faith groups available (see **Resources & Recommended Reading**). If a person is unable or unwilling to participate in a way that does not distract others, it may be best to ask them to leave the session.

Breaks!

Remember, transgender-related content can be cognitive and emotionally challenging for participants. It can be very helpful to plan for a 10-minute break after about every 75 minutes of teaching time. Beyond that, participants will often lose their focus and be unable to absorb new material/information.

How Do I Create an Affirming PowerPoint?

PowerPoint is ubiquitous, and many facilitators feel more comfortable knowing that they have the information they need on slides in case they get stuck. That said, PowerPoint presentations are not always particularly engaging—especially for those who are not visual or auditory learners. A few thoughts if you do decide to use PowerPoint:

- Make sure that any images you include as a part of the presentation represent the breadth and depth of the transgender community. Representing various types of diversity is essential. (Also, make sure that you have permission to use any images you select—otherwise you risk accidentally "outing" someone in your training.)

- Avoid putting all of the text onto the slides. It is more useful to create a PowerPoint that uses talking points and anchors rather than trying to capture every word that you intend to say during the training. This will help keep your participants engaged and help you to distill the content to key points.

- Include activity instructions for the lessons that you choose. Many participants greatly appreciate the opportunity to re-read prompts or directions when they get stuck during an activity. This will be particularly helpful for participants who have an easier time reading instructions than remember the verbal prompts.

PARTICIPANT HANDOUT

Glossary of Transgender Terms

This is a glossary of some of the more common terms that are used when discussing transgender identities and experiences. Definitions and preferred terms will vary by location and group.

Affirming:
The unequivocal support for an individual person's gender identity or expression, regardless of the biological sex they were assigned at birth; the systematic support to ensure that transgender people and communities are fully represented, included, valued and honored.

Affirming Pronouns:
Refers to the most respectful and accurate pronouns for a person, as defined by that person. This is also sometimes referred to as "preferred gender pronouns," although this phrasing is increasingly outdated. To ascertain someone's affirming pronouns, ask: "What are your pronouns?"

Agender:
A person who does not identify as having a gender identity that can be categorized as male or female, and sometimes indicates identifying as not having a gender identity.

AG/ Aggressive:
A term used to describe a female-bodied and identified person who prefers presenting as masculine. This term is most commonly used in urban communities of color.

Biological Sex:
A person's combination of genitals, chromosomes and hormones, usually categorized as "male" or "female" based on visual inspection of genitals via ultrasound or at birth. Many assume that a person's gender identity will be congruent with their sex assignment. Everyone has a biological sex.

Bigender:
A person who experiences gender identity as two genders at the same time, or whose gender identity may vary between two genders. These may be masculine and feminine, or could also include non-binary identities.

Butch:
A term used to describe a masculine person or gender expression.

Cisgender: (pronounced /sis-gender/)**:**
An adjective to describe a person whose gender identity is congruent with (or "matches") the biological sex they were assigned at birth. (Some people abbreviate this as "cis").

Coming Out:
The process through which a transgender person acknowledges and explains their gender identity to themselves and others.

(Anti-Transgender) Discrimination:
Any of a broad range of actions taken to deny transgender people access to situations/places or to inflict harm upon transgender people. Examples of discrimination include: not hiring a transgender person, threatening a gender non-conforming person's physical safety, denying a transgender person access to services, or reporting someone for using the "wrong" bathroom.

Gender Binary:
The idea that gender is strictly an either/or option of male/men/masculine or female/woman/feminine based on sex assigned at birth, rather than a continuum or spectrum of gender identities and expressions. The gender binary is often considered to be limiting and problematic for all people, and especially for those who do not fit neatly into the either/or categories.

Femme:
A term used to describe a feminine person or gender expression.

Femme Queen:
A term used to describe someone who is male bodied but identifies as and expresses feminine gender. Used primarily in urban communities, particularly in communities of color and ballroom communities.

Gender Conforming:
A person whose gender expression is perceived as being consistent with cultural norms expected for that gender. According to these norms, boys/men are or should be masculine, and girls/women are or should be feminine. Not all cisgender people are gender conforming and not all transgender people are gender non-conforming. (For example, a transgender woman may have a very feminine gender expression).

Gender Dysphoria (GD):
The formal diagnosis in the American Psychiatric Association's *Diagnostic and Statistical Manual, Fifth Edition (DSM 5),* used by psychologists and physicians to indicate that a person meets the diagnostic criteria to engage in *medical transition*. In other words, the medical diagnosis for being transgender. Formerly known as *Gender Identity Disorder (GID)*. The inclusion of Gender Dysphoria as a diagnosis in the DSM 5 is controversial in transgender communities because it implies that being transgender is a mental illness rather than a valid identity. On the other hand, since a formal diagnosis is generally required in order to receive or provide treatment in the US, it does provide access to medical care for some people who wouldn't ordinarily be eligible to receive it.

Gender Expression:
A person's outward gender presentation, usually comprised of personal style, clothing, hairstyle, makeup, jewelry, vocal inflection and body language. Gender expression is typically categorized as masculine or feminine, less commonly as androgynous. All people express a gender. Gender expression can be congruent with a person's gender identity, but it can also be incongruent if a person does not feel safe or supported, or does not have the resources needed to engage in gender expression that authentically reflects their gender identity.

Genderfluid:
A person whose gender identity or expression shifts between masculine and feminine, or falls somewhere along this spectrum.

Gender Identity:
A person's deep-seated, internal sense of who they are as a gendered being—specifically, the gender with which they identify themselves. All people have a gender identity.

Gender Marker:
The marker (male or female) that appears on a person's identity documents (e.g., birth certificate, driver's license, passport, travel or work visas, green cards, etc.). The gender marker on a transgender person's identity documents will be their sex assigned at birth until they undergo a legal and logistical process to change it, where possible.

Gender Neutral:
A term that describes something (sometimes a space, such as a bathroom; or an item, such as a piece of clothing) that is not segregated by sex/gender.

Gender Neutral Language:
Language that does not assume or confer gender. For example "person" instead of " man" or " woman."

Gender Non-Conforming:
A person whose gender expression is perceived as being inconsistent with cultural norms expected for that gender. Specifically, boys/men are not masculine enough or are feminine, while girls/women are not feminine enough or are masculine. Not all transgender people are gender non-conforming, and not all gender non-conforming people identify as transgender. Cisgender people may also be gender non-conforming. Gender non-conformity is often inaccurately confused with sexual orientation.

Genderqueer:
A person whose gender identity is neither male nor female, is between or beyond genders, or is some combination of genders.

Intersex or Disorder of Sex Development (DSD):
A category that describes a person with a genetic, genital, reproductive or hormonal configuration that results in a body that often cannot be easily categorized as male or female. Intersex is frequently confused with transgender, but the two are completely distinct and generally unconnected. Participants may be more familiar with the term *hermaphrodite, which is considered outdated and offensive*

LGBTQ:
An acronym commonly used to refer to Lesbian, Gay, Bisexual, Transgender, Queer and/or Questioning individuals and communities. LGBTQ is often erroneously used as a synonym for "non-heterosexual," which incorrectly implies that transgender is a *sexual orientation*.

Medical Transition:
A long-term series of medical interventions that utilizes hormonal treatments and/or surgical interventions to change a person's body to be more congruent with their gender identity. Medical transition is the approved medical treatment for *Gender Dysphoria*.

Microaggressions:
Small, individual acts of hostility or derision toward transgender or gender non-conforming people, which can sometimes be unintentional. Examples of microaggressions include: use of non-affirming name or pronouns, derogatory language, asking inappropriate or offensive questions, and exhibiting looks that reveal distaste or confusion.

Non-Binary:
A continuum or spectrum of gender identities and expressions, often based on the rejection of the gender binary's assumption that gender is strictly an either/or option of male/men/masculine or female/woman/feminine based on sex assigned at birth. Words that people may use to express their non-binary gender identity include "agender," "bigender," "genderqueer," "genderfluid," and "pangender."

Pangender:
A person who identifies as all genders.

(Anti-Transgender) Prejudice:
An individual's negative attitudes, beliefs, or reactions to transgender people. Examples of anti-transgender prejudice include: believing that transgender people are mentally disturbed, being uncomfortable sharing space with a transgender person, or thinking that transgender people should not be allowed to use public bathrooms.

Pubertal Suppression:
A low-risk medical process that "pauses" the hormonal changes that activate puberty in young adolescents. The result is a purposeful delay of the development of secondary sex characteristics (e.g. breast growth, testicular enlargement, facial hair, body fat redistribution, voice changes, etc.). Suppression allows more time to make decisions about hormonal interventions and can prevent the increased dysphoria that often accompanies puberty for transgender youth.

Questioning:
A person who is exploring or questioning their gender identity or expression. Some may later identify as *transgender* or *gender non-conforming*, while others may not. Can also refer to someone who is questioning or exploring their sexual orientation.

Same-Gender Loving A label sometimes used by members of the African-American/Black community to express an alternative sexual orientation without relying on terms and symbols of European descent. The term emerged in the early 1990's with the intention of offering Black women who love women and Black men who love men a voice, a way of identifying and being that resonated with the uniqueness of Black culture. (Sometimes abbreviated "SGL.")

Sex Assigned at Birth:
The determination of a person's sex based on the visual appearance of the genitals at birth. The sex someone is labeled at birth.

Sexual Orientation:
A person's feelings of attraction (emotional, psychological, physical, and/or sexual) towards other people. A person may be attracted to people of the same sex, to those of the opposite sex, to those of both sexes, or without reference to sex or gender. And some people do not experience primary sexual attraction, and may identify as asexual. Sexual orientation is about attraction to other people (external), while *gender identity* is a deep-seated sense of *self* (internal). All people have a sexual orientation that is separate from their biological sex, gender identity and gender expression.

Social Transition:
A transgender person's process of a creating a life that is congruent with their gender identity, which often includes asking others to use a name, pronoun, or gender that is more congruent with their gender identity. It may also involve a person changing their gender expression to match their gender identity.

Trans:
This is sometimes used as an abbreviation for "transgender."

Transgender:
An adjective used to describe a person whose gender identity is incongruent with (or does not "match") the biological sex they were assigned at birth. "Transgender" serves an umbrella term to refer to the full range and diversity of identities within transgender communities because it is currently the most widely used and recognized term.

(Transgender) Ally:
A cisgender person who supports, affirms, is in solidarity with, or advocates for transgender people.

Transgender men and boys:
People who identify as male, but were assigned female at birth. Also sometimes referred to as transmen.

Transgender women and girls:
People who identify as female, but were assigned male at birth. Also sometimes referred to as trans women.

Transexual/Transsexual:
This is an older term that has been used to refer to a transgender person who has had hormonal or surgical interventions to change their bodies to be more aligned with their gender identity than the sex that they were assigned at birth. While still used as an identity label by some, "transgender" has generally become the preferred term.

Two Spirit:
A term used by Native and Indigenous Peoples to indicate that they embody both a masculine and a feminine spirit. Is sometimes also used to describe Native Peoples of diverse sexual orientations, and has nuanced meanings in various indigenous sub-cultures.

AVOIDING OUTDATED & OFFENSIVE TERMINOLOGY

...

The following terms are generally considered to be outdated, offensive or derogatory when discussing people who are, or are perceived to be, transgender or gender non-conforming. And as noted in the lesson, usage and preferred terms can vary by audience and community. This is not an exhaustive list.

- Tranny, or Trannie
- Hermaphrodite
- Transvestite
- Transgendered
- Transgendering
- Transgenders
- It
- She-Male, or He-She
- "The Surgery"
- Pre-Op, or Post-Op
- Deviant
- Fooling, or Deceiving
- "Real" sex
- Sex Change
- Cross-Dressing

Instead of saying this:	Say this:
"Real" sex, "real" gender, genital sex	Sex assigned at birth
A transgender	Transgender person, or, Person who is transgender
Transgenders	Transgender people, or, People who are transgender
Transgendered	Transgender
FTM, used to be a woman, born a female	Transgender man, or, Transman
MTF, used to be a man, born a male	Transgender woman, or, Transwoman
Sex Change, The Surgery, Transgendering, pre-operative, post-operative	Medical Transition
Hermaphrodite	Intersex person or Person who is intersex
Sexual preference, homosexual	Sexual orientation

REMEMBER

It is very likely that these terms and definitions will continue to evolve over time.
Check out **www.teachingtransgender.com** for updated references and resources.

GETTING STARTED:
Opening Activities

The way you start off the training will set the tone for the rest of the training session. Introductions and opening activities are two specific strategies that can help get the training off to a good start.

Why Introductions?

Depending on the duration of the training, you may wish to start by having participants introduce themselves to the group. This will provide you with the opportunity to learn more about your participants so that you can tailor your content as you go, and it will give participants the opportunity to network or connect with each other. Some good starter questions to consider are:

- What is your name?
- What is your organization/role at the organization?
- What pronoun is most affirming for you? (See note about asking for pronouns on page 51)
- What is one thing that you hope to learn today?
- What prompted you to sign up for today's training?

Why Opening Activities?

We have probably all been in trainings where we have heard a facilitator use the phrase "ice breaker" and we have groaned to ourselves, wondering what sort of cliché or embarrassing activity we were going to have to muddle through. Thankfully, opening activities don't always have to follow that pattern. From a facilitator's standpoint, opening activities serve an important role in effective trainings—particularly with topics that are new or intense, or in conjunction with teaching methods that involve affective content. Specifically, opening activities provide opportunities for participants to become familiar and comfortable with the facilitator, each other, and the general topic before beginning the in-depth portion of a lesson. Opening activities can also be useful for facilitators to quickly get a sense of group dynamics and baseline levels of knowledge. We have included three opening activities here:

1 Snapshots: An individual activity for sessions where time is limited and you want to quickly understand participants' baseline knowledge and questions. (This activity is completed as participants arrive and settle into the training.)

2 Find Someone Who...: An interactive activity that asks participants to introduce themselves to each other and introduces the idea of learning about transgender people.

3 Thinking About Gender Messages: A group activity that has participants out of their seats and thinking about how gender has affected their own lives.

1

SNAPSHOTS:
Assessing Participants' Pre-existing Knowledge

...

Overview & Rationale

Using index cards as an "entrance" activity, this opening lesson gives facilitators a quick understanding of participants' existing knowledge, particularly any misinformation or myths that they have about transgender people. Facilitators can then weave the requested information and correct misinformation or inappropriate terminology during the training without having to call participants out individually.

Audience

This activity works well with audiences when there is adequate physical space and participants can write. This works well with groups of all sizes.

Objectives

By the end of this lesson, participants will be able to:
- Identify 1 piece of information that they already know about transgender people.
- Identify 1 question they have about transgender people

Background Knowledge for Facilitators

A foundation and general knowledge about transgender, non-binary and gender non-conforming people will be useful. (See **Handling Frequently Asked Questions** and **Understanding Transgender People's Experiences** on pages 23 and 14.)

Time

- Preparation: 2 minutes
- Implementation: 10–15 minutes

Materials

- Index cards – 1 for each participant, with a few to spare
- Writing implements – 1 for each participant
- Easel paper or PowerPoint, computer and projector

Preparation

- Write the Activity Prompt on easel paper or PowerPoint slide

Procedure

Hand out index cards to each of the participants as they arrive.

1. Activity Prompt: Direct participants to write 1 thing they know about transgender people on one side of the card. On the other side of the card, direct participants to write 1 question they have about transgender people.

2. Assure participants that it is not necessary to worry about how to phrase the information or questions. Direct participants not to write any identifying information on the cards to ensure anonymity. Once the participants have completed their cards, collect them.

3. When planning the rest of your training session, build in 5 minutes for you to review the content of the cards while participants are working on other activities or during a break. (If using **Lesson 4: Wait, What?! Understanding Transgender Terminology,** on page 71, you will have time to review the cards while participants are working on the handout). Alternately, you can collect the responses in one session, and use them in the next one.

   Knowledge cards: Make note of any cards that contain significant misinformation so that the correct information can be given out during the session.

   Question cards: Separate out any cards with duplicate questions. Make note of any questions that are not likely to be addressed in the session's content and set these cards aside to be answered at the end of the session.

4. Optional: Save the cards for the end of the training and ask participants to volunteer their answers to the group. This can be a great way of assessing the knowledge acquired during the training, and enables participants to demonstrate what they have learned.

TIPS
FOR FACILITATORS

This activity works best when participants are prompted to complete the task as they enter and get settled into the room. It is also useful as a starting activity when you are concerned that some participants may arrive late. This prevents the activity from using time that could be used for teaching content.

• • •

After reading the cards, it will be useful to interweave the correct information during the session whenever possible. This is particularly important to correct misinformation and dispel myths about transgender, non-binary and gender non-conforming people.

• • •

Some questions may be unclear or confusing, and it is important not to ask participants to reveal themselves as having written particular questions. Instead, state that you are not exactly sure what the question is asking, but that you think it is asking "_____" and answer accordingly.

② FIND SOMEONE WHO...

Overview & Rationale

Using a "getting to know you" activity, this icebreaker provides a fun and interactive way to begin a conversation around transgender topics and helps to build comfort among participants. It can also provide facilitators with a quick understanding of participants' existing knowledge of transgender people and themes, opening opportunities to add to that knowledge as the activity progresses.

Audience

This activity works well with audiences where there is enough physical space to move around the room. This activity works best with groups of 20-25 people, but can work with groups of 10-50 people.

Objectives

By the end of this lesson, participants will be able to:
- Be able to identify at least two other participants by name
- Report an increased sense of comfort with their fellow participants

Background Knowledge for Facilitators

Facilitators should be able to explain and provide one example for each of the transgender-specific items on the *Find Someone Who...* handout, in case there are questions. See also **Adaptations for Accessibility on** page 46.

Time

- Preparation: 5 minutes for stickers (optional)
- Implementation: 10-15 minutes

Materials

- *Find Someone Who...* handout (1 per participant)
- Writing implements - 1 for each participant
- Stickers (optional)
- Prizes (optional)

Preparation

- Make copies of the *Find Someone Who...* handout.
- Since this activity requires physical movement and may not be equally accessible to all, be sure to review the list of adaptations in the **Adaptations for Accessibility** section of this book (on page 46) prior to implementing this activity.
- *Optional:* If during the training you will be facilitating a lesson that requires breaking participants up into small groups, you may wish to place stickers on the *Find Someone Who...* handouts in advance of the training. For example, if you will need 5 small groups, you can use 5 stickers, placing one of the stickers on the top of the page of each sheet. When the time comes to break the participants into small groups, you can direct them back to their *Find Someone Who...* handouts.

Procedure

OPTION 1:

As participants enter the room, direct them to the *Find Someone Who...* handout and ask them to begin the activity once they have settled in. You may have to provide additional encouragement for participants to get started. Continue to direct participants to the handout and activity as they arrive. Allow the activity to run until most people have had a chance to have most of their sheet signed by their peers, or as time allows. When time for the activity has elapsed, ask participants to return to their seats. Lead a short discussion, using the questions provided.

OPTION 2:

1. Wait until all of the participants have arrived and explain that you will be initiating a brief activity to help everyone get acquainted. Distribute the *Find Someone Who...* handout, face down. Make sure each participant has a pen or pencil. Instruct participants not to turn over the handout until you give the signal.

2. Explain that, when you give the signal, participants will have about 10 minutes to move about the room. They should introduce themselves to someone, and ask that person one of the questions on the handout. If the person can answer it, they sign their initials next to that question. Each person can sign a participant's sheet only once, so there may be an element of strategy involved in figuring out which questions are such that it may be easier or more difficult to find someone who can answer them. The object is to have one's sheet completely filled with a different person's initials next to each question, before time is called.

3. Ask participants if they have any questions about the activity. Tell participants they'll have only a short time to do this (allow 5-15 minutes, depending on the size and enthusiasm of the group), and must sit down when time is called or when their sheet is complete, whichever comes first.

4. Give the signal to start. Move about the room in case there are any questions about the procedure or about the questions on the handout.

5. When time for the activity has elapsed, ask participants to return to their seats. Lead a short discussion, using the questions provided.

Discussion Questions:

- What was it like to participate in the activity?
- Were there any questions such that it was very easy to find people who could answer them? Which ones?
- Were there any questions such that it was more difficult to find people who could answer them? Which ones?
- Were you surprised by the amount of information you and other participants already know about transgender people and themes? Were there any terms or questions that you are still unsure about?
- What transgender topics or ideas has this activity made you think about, that you'd very much like to learn more about?

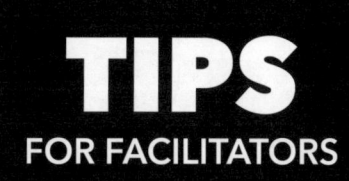

TIPS FOR FACILITATORS

When conducting this activity as a pre-session starter, it works best to prompt participants as they enter and get settled into the room. You may also wish to have music playing to help create a more sociable atmosphere.

• • •

For smaller groups of 20 or less, the facilitator may allow each person to sign the same handout twice, allow less time for completion, or other similar modifications.

• • •

Some groups respond well to the incentive of a small prize for the participant who successfully completes their sheet first, or to all those who complete their sheets within the allotted time. Facilitators who have access to organizational giveaways like pens or stress balls, or to very low-cost items like wrapped pieces of candy or party-favor-style toys, can reward the winners.

PARTICIPANT HANDOUT

Find Someone Who...

Go around to the other participants in the room, and find someone for whom the statement is true. Have that person write their initials next to the item. You may have a person sign only ONE item on the sheet (no duplicates). Once you have completed all of the items, return to your seat and await further instructions.

_____ Is currently wearing socks that are not black or brown

_____ Can name two famous transgender people

_____ Traveled more than 30 minutes to get to here today

_____ Has heard someone say something complimentary about a transgender person

_____ Is an only child

_____ Has a transgender friend or relative

_____ Grew up more than 5 hours from here

_____ Has read a book with a transgender character

_____ Is a dog lover

_____ Has ever gone skydiving or bungee jumping

_____ Has heard someone say something prejudiced about a transgender person

_____ Has a red or green car

_____ Prefers soccer or baseball over football or hockey

_____ Has met someone who identifies as transgender

_____ Is a cat lover

_____ Knows the weather forecast for the next three days

_____ Has seen a movie or TV show with a transgender character

_____ Loves to garden

_____ Has ever spoken up on a transgender person's behalf

_____ Has traveled outside of the United States

_____ Knows how to pronounce the word "cisgender"

_____ Can name 5 Bon Jovi songs

_____ Has seen a documentary about a transgender person

3
THINKING ABOUT
GENDER MESSAGES

• • •

Overview & Rationale

In this opening activity, participants will briefly share ideas about their first recollections of receiving messages about gender. This will provide a basis for developing a common focus and group teamwork, and will introduce a fun element into learning.

Audience

This activity works well with audiences where there is enough physical space to move around the room. This activity works best with groups of 10-24 people, but can work with groups up to 50 people when facilitated carefully.

Objectives

By the end of this lesson, participants will be able to:
- Identify at least 1 message about gender they received from their parents, family or caregivers while growing up
- Describe at least 1 message about gender they received from their peers while growing up
- Describe at least 1 message about gender they received from the media while growing up

Background Knowledge for Facilitators

Facilitators should be well versed in cultural messages related to gender, gender norms and gender roles, and be able to explain the examples provided in the activity prompt questions.

Time

- Preparation: 5 minutes
- Implementation: 15-20 minutes, depending on size of group.

Materials

- A koosh ball
- A bell (optional)

Preparation

- Read through and review the lesson, and choose a koosh Ball or Concentric Circle format.
- Since this activity requires physical movement and may not be equally accessible to all, be sure to review the list of adaptations in the **Adaptations for Accessibility** section of this book (on page 46) prior to implementing this activity.

Procedure for Option 1 – Koosh Ball

1. Tell the group they will be participating in a short activity as an opening exercise. Explain the directions for this activity before beginning:

    - The facilitator will pose a question, and then toss the koosh ball to someone in the circle. When that person catches it, it is their turn to quickly answer the question using only a few words or a brief phrase. After answering, they then throw the ball to another person in the group.

    - When that person catches it, it is their turn to answer the question in the same manner. Anyone may elect to "pass" and answer the question later or not at all.

    - The goal is for each person to have a turn, and for the question to be answered quickly by everyone in the group when it is their turn (when they catch the koosh ball). After everyone has had a turn, the last participant to have a turn will toss the ball back to the facilitator, and the facilitator will introduce a new question and the process begins again.

    - During the activity, others are instructed to listen carefully to everyone's responses. Only one person may speak at a time—the person holding the koosh ball.

2. After all of the activity prompts have been completed, have everyone return to their seats for a large group discussion. Lead a short discussion using the questions and talking points provided.

Procedure for Option 2 – Concentric Circles

1. Tell the group that they will be participating in a short activity as an opening exercise.

2. Ask participants to count off by 2's. Instruct the 1's to form a circle in the center of the room. Once they have formed the circle, ask everyone to turn around and face the outside of the room so that their backs are to each other. Then instruct the 2's to form a circle around the first circle, so that each 1 is paired with and facing a 2. If there is an odd number of people ask for a 1 to volunteer to join a current pair.

3. Explain the directions for this activity before beginning:

    - The facilitator will pose a question for each pair to discuss for about 4 minutes. Each person in the pair should share their response.

    - After 4 minutes the facilitator will ring a bell or flash the lights. At this time, the 2's will move clockwise so that they are standing across from the next 1. (The 1's will remain in the same spot.) Once everyone has found their new partner, the facilitator will read off another statement. This will repeat several times until all the questions have been read and discussed.

4. After all of the activity prompts have been completed, have everyone return to their seats for a large group discussion. Lead a short discussion using the questions and talking points provided.

Activity Prompt Questions:

1. **What is one message you received about gender while growing up from your parents/family? If the group needs examples, provide these.**
   Examples:
   - *"Boys will be boys"*
   - *"Girls like the color pink."*
   - *"Children can and should play with whatever toys they enjoy."*
   - *"Children can grow up to be whatever they wish, regardless of their gender."*

2. **What is one message you received about gender while growing up, from peers? Again, provide examples if needed.**
   Examples:
   - *"Men who have many partners are 'studs'; women who have many partners are 'sluts.'"*
   - *"Boys don't cry."*

3. **What is one message you received about gender from the media as you were growing up? Again, provide examples if needed.**
   Examples:
   - *"There are 'boy's toys' and 'girl's toys.'"*
   - *"Women are more focused on family; men are more focused on career."*
   - *Certain networks or magazines promote gender equality.*

Post- Activity Discussion Questions:

a. What common themes did you hear as everyone shared? What differences?

b. What insights did you gain into the topic of gender from this brief activity?

c. Were any of the questions easier, or more challenging, to answer quickly?

d. What do you hope to learn from the more in-depth lesson we're about to begin?

Talking Points for Post-Activity Discussion:

- Gender is all around us, and many of us receive our first messages about gender when we are very young.
- These messages may embody stereotypes deeply ingrained in society, or they may challenge such stereotypes.
- Thinking back to the messages we remember first receiving, and sharing commonalities and differences, can help us find common ground and perhaps even share some lighthearted moments or fun which can help us then be ready to tackle deeper ideas about gender and gender identity.

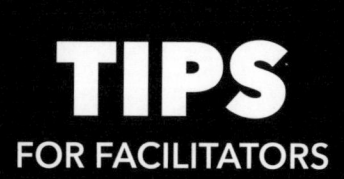

TIPS FOR FACILITATORS

It is important to note that the Concentric Circles option can become a rather loud activity. Keep in mind that some participants may have a harder time hearing in this setting.

• • •

If you choose the Koosh Ball option, it can be helpful to validate in advance that not all participants are good at throwing or catching a ball. Keep in mind that not all participants will have the mobility or dexterity to use the ball.

Transgender "101"

WHO Are Transgender People?

By Jennifer Finney Boylan
Author and Professor

• • •

My mother used to say: *"It is impossible to hate anyone whose story you know."*

In teaching transgender issues, it's important to understand the facts, both scientific and cultural, that make us who we are. But it's easy, sometimes, when we wax rhapsodic with gender theory, to forget that we are talking about the lives of real individuals, men and women who are trying to live their lives with courage and grace, often against very long odds. And so, among the best ways of coming to an understanding of trans experience is hearing the actual stories of trans people, and to understand through their tales that being trans is just another way of being human.

A particularly challenging truth for those who wish to be our allies is that there are hundreds and hundreds of different ways of "being" trans, and that even trans people themselves don't often agree on what the issues are, or ought to be. Some of us see ourselves on a quest to defy binary cultural expectations of gender expression. Some of us see ourselves as men and women with a set of unique birth defects that can be addressed through the intervention of the medical community. Others experience gender as a kind of performance, and are interested in the ways that transgressing gender can provide cultural commentary—not to mention a kind of joyful, theatrical experience. And still others don't have words to describe themselves, or the journey that they are on, and follow no one's path—or theory—but their own.

It can be bewildering for others to try to put their arms around the many different kinds of trans experience. Learning about our stories—and the rich diversity of our lives—we will come a little closer to the time when trans experience begins to feel more commonplace, and we start to be a little more familiar to others.

Understanding the many ways there are of being trans, in fact, is really just subset of an education in the many ways there are of being human. It's not just trans people who are trying to move beyond the binary— it's all of us. Each of us is on a journey to find our own truth, a truth that more often than not lies somewhere between the poles of human experience.

As Oscar Wilde once observed, *"Be yourself. Everyone else is already taken."*

WAIT ... WHAT?!
Understanding Transgender Terminology

...

Overview & Rationale

Although terminology about biological sex, sexual orientation, gender identity and gender expression is becoming increasingly common in the popular media and everyday life, these terms and their definitions—and scope—may still be confusing. This lesson provides participants with an introduction to the concepts of biological sex, gender identity, gender expression, and sexual orientation, and helps to clarify the meanings of the terms that will be used in the remainder of the training.

Audience

This lesson is designed as a foundational lesson for all target audiences within this book. This activity works best with groups smaller than 35, but can be modified for use with larger audiences by limiting discussion.

Objectives

By the end of this lesson, participants will be able to:
- Explain the difference between biological sex, gender identity, gender expression and sexual orientation
- Correctly define "transgender" and "gender non-conforming"
- Identify 2 words or phrases that are considered to be derogatory to transgender people and should be avoided

Background Knowledge for Facilitators

A throughout review of the **Navigating Transgender Terminology, Tips for Teaching Transgender Terminology** and **The SIEO Model** pieces in the **Foundations & Best Practices for Facilitators** section will be particularly useful in facilitating this lesson.

Time

- Preparation: 3 minutes
- Implementation: 45 minutes, (depending on group and facilitation)

Materials

- Copies of the *Understanding Transgender Terminology* handout (one per participant)
- Copies of the *Glossary of Terms* on page 53 (one per participant)
- Easel Paper or PowerPoint slide that lists correct answers
  (See www.teachingtransgender.com/printables for a downloadable slide. PW: TTTprep15).

Preparation

- Make copies of the handouts
- Prepare the PowerPoint or easel paper sign that lists the correct answers, so that participants can compare their own answers with those on the list of correct answers

Procedure

Hand out index cards to each of the participants as they arrive.

1. Explain that: In this first portion of the training, we will be reviewing some common terms that are used when discussing transgender and gender non-conforming youth. You may be familiar with some of these terms, but since different people use the terms in different ways, we want to make sure that we are all working with the same definitions.

2. Distribute the *Understanding Transgender Terminology* handout. Instruct participants to complete the handout by working together with 2-3 people around them to figure out the correct answers. (It can be useful to explain that you will provide the correct answers and explanations after they have had a chance to complete the handout.)

3. After about 10-15 minutes bring the participants back to the large group. Explain that you are going to display the list of correct answers, and then after everyone has had a chance to check their answers you will provide explanations for each of the definitions. (See the *Understanding Transgender Terminology: Facilitator's Guide* for the correct answers and talking points for each term).

4. Ask participants if they have any questions about these concepts or terms. Validate that this is a lot of information in a short period of time, and that it can be confusing or overwhelming.

5. Explain that there are some terms that are derogatory and offensive and should never be used and that you are passing out the *Glossary of Terms* handout, which includes a grid that explains affirming alternatives.

6. Conclude the conversation with these final talking points:

    Wrap Up Talking Points:
    - Every person in the room, and every person who is born, has a biological sex, a gender identity, and a gender expression. This combination is what comprises a person's gender. All people also have a sexual orientation that is separate from gender identity. Sexual orientation is attraction to and desire to have relationships with other people.
    - Transgender people also have a sexual orientation that is separate from their gender identity. Transgender people can have any and all of these sexual orientations. It is important to remember that all transgender people also have a sexual orientation.

Evaluation Questions

✔ Explain the difference between biological sex, gender identity, gender expression and sexual orientation.
✔ Define the terms: "transgender" and "gender non-conforming"
✔ What are 2 transgender-related words or phrases that are considered to be derogatory and should be avoided?

SOURCE: This handout is a modified version from: Green, E.R. & Perry, J.R. (2014). *Safe & Respected: Providing Culturally Competent Services for Transgender and Gender Non-Conforming Youth in ACS Care (Training Curriculum).* New York: New York City's Administration for Children's Services. Used with permission.

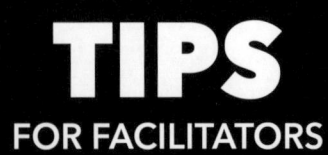

TIPS FOR FACILITATORS

Terminology can be particularly challenging and confusing for participants, largely because many of the terms that are presented and explained in this activity are new terms and concepts. Participants may feel overwhelmed by this activity, and it will be useful to validate their experience. Follow the **Tips for Teaching Transgender Terminology** to help participants absorb as much information as they can.

• • •

This lesson tends to evoke the most questions from participants. These questions are often motivated by a desire to genuinely understand the topic and connect this new information to their previous knowledge. Careful facilitation of the discussion and setting clear boundaries about the amount of time available for Q&A will be helpful.

• • •

Since discussions of transgender people in popular media tend to dwell on medical transition, participants may have questions about the specifics of how transition works from a medical or biological standpoint. It is appropriate to state that this lesson does not focus on surgical or hormonal transitions, and that such a focus is outside the scope of this training.

Understanding Transgender Terminology:
FACILITATOR'S GUIDE

(See explanations and talking points for each of these answers on the next page).

> A: Cisgender
> B: Gender Non-Conforming
> C: Biological Sex
> D: Gender Dysphoria
> E: Medical Transition
> F: Sexual Orientation
> G: Heterosexual
> H: Transgender woman
> I: Transgender
> J: Transgender man
> K: Sex Assigned at Birth
> L: Pubertal Suppression
> M: Gender Expression
> N: Gender Identity

1. __F__ (Example) — A person's sexual, emotional, physical and psychological attraction to other people.
2. __C__ — A person's combination of genitals, chromosomes and hormones.
3. __K__ — The sex that someone is labeled at birth, usually based on the appearance of their genitals.
4. __N__ — A person's deep-seated internal sense of their own gender.
5. __A__ — A term used to describe a person whose biological sex and gender identity are congruent, or "match."
6. __I__ — A term used to describe a person whose biological sex and gender identity are incongruent, or do not "match."
7. __M__ — The gendered way that a person dresses or presents themselves.
8. __B__ — A term used to describe a person whose gendered appearance does not conform to traditional masculinity or femininity.
9. __H__ — The affirming way to refer to a person who identifies as a woman but was assigned male at birth.
10. __J__ — The affirming way to refer to a person who identifies as a man but was assigned female at birth.
11. __E__ — The approved medical process of changing one's body to be more aligned with their gender identity.
12. __L__ — An approved medical process used to delay puberty for transgender children.
13. __D__ — The medical diagnosis for being transgender, formerly known as Gender Identity Disorder.

1. **(F) Sexual Orientation:** Sexual orientation is a person's sexual, emotional, physical and psychological attraction to another person. Heterosexual people are usually attracted to people of a different gender, gay men are attracted to men, and lesbians are attracted to women. Bisexual people are attracted to people of the same and different genders. Transgender is not a sexual orientation.

2. **(C) Biological Sex:** Biological sex is a person's combination of sex organs, chromosomes, and hormones. In most cases, people are assigned either 'female' or 'male' at birth.

3. **(K) Sex Assigned at Birth:** The biological sex that someone is assumed to be at birth, usually based on a visual assessment of their genitals. This is what is recorded on a person's birth certificate.

4. **(N) Gender Identity:** Gender identity is a person's deep-seated, felt sense of gender, or how a person feels on the inside, regardless of what their body looks like. Most people's gender identity is congruent with or "matches" their biological sex, but some people's gender identity is incongruent with or does not "match" the sex that they were assigned at birth.

5. **(A) Cisgender:** (Pronounced /sis-gender/). This is a term used to describe a person whose gender identity is congruent with or "matches" their biological sex. Most people are cisgender.

6. **(I) Transgender:** A term used to describe people who experience a disconnect between their biological sex and their gender identity. Which is to say, their biological sex and gender identity are incongruent, or their gender identity is not what we would usually expect based on their biological sex. The term "transgender" is most often used to refer to the entire community of people who experience this disconnect between gender identity and biological sex, and "transgender" is sometimes shortened to "trans." Generally speaking, "transgender" is the best term to use, unless a person uses a different term to describe their identity. In that case, it is appropriate to mirror the language they use.

7. **(M) Gender Expression:** Gender expression is what we call the ways in which people outwardly communicate their gender to others. These cues can include hairstyle, clothing choices/style, make-up, tattoos, piercings, facial hair, walking gait, vocal pitch, etc. Some aspects of gender expression, such as clothes and haircut, are matters of choice. Other aspects such as vocal pitch and walking gait are more innate. These cues are usually categorized as "masculine" or "feminine." When people assume that someone is not heterosexual, they are often responding to a person's gender expression, rather than their sexual orientation, because expression is what is visible, while orientation is internal.

8. **(B) Gender Non-Conforming:** A term referring to people whose gender expressions do not conform with the traditional norms for what is expected of their sex assigned at birth. Not all gender non-conforming people identity as lesbian, gay, bisexual or transgender, although some gender non-conforming people do. Gender non-conforming people are the primary targets of homophobia (prejudice toward LGB people) because people assume they are not heterosexual.

9. **(H) Transgender Woman:** People who identify as female but were assigned male at birth are most respectfully referred to as "transgender women," or simply "women." When referring to someone, it is always most appropriate to use the language that affirms their gender identity. For a transgender woman, this includes using female pronouns, her chosen (preferred) name, and referring to her as a woman (not by the sex she was assigned at birth).

10. **(J) Transgender Man:** People who identify as male but were assigned female at birth are most respectfully referred to as "transgender men," or simply "men." When referring to someone, it is always most appropriate to use the language that affirms their gender identity. For a transgender man, this includes using male pronouns, his chosen (preferred) name, and referring to him as a man (not by the sex he was assigned at birth).

11. **(E) Medical Transition:** Many people have likely heard the term "sex change" or "sex reassignment surgery" associated with a transgender person who has had genital surgery. Sex change and sex reassignment surgery are terms that are outdated and offensive. The appropriate term is "medical transition," which refers to the range of hormonal and surgical treatments that treat Gender Dysphoria. While many transgender people desire to medically transition, not all do.

12. **(L) Pubertal Suppression:** A medical process that delays the onset of puberty in transgender youth. This is an approved medical treatment that safely provides time for transgender young people and their caregivers and providers to determine whether to administer cross-sex hormones at the start of puberty, so that their bodies do not develop secondary sex characteristics that are incongruent with their gender identity.

13. **(D) Gender Dysphoria:** This is the medical diagnosis in the DSM 5 (Diagnostic and Statistical Manual) that describes the intense and persistent discomfort transgender people feel because of the disconnect between their biological sex and their gender identity.

PARTICIPANT HANDOUT

understanding Transgender Terminology

Read each of the definitions below, and match them with the correct term from the top of the page.

> A: Cisgender
> B: Gender Non-Conforming
> C: Biological Sex
> D: Gender Dysphoria
> E: Medical Transition
> F: Sexual Orientation
> G: Heterosexual
> H: Transgender woman
> I: Transgender
> J: Transgender man
> K: Sex Assigned at Birth
> L: Pubertal Suppression
> M: Gender Expression
> N: Gender Identity

1. __F__ (Example) — A person's sexual, emotional, physical and psychological attraction to other people.

2. _____ A person's combination of genitals, chromosomes and hormones.

3. _____ The sex that someone is labeled at birth, usually based on the appearance of their genitals.

4. _____ A person's deep-seated internal sense of their own gender.

5. _____ A term used to describe a person whose biological sex and gender identity are congruent, or "match."

6. _____ A term used to describe a person whose biological sex and gender identity are incongruent, or do not "match."

7. _____ The gendered way that a person dresses or presents themselves.

8. _____ A term used to describe a person whose gendered appearance does not conform to traditional masculinity or femininity.

9. _____ The affirming way to refer to a person who identifies as a woman but was assigned male at birth.

10. _____ The affirming way to refer to a person who identifies as a man but was assigned female at birth.

11. _____ The approved medical process of changing one's body to be more aligned with their gender identity.

12. _____ An approved medical process used to delay puberty for transgender children.

13. _____ The medical diagnosis for being transgender, formerly known as Gender Identity Disorder.

IMAGINING Transgender

Overview & Rationale

This affective activity is based on Brian McNaught's (2011) classic guided imagery, in which heterosexual participants are asked to imagine they are growing up in a world in which everyone else is gay. In this version, participants are asked to imagine what their world might be like if they were transgender. Through this process, participants will develop a better understanding of the interpersonal struggles that many transgender people face while coming out. By empathizing with people whose experiences are different than their own, participants will be better prepared to act as transgender allies.

Audience

This lesson works well with people who are relatively new to learning about transgender people and for more advanced participants who have a strong knowledge base but will benefit from empathy-based activities. This activity works well with groups of 50 people or less, but if facilitated carefully, can work with larger groups.

Objectives

By the end of this lesson, participants will be able to:
- Name at least 2 challenges many transgender people experience before and after coming out.
- Identify 3 emotions a transgender person might experience during their coming out experience.

Background Knowledge for Facilitators

It will be useful for facilitators to have a strong empathetic understanding of the challenges that transgender and gender non-conforming people face. Experience and/or confidence in facilitating highly affective content will also be useful.

Time

- Preparation: 10 minutes
- Implementation: 30 minutes

Materials

None needed.

Preparation

Read through the Imagining Transgender scenarios in their entirety, and select the youth or adult scenario (based on your target audience). Practice reading the scenario out loud.

Procedure

1. Explain to participants that for this activity, you will be leading them through a guided imagery exercise. If possible, it may be useful to dim the lights.

2. Slowly, read the selected scenario aloud to the participants from the *Imagining Transgender Facilitator Guide*. Pause frequently to allow participants to think through the various aspects of the scenario.

3. After a minute or so of silence, explain that you will discuss the activity in greater depth momentarily but that first you would like to ask each of the participants to share one word that describes how they would be feeling at the end of the day that you have all just imagined. Ask for a volunteer to go first. Participants may respond in turn, or speak as they feel ready.

4. After everyone has shared their word, lead the group in discussion using the questions and talking points on the *Imagining Transgender Facilitator Guide*.

5. If using as a standalone lesson, conclude by explaining that: This activity has given us a brief glimpse into what many transgender people experience on a consistent basis, and while there are many transgender people who live happy and fulfilling lives, there are often unique challenges they must overcome to achieve that happiness.

6. Then, ask participants to identify 1 emotion or feeling they are aware of experiencing, and have each participant share their emotion/feeling using 1 word. (Note: This works best when participants are restricted to 1 word—otherwise they may want to explain why, which changes the tone and lengthens the activity). After all participants have shared their word, acknowledge the range of feelings and emotions in the room, and thank people for sharing and participating.

Evaluation Questions

✔ What are 2 challenges that transgender people might experience before and after coming out?

✔ What are 3 emotions that transgender people might commonly feel while navigating being transgender or coming out as transgender?

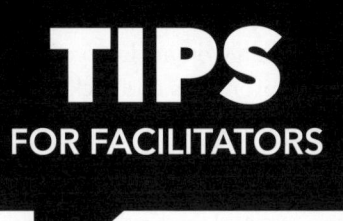

TIPS FOR FACILITATORS

This opening activity works specifically to elicit an affective and emotional response from participants, and can result in their experiencing strong feelings. Some participants may cry, others may report feeling overwhelmed. While these responses are appropriate for this activity, the high levels of emotions can and will affect the tone of the training, and may influence the group dynamics. In addition to allowing participants to process their responses, it can also be useful to name and validate this experience as strategic and intentional as a way of giving a brief glimpse into the intensity of transgender people's experiences.

• • •

Because this activity is an affective-based one that can elicit a strong emotional response, it may not work as well with groups who are especially hostile or resistant to learning about transgender people.

• • •

This opening activity can also be used as an exercise during a longer training, particularly if it seems as though participants are having a hard time personally connecting with the content you are facilitating. This will be most effective when combined with other lessons that offer concrete action points on how to be an affirming ally or advocate, so that participants have clear next steps on how to move forward.

• • •

When facilitating this activity, it is not unusual for the facilitator to have a strong emotional response while reading the imagery. For some, it can be hard to read this aloud without feeling overwhelmed, speaking in a wavering voice or wanting to cry. It will be helpful for facilitators to read the imagery aloud to themselves prior to implementing this in a group. If strong emotions surface during the group reading, it can be helpful to explain to participants that even though you have read this before, you still find it to be very powerful and moving. Indicate that you understand that they may also be having strong responses to the story, and that it is a normal part of this activity.

IMAGINING TRANSGENDER (ADULT)

I would like you to imagine with me... an average day as a transgender person who is in the process of coming out. Please close your eyes and follow along.

If you currently identify as a woman, then imagine that everywhere you go, the people around you treat you as if you are man. You are expected to act and dress like a man. Everyone refers to you using male pronouns and nicknames . . . he, him, his, mister, buddy, dude, or sir. Even though you know in your heart and mind that you are a woman, everyone around you sees you as a man and acts accordingly. You are expected to use the men's bathrooms, locker rooms, and changing rooms.

If you currently identify as a man, then imagine that everywhere you go, the people around you treat you as if you are a woman. You are expected to act and dress like a woman. Everyone refers to you using female pronouns and nicknames . . . she, her, miss, girl, lady, or ma'am. Even though you know in your heart and mind that you are a man, everyone around you sees you as a woman and acts accordingly. You are expected to use the women's bathrooms, locker rooms, and changing rooms.

[pause]

This mislabeling of your gender happens in the morning when the attendant at the gas station says hello. It happens when the clerk at the coffee shop says good morning, and asks what they can get you. It happens when the front desk person greets you, on your way into your office.

While you are at work, your co-workers refer to you using the wrong gender language. They use the wrong pronouns, and they expect you to conform to traditional gender roles. You know that they don't mean anything by it—they don't even know how you identify. But still, the constant misgendering wears you down. Every day, you plan for the day when you will tell them how you identify and want to be addressed, but you keep putting off that day because you are nervous that they won't support you, that they will treat you differently, or that you might lose your job.

[pause]

After a long day at work, you decide to go to the gym. Before you go, you wait for everyone else to leave work so that you can change into your gym clothes with no one else in the bathroom (the locker room at the gym is out of the question). While at the gym, you choose exercises that might help disguise the parts of your body that are most uncomfortable for you.

After you leave the gym, you stop by the grocery store, the pet store, and the pharmacy. In each place, as you interact with the cashiers, they refer to you using the wrong gender language.

[pause]

Afterwards, you go to the restaurant where you are meeting your partner for dinner. In hopes of getting a better tip, the person serving your table tries to be friendly with you, and makes a joke that presumes your gender. Your partner sees that this bothers you, but knows that there is nothing that they can say to make it better and changes the subject.

[pause]

After dinner, you go home and change out of your clothes. You glance in the mirror, and are immediately frustrated and disappointed when you don't recognize the person looking back at you in the mirror. Every time you look in the mirror, you are surprised by your reflection because it doesn't match the image that you have of yourself in your mind's eye. You quickly glance away from the mirror and block the thoughts out of your mind.

[Pause]

Take a moment now to reflect on how you're feeling. When you feel ready, please open your eyes. Once everyone is ready, we will discuss this scenario as a group.

IMAGINING TRANSGENDER (YOUTH)

I would like you to imagine with me... an average day as a young person who is transgender, around the age of 7 years old. Please close your eyes and follow along.

If you currently identify as a woman, please imagine that everywhere you go, the people around you treat you as if you are a little boy. You are expected to act and dress like a boy. Everyone refers to you using male pronouns and nicknames . . . he, him, his, little man, buster, champ, or son. Even though you know in your heart and mind that you are a girl, everyone around you insists that you are a boy and demands you act accordingly.

If you currently identify as a man, please imagine that everywhere you go, the people around you treat you as if you are a little girl. You are expected to act and dress like a girl. Everyone refers to you using female pronouns and nicknames . . . she, her, sweetie, girlie, or darling. Even though you know in your heart and mind that you are a boy, everyone around you insists that you are a girl and demands you act accordingly.

[pause]

When you get out of bed in the morning, you survey your closet and aren't happy with any of the clothing options you see. These clothes make you feel really uncomfortable and upset when you wear them. Your parents tell you to hurry up and get dressed, so you pick the clothes that are least uncomfortable—they make you feel more like yourself.

When you get on the bus in the morning, some of the other kids tease you. They say mean things like "What are you, gay or something?" and "Why do you dress like that?" Other kids ignore you. You feel isolated and alone. Once you get to school, you are asked to line up by gender and you consistently get yelled at for where you go, and the teacher tells you to stop causing problems and to get in the "correct" line or they will call your parents. During recess, the other kids group together by activity, but you have a hard time choosing—when you do what you really want to do, it results in more teasing. You are sad, frustrated, and confused.

[pause]

Imagine now that you are 14. For the past few years, your body has been changing in ways that are profoundly uncomfortable. You are starting to have sexual feelings and fantasies, which are confusing because it feels good, but also feels uncomfortable. You have asked your close friends questions to see if they have similar feelings, but so far no one else has had a similar experience. At the same time, everyone else is suddenly interested in hooking up and dating, and that feels overwhelming. Sometimes you feel like you should just hook up/date so that people will stop harassing you about whether or not you are gay, and besides, you really want to be in a relationship... but things are so overwhelming. You know that you are attracted to one gender, but think that you might also be attracted to the other gender. Maybe all of this discomfort is because you are gay. You seek out information online about being gay, but somehow it doesn't seem to fit. You found a transgender teen support forum, and a lot of what is you find there makes sense, but it is super scary.

You wish that someone could understand where you are coming from, explain why you feel this way, and help you figure out how to make it stop feeling so bad. You can't talk to your parents about this.

Over the years, you have noticed your parents saying little things here and there about how transgender people are freaks, and how they would never let their kid do that. You are afraid of how they will react if you tell them, and life is hard enough as it is. You don't want to risk their rejecting you because you just aren't sure that you will be able to handle it. Besides, you know that your parents are struggling for money, and dealing with your aging grandparents and your siblings—you don't want to add to their burden when they are already so stressed out.

Every day starts to feel like a battle, and you are exhausted. You are feeling increasingly depressed and start looking for things to help make you feel better. You consider experimenting with drinking and drugs, or maybe cutting—anything that might help. You saw the "it gets better" videos online, but frankly you just can't see how that can possibly be true for you.

[Pause]

Take a moment now to reflect on how you're feeling. When you feel ready, please open your eyes. Once everyone is ready, we will discuss these scenarios as a group.

IMAGINING TRANSGENDER:
FACILITATOR'S GUIDE

Post-Reading Discussion Questions:

1. **What feelings came up for you as you listened to this story? Specifically, what might you be feeling if this was your consistent experience in the world?**

    Common responses: Anger, frustration, depression, sadness, hopelessness, invisibility.

2. **Based on your experience imagining this scenario, what might be some of the hard parts of being transgender?**

    Common responses: The persistence across settings, the lack of support, the ongoing effects of not feeling safe or affirmed, constantly having to fight to be seen.

3. **What might be some examples of places in the story where an ally could have intervened to provide support?**

    Examples (Adult Scenario):
    - A co-worker could advocate proactively for transgender-affirming policies and practices
    - Store workers could have used gender-neutral language (instead of gendering)
    - The partner could have made it a point to provide an affirming correction to the waitstaff, or provided a reassuring comment

    Examples (Youth Scenario):
    - The parents could have provided gender-neutral or affirming clothing options and consistently stated their unconditional love
    - Peers could have stood up against gender-based bullying and made it a point to connect
    - The teacher could have used non-gender-based dividing techniques
    - Your school's sexuality education could have been transgender-inclusive
    - Someone might have noticed the depression and reached out with support

4. **Based on your experience imagining this scenario, what might be some the ways that having strong transgender allies in a person's life could be beneficial?**

    Examples:
    - Providing an empathetic ear so they can vent frustrations
    - Having someone else speak up on their behalf
    - Running interference to help smooth out potentially challenging situations in advance
    - Providing unconditional love and acceptance to offset negativity and prejudice
    - Reminders of value and worth

"ARE YOU A BOY OR A GIRL??"
Transgender In Childhood

Overview & Rationale

In this lesson, participants will watch two video clips of transgender children (Ryan Whittington & Jazz Jennings), participate in a guided discussion to help gain greater understanding of how transgender identity emerges in children, and explore implications for other transgender children. This lesson uses the recent media coverage of transgender children and specifically helps participants process the underlying messages and overall concepts.

Audience

This lesson works well with people who work with children and families (teachers, school staff and administrators, early childhood educators, counselors and therapists, healthcare providers, human service providers, and others) and with parent/family groups. This lesson works best with groups of 35 participants or less, but if facilitated carefully can be used in groups of up to 50.

Objectives

By the end of this lesson, participants will be able to:
- Name 2 actions a transgender child will perceive as affirming their gender identity.
- Describe 2 positive outcomes that result from a transgender child being affirmed and
- Describe 2 potential negative outcomes that might occur if a transgender child is not affirmed.

Background Knowledge for Facilitators

It will be useful for participants to be familiar with the stories of multiple transgender children, beyond those in the linked clip. Additional information about pubertal suppression and medical transition options for youth will also be helpful when fielding questions. Facilitators are also encouraged to watch the follow-up video and series (linked below) about Jazz's experiences and review the most up-to-date information from Jazz's website.

Time

- Preparation: 15 minutes
- Implementation: 45–60 minutes

Materials

- Computer with Internet access
- Projector and speakers
- "I Am Jazz" video clip (Play through minute 11:00)
  (Available for free online at: www.transkidspurplerainbow.org/featured/i-am-jazz-a-family-in-transition/)
- "Ryland's Story" video clip
  (Available for free online at: http://www.youtube.com/watch?v=yAHCqnux2fk)

Preparation

- Preview the videos in full, prior to session
- Watch the follow-up to Jazz's story, her TLC series "I am Jazz" and review recent updates on Jazz's website (http://www.tlc.com/tv-shows/i-am-jazz/ and http://www.transkidspurplerainbow.org)
- Review Pubertal Suppression overview: http://www.imatyfa.org/permanent_files/pubertyblockers101.html
- Download/pre-load the clips for use during the presentation

Procedure

1. Explain that: We will be watching two brief documentaries about the experiences of transgender children. We will start with a video about a young boy named Ryland and we will then take some time to discuss it before we move on to our second clip of a young girl named Jazz.

2. Show clip of Ryland and facilitate discussion using the following questions. (See *Ryland & Jazz: Facilitator's Guide* for the questions and guidance on talking points for each.)

3. Show clip of Jazz and facilitate discussion using the following questions. (See *Ryland & Jazz: Facilitator's Guide* for the questions and guidance on talking points for each.)

4. After discussing both clips, move to the concluding questions. (See *Ryland & Jazz: Facilitator's Guide* for the questions and guidance on talking points for each.)

Evaluation Questions

✔ What are 2 actions that a transgender child may perceive as affirming their gender identity?

✔ What are 2 positive outcomes that result from affirming a transgender child?

✔ What are 2 potential negative outcomes that might occur if a transgender child is not affirmed?

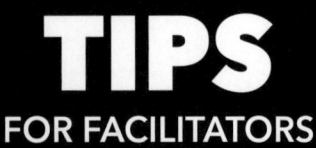

TIPS FOR FACILITATORS

This lesson plan is particularly effective at helping people to understand that being transgender is not a "choice," but in some ways by focusing on transgender children with very clear narratives, this lesson may also lead participants to believe that these types of narratives are the only or most valid ones. It is important to remind participants that there are other presentations of being transgender that are equally valid and important to recognize. Not all transgender people present this degree of persistence, insistence and consistency—but that does not mean that their gender identities are any less valid.

• • •

Some participants may feel that Jazz's parents caused her identity or pushed her into being transgender. This is often because participants struggle with the idea that this can emerge so young, and are uncomfortable that Jazz's parents were affirming of her/did not try to discourage her from being a girl. It is important to help participants understand the negative consequences that happen for transgender children who are not affirmed, and remind participants that it is not possible to change someone's identity.

Ryland & Jazz:
FACILITATOR'S GUIDE

Discussion Questions & Guide for "Ryland's Story" clip:

1. **At what age did it become clear that Ryland identified as a boy, and how did he communicate that to his parents?**

   - *Talking Points:* Ryland's identity became clear when he was a few years old and learned to speak after receiving his cochlear implants, when he stated directly that he was a boy. As he continued to age, he showed increased signs of being a boy—in particular, he wanted to cut off his hair, experienced increasing shame, and didn't understand why God made him that way.

2. **In what ways did Ryland's parents communicate their affirmation to Ryland?**

   - *Talking Points:* His parents switched to male pronouns, changed his wardrobe to male clothing, changed his bedroom, sent a letter to friends and family explaining Ryland was a boy, and put together this video for people to better understand why they chose to support Ryland.

Discussion Questions & Guide for "I am Jazz" clip:

3. **How does Jazz describe herself and her identity?**

   - *Talking Points:* Jazz explains that she has a girl brain and a boy body. She states that she has always identified as a girl, as long as she can remember.

4. **At what age did it become clear that Jazz identified as a girl?**

   - *Talking Points:* Jazz displayed feminine characteristics from the time that she was very young, and continued to display them more as she grew older. At her 5th birthday party, she was allowed to wear the bathing suit that was most affirming for her. Jazz identifies that she has experienced gender dysphoria from when she was very young.

5. **Jazz's family is a great example of affirming a transgender young person's gender identity. What are some of the ways in which Jazz's family affirmed her?**

   - *Talking Points:* Jazz's family calls her by the name that she prefers, consistently refers to her using female pronouns, provides her with female clothing, treats her like a girl, prioritizes Jazz's happiness, has sought out the expertise of gender professionals, and advocates for Jazz in school, sports and other aspects of her life.

6. **In what ways do you think that Jazz's experience might have been different if her family had not affirmed her gender identity?**

   - *Talking Points:* Jazz would have been very likely to experience significant depression, anxiety, increased gender dysphoria, and the possibility of self-harm including suicidal attempts and/or drug/alcohol abuse, increased social isolation, and a hard time making friends and connecting with others.

7. Jazz is a very self-confident young person, and her ability to articulate her identity shows that she is clearly very well-accustomed to explaining herself to adults. This is a great example of a specific resiliency that Jazz has developed. What other resiliencies do we see in Jazz?

    - *Talking Points:* Jazz is very self-confident, she has high self-esteem, she has a positive relationship with family and peers, and she can advocate for herself and what she wants.

8. Jazz's family clearly has a lot of economic and other privileges. What do you think might have been different for Jazz if her family was less privileged?

    - *Talking Points:* Jazz's parents likely would not have had the same amount of time to dedicate to advocating for and supporting Jazz, they likely would not have had access to resources to take Jazz to so many gender specialists, they would have been less able to have Jazz change schools, and they may have had a harder time accepting Jazz (or handling the stress related to having a transgender child).

Culminating Discussion Questions & Guide

9. After seeing both of the video clips, in what ways are Ryland and Jazz's experiences similar?

    - *Talking Points:* Both Ryland and Jazz's gender identities emerged at a very young age, both have parents who found a path towards affirmation, both have parents who are willing to advocate for them, both have parents who have chosen to be public about their journeys, and above all, both Ryland and Jazz are happy, well-adjusted children who are clearly respected and well loved.

10. As noted in the Jazz video clip; sometimes a young person's transgender identity emerges at an early age with consistency and clarity, while for others it may emerge later and with less clarity. Both Ryland and Jazz are examples of early emergence and clarity. What do you think might be some of the challenges for young people whose identities become clear later in adolescence or present with less consistency or clarity?

    - *Talking Points:* One of the main challenges that transgender adolescents, teens and adults may experience differently is that people may be less likely to believe a person who says that they are transgender if they have not exhibited gender non-conforming behaviors or expression throughout their lifetime. This is particularly true with the increasing number of transgender children appearing in the media.

11. After watching these clips, what recommendations would you have for family members, friends and teachers of gender non-conforming children?

    - *Talking Points:* It is essential to the mental, emotional and physical well-being of all young people that they are affirmed, regardless of their gender identity or expression. Affirmation includes creating gender-neutral environments and encouraging all children to challenge limiting gender stereotypes. Individual-level supports include making sure to use affirming names and pronouns for all children, and helping other children accept and understand differences.

WHAT DOES NON-BINARY MEAN?
Understanding and Supporting People Who Have Non-Binary Gender Identities

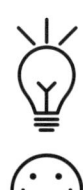

Overview & Rationale

While many people are gaining greater awareness of transgender people who transition from one gender to another, most people are still largely unfamiliar with people whose gender identities are non-binary. This lesson provides participants with an intermediate-level understanding of the concept of non-binary gender identities, the identities and experiences of people who have non-binary gender identities, and the challenges they may face.

Audience

This lesson is designed for audiences who have a solid understanding of basic transgender terminology and themes. This activity works best with groups of 35 participants or less.

Objectives

By the end of this lesson, participants will be able to:
- Correctly define "non-binary gender identity"
- Identify 2 challenges people with non-binary gender identities may face
- Demonstrate 1 example of gender-neutral language use

Background Knowledge for Facilitators

Facilitators will need to have a solid understanding of the terms used to describe transgender and the identities and experiences of people who have non-binary genders. They will also need to feel comfortable explaining identities that are often inherently complex. Facilitators may find it helpful to watch the full *Three to Infinity: Beyond Two Genders* documentary to increase understanding of the identities and experiences of people who have non-binary gender identities, prior to facilitating this lesson.

Time

- Preparation: 25 minutes
- Implementation: 75 minutes

Materials

- Copies of *Non-Binary Gender Terms* handout (1 per participant)
- *Three to Infinity: Beyond Two Genders* documentary
- Computer, projector, speakers
- Easel paper and markers
- Tape

Preparation

- Make copies of the handout.
- Review the full explanations of the terms and definitions provided in the **Navigating Transgender Terminology** on page 5, the **Tips for Teaching Transgender Terminology** on page 10, and the **Understanding Intersecting Identities & Oppressions** section on page 20.
- Preview the Three to Infinity clips from Procedure step 5, and review the cast bios on www.threetoinfinity.com/about/
- Using easel paper and a marker, write each of the following impact areas at the top of 6 separate sheets of easel paper: (1) family and social relationships, (2) dating and sexual relationships, (3) accessing education, (4) seeking role models, (5) navigating health care, and (6) typical day/everyday life.
- Using the examples below, write out the corresponding example for each of the posters, so that each poster has a sample response.

Examples:

(1) Family & Social Relationships: Having family say their identity is a phase
(2) Dating & Sexual Relationships: Having to explain a non-binary identity to a potential new partner
(3) Accessing Education: Having teachers not use gender neutral pronouns
(4) Seeking Role Models: No well-known celebrities who are non-binary
(5) Navigating Healthcare: Only two gender marker choices on intake forms
(6) Typical Day/Everyday Life: Being persistently misgendered

Procedure

1. Introduce the lesson by explaining that it is about people who have non-binary identities, specifically transgender people whose gender identity is outside the gender binary, and will explore some of the challenges that people who have non-binary identities may face.

2. Use the following talking points to explain what a non-binary gender identity means:
   - The gender binary is what says people must be *either* men or women.
   - Like transgender people, people who have non-binary identities have a gender identity that is incongruent with the sex they were assigned at birth. People who have non-binary identities have gender identities that are more fluid or fall outside of the male/female binary.
   - People who have non-binary gender identities may have some experiences and needs in common with their transgender peers who identify within the gender binary. Some people who have non-binary gender identities also have some experiences and needs that are different from other transgender and cisgender people.
   - People who have non-binary identities are generally considered a subset of the transgender community, but not all people who have non-binary identities identify as transgender.
   - While the Western world operates under a binary gender system, in other cultures and times in human history, there have been communities that recognize more than two genders.

3. Distribute the *Non-Binary Gender Terms* handout and invite participants to take about 5 minutes to review the terms and definitions that are used to by some people to describe their identities and experiences. If participants are struggling to understand the terms, it can be helpful to reassure participants that learning about non-binary identities can feel complicated and overwhelming.

4. Explain that in order to help participants better understand what it means to have a non-binary gender identity, we will be viewing part of a documentary called *Three to Infinity: Beyond Two Genders* in which people explain a bit about their identities and selves.

5. Play the following two clips from the film [Times listed are for the 84 minute version]:
   - Start to Minute 7:00 (to the church scene)
   - Minute 33:00 (ferry arriving) to Minute 41:00 (to the ferry leaving)

6. Lead a brief discussion about the film clip, using the following discussion questions:
   - Regarding the first clip that we watched, what were some of the ways in which the people in the film described their gender?
   - How did these people describe gender as a whole?
   - In the second clip that we watched, what does Jonnie's mother say about being transgender/non-binary as a Black child?
   - What are some other possible effects of intersecting identities on people who have non-binary identities and experiences?

7. Explain that, since accepting the idea that some people have non-binary gender identities can be challenging for many people to grasp or respect (even for some people who are transgender), people who have non-binary identities often experience higher rates of marginalization and discrimination. Explain the talking points below:
   - In the National Transgender Discrimination Survey (Grant et al., 2011), over 13% of the respondents indicated a non-binary identity and wrote in their own identity labels. In this sample, the people who have non-binary gender identities were more likely to be younger, well-educated and multi-racial (and less likely to be white; Harrison et al., 2012).
   - When compared with transgender participants who did not indicate a non-binary identity, the non-binary respondents were more likely to have experienced:
     - physical assault (32% non-binary vs. 25% transgender),
     - sexual assault in K–12 education (16% non-binary vs. 11% transgender),
     - harassment by police (31% non-binary vs. 21% transgender),
     - unemployment (76% non-binary vs. 56% transgender).

8. Explain that the group will now participate in an activity to help them think about the challenges people who have non-binary gender identities might face. Direct participants' attention to the easel paper and point out that each piece of paper has a different heading and example.

9. Break participants up into 6 small groups, assign each of the groups a poster at which to start, and give each group 1-2 markers. Explain that each group will have a few minutes at each poster to brainstorm challenges that people who have non-binary gender identities may face in that particular area or setting. Have participants spend about 4 minutes at each poster and then direct them to move clockwise to the next sheet.

10. After all groups have had the chance to write on each of the posters, provide about 5 minutes for participants to circulate to all of the posters and review the resulting lists. Once participants have returned to their seats, lead them in a short discussion using the questions below:
    - Which areas had many challenges?
    - Did some areas seem like they might present fewer challenges?
    - How do you think experiencing barriers in these areas, or expecting to experience these barriers, might affect people who have non-binary identities?
    - Beyond focusing on the challenges, what are some possible positive aspects of having a non-binary gender identity?
    Examples:
    - Getting to use language and terms to describe their most authentic self rather than trying to fit themselves into the pre-existing binary model
    - The person has the chance to build community with others who share their experiences.

11. Explain that consistently using gender-neutral language is one way to increase support for people who have non-binary gender identities. Instruct that as a closing activity for the lesson, participants are going to spend a few minutes practicing using gender-neutral language and pronouns. Ask participants to use the back of their handout sheet to write out three sentences (on any topic) that uses gender-neutral pronouns or language. Allow about 5 minutes to write the sentences and then ask for each participant to share one of the sentences that they wrote with the group.

    Examples:
    - "Dylan went to their car to get their lunch."
    - "Santi's parents want to know when Santi will be coming home from school"
    - "The person waiting in line was humming my favorite Bon Jovi song, and the song is now stuck in my head!"
    - "Ze's partner is going to be arriving in about 15 minutes."

Evaluation Questions

✔ Define the term "non-binary gender identity."

✔ What are 2 challenges people who have non-binary gender identities may face?

✔ What is 1 example of a word or phrase that is gender neutral?

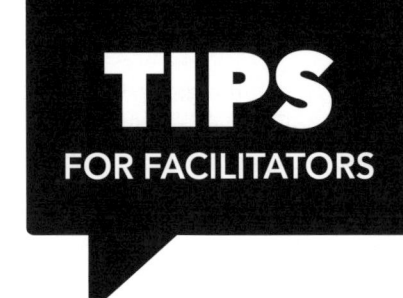

Participants may feel confused or uncomfortable with the variety of words people use to describe their gender. They may also express some resistance to using pronouns that differ from the ones they are used to using. Facilitators can help participants think about ways in which language is powerful and important, especially when it comes to describing oneself.

• • •

Terminology can be particularly challenging and confusing for participants, if many of the terms that are presented and explained in this activity are new to them. Participants may feel overwhelmed by this activity, and it will be useful to validate their experience. Please see the glossary of some of the more common terms that are used when discussing non-binary gender identities and experiences in the **Navigating Transgender Terminology** section of this book. Definitions and preferred terms will vary by location and group. See also the additional information on this topic in the section **Understanding Transgender People's Experiences.**

• • •

Since discussions of transgender people in popular media rarely include the experiences of people who have non-binary gender identities, participants may be unfamiliar with this concept. Participants may pose questions about the validity of non-binary gender identities, or challenge the idea that these identities exist. It is appropriate to refocus discussion on the importance of treating each person with respect, and using the terminology and pronouns they use to describe themselves. This is an important way to confer dignity and respect even if—perhaps especially if—participants are unaccustomed to these terms and pronouns.

Citation:
Shavelson, L. (2015). Three to Infinity: Beyond Two Genders. Photowords Films.

PARTICIPANT HANDOUT

Non-Binary Gender Terms

Gender Binary:
The idea that gender is strictly an either/or option of male/men/masculine or female/woman/feminine based on sex assigned at birth, rather than a continuum or spectrum of gender identities and expressions. The gender binary is often considered to be limiting and problematic for all people, and especially for those who do not fit neatly into the either/or categories.

Non-Binary:
A continuum or spectrum of gender identities and expressions, often based on the rejection of the gender binary's assumption that gender is strictly an either/or option of male/men/masculine or female/woman/feminine based on sex assigned at birth.

Agender:
A person who does not identify as having a gender identity that can be categorized as male or female, and sometimes indicates identifying as not having a gender identity.

Bigender:
A person who experiences gender identity as two genders at the same time, or whose gender identity may vary between two genders. These may be masculine and feminine, or could also include non-binary identities.

Genderfluid:
A person whose gender identity or expression shifts between masculine and feminine, or across this spectrum.

Genderqueer:
A person whose gender identity is neither male nor female, is between or beyond genders, or is some combination of genders.

Pangender:
A person who identifies as all genders.

Two Spirit:
A term used by Native and Indigenous People to indicate that they embody both a masculine and a feminine spirit. Is sometimes also used to describe Native Peoples of diverse sexual orientations, and has nuanced meanings in different indigenous sub-cultures.

What about pronouns?

Some people who have non-binary gender identities refer to themselves using pronouns that are gender-neutral, or that do not have binary assumptions about gender built in. Gender-neutral pronouns include "they/them/theirs" or "ze/hir/hirs." There are many other pronouns people may use. It is appropriate, respectful, and necessary to use the pronouns each individual person finds most affirming (which is also true of cisgender people). If you are unsure, observe the pronouns a person and those close to them use. Or, if necessary, ask them politely.

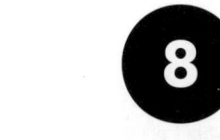

MYTH OR FACT?
Stats & Stereotypes

Overview & Rationale
Through the use of an interactive worksheet and facilitator-led discussion, this lesson names and corrects several common stereotypes and misbeliefs about transgender people, while also providing factual information about the barriers and prejudice that many transgender and gender non-conforming people face. The handout format allows participants to think through the various statements at their own pace and work together to build collaborative knowledge among the members of the group.

Audience
This lesson works well as a foundational activity for those who are new to learning about transgender people and as a refresher/comprehension check for more advanced participants who have pre-existing knowledge. This activity works best with groups of 20 people or less, but if facilitated using the alternative adaptations it can work well with groups of up to 50.

Objectives
By the end of this lesson, participants will be able to:
- Name 2 common stereotypes about transgender people and explain why the information is false.
- Name 2 negative outcomes that occur for transgender people who experience rejection or hostility because of their identity.

Background Knowledge for Facilitators
In preparing for this lesson, it will be useful to become familiar with the *Injustice at Every Turn: Findings of the National Transgender Discrimination Survey,* which provides detailed information on transgender people's experiences of prejudice and discrimination (available for free online at: www.endtransdiscrimination.org) and the other references cited in the *Myth or Fact? Answer Key.*

Time
- Preparation: 15 minutes
- Implementation: 45 minutes

Materials
- *Myth or Fact?* handout (1 per participant)
- *Myth or Fact? Answer Key* handout (1 per participant)
- Optional: 5X8 index cards, or 2 differently colored index cards
- Optional: PowerPoint, computer & projector

Preparation
- Make copies of the handouts
- Thoroughly review the talking points for each of the questions provided on the *Myth or Fact? Answer Key*
- Hang "Myth" and "Fact" signs on either side of the room, ideally using a different color for each sign, and prepare the training space so that participants can move from one sign to the next.
- Alternate/Adaptation: Label the 5X8 index cards so that one side says "Myth" and the other side says "Fact" (1 per participant). Alternatively, use blank index cards that match the colors of the Myth/Fact signs.
- If using, download the PowerPoint with the questions and answers/citations from www.teachingtransgender.com/printables PW: TTTprep15

Procedure

1. Explain that: For this activity, we will be exploring some common stereotypes and myths about transgender people, and we will learn more about transgender people's experiences of prejudice and discrimination.

2. Direct participants to work independently to read each of the statements on the handout, and determine whether or not they think that the statements listed are myths or facts. Explain that they will have about 15 minutes to read through and complete the handout and that all present will review the results after everyone has had a chance to finish the handout. When the allotted time has almost passed, provide participants with a 3-minute warning and ask them to continue working to get through as many of the statements as they can.

3. Once everyone has had a chance to complete the handout, ask participants to gather in the center of the training space. Explain that, for each of the questions, participants will be asked to move to the side of the room with the Myth or Fact sign that reflects their given response. [Alternate/Adaptation for Accessibility: Explain that for each of the questions, participants will be asked to raise their Myth or Fact sign (or colored card) to reflect their given response.]

4. For each of the questions, ask for a few volunteers to explain why the statement is a myth or a fact. If the participants have selected the wrong answer or their reason is inaccurate, provide the correct answer and explain why it is the correct response using the talking points provided on the *Myth or Fact? Answer Key*. (Optional: Use the PowerPoint to have each of the questions on screen and then advance it to the correct answer with the rationale after everyone has had the chance to move to/share their selected answers.)

5. After reviewing all of the questions and responses, pass out the *Myth or Fact? Answer Key* so that participants have the correct answers, rationale and references in print form. Allow participants to ask additional clarifying questions as needed.

6. If using this as a standalone lesson, conclude the activity by asking participants to share which of the statements/answers was most surprising to them and explain why. Summarize the discussion by explaining that there are ample myths and misinformation about transgender people, and that it is important that we continue to question information to determine whether it is factual and affirming

Evaluation Questions

✔ Name 2 common stereotypes about transgender people and explain why these stereotypes or information is false.

✔ Describe 2 negative outcomes that occur for transgender people who experience rejection or hostility because of their identity.

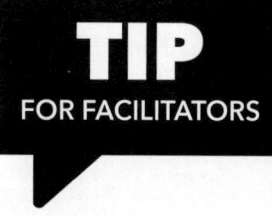

During Step 4, it is essential to ask participants to explain their responses and why they chose them because it requires participants to explain their rationales behind their responses. This will help ensure that participants are processing the information correctly, and will help you to understand their perspectives so that you can adjust your talking points accordingly. It also provides participants with the opportunity to hear from their peers, and to evaluate other people's responses.

NOTE: This activity is a modified version taken from: Green, E.R. & Perry, J.R. (2014). *Safe & Respected: Providing Culturally Competent Services for Transgender and Gender Non-Conforming Youth in ACS Care (Training Curriculum)*. New York: New York City's Administration for Children's Services. Used with permission.

MYTH OR FACT?
ANSWER KEY & REFERENCES

• • •

1. **MYTH** or FACT: Transgender is an extreme presentation of a homosexual sexual orientation.

    Transgender is not a sexual orientation. "Sexual orientation" refers to those to whom a person is physically, psychologically, emotionally or sexually attracted (e.g., who they want to be in a relationship with). "Transgender" refers to a person's gender identity as being incongruent with their biological sex, (e.g., who they are as a gendered being does not match the sex they were assigned at birth). All people have a both a gender identity and a sexual orientation.

    Source: American Psychological Association (APA). 2014. *Answers to your questions about transgender people, gender identity and gender expression.* Available online at: http://www.apa.org/topics/lgbt/transgender.aspx

2. **MYTH** or FACT: Mental health counseling can be successful in helping a transgender or questioning person change their gender identity to be consistent with the sex that they were assigned at birth.

    There is no counseling that can "fix" or "change" a person's gender identity. Attempts to do so have consistently been shown to be psychologically damaging and harmful. International experts, including the American Psychiatric Association, have determined that being transgender and/or gender non-conforming is not a mental illness. Any counseling related to being transgender should be done to provide affirmation and support in helping a person to manage stress related to discrimination and make decisions related to medical transition.

    Source: American Medical Association (AMA). 2014. AMA Policies on GLBT Issues. Available online at: http://www.ama-assn.org/ama/pub/about-ama/our-people/member-groups-sections/glbt-advisory-committee/ama-policy-regarding-sexual-orientation.page?

3. **MYTH** or FACT: Anyone under the age of 18 is developmentally and psychologically too young to know who they are or what they want, and are quite likely to change their mind about their gender identity down the line.

    By 3–4 years old, children have a strong sense of their gender identity, and the average age for a transgender young person verbalizing that their gender identity is incongruent with their biological sex is around 10–11 years old. Psychological experts have repeatedly determined that the best course of action for transgender and gender non-conforming youth is to affirm their gender identity and expression (Spack 2012). When accompanied by screenings by transgender-culturally competent mental health professionals, leading medical experts recommend interventions, (including delaying puberty and/or medical transition), to help reduce unnecessary stress, dysphoria, and medical interventions later in life (WPATH, 2012). Follow-up studies have shown that 100% of youth who were treated with pubertal suppression stayed on treatment and initiated cross-sex hormones as their next stage of treatment (de Vries, 2012). In a follow-up study that tracked that same group into adulthood, none of the people reported regret, and all experienced positive outcomes and general well-being (de Vries, 2014).

    Sources:

    de Vries, A. L. C., et al. (2014). Young adult psychological outcome after puberty suppression and gender reassignment. *Pediatrics,* DOI: 10.1542/peds.2013-2958

    de Vries, A. L. C., et al. (2011). Puberty suppression in adolescents with Gender Identity Disorder: A prospective follow-up study. *Journal of Sexual Medicine,* 1 (8), 2276-2283.

    Spack, N., et al. (2012). Children and Adolescents with Gender Identity Disorder Referred to a Pediatric Medical Center. Pediatrics, 129(3), 418-425.

    World Professional Association for Transgender Health. (2012). Standards of Care, v7. Retrieved from: http://www.wpath.org/site_page.cfm?pk_association_webpage_menu=1351&pk_association_webpage=3926

4. **MYTH** or FACT: Many transgender women are prostitutes, who are tricking straight men into having gay sex.

There are persistent stereotypes that all transgender women are sex workers, and that transgender women are "pretending" to be women to purposely deceive others about their history, particularly as it relates to engaging in sexual contact with heterosexual men. This stereotype is frequently seen in the media, and is often used as the punchline of a joke, as a central theme in syndicated shock/reveal type television shows, or as a plot twist—particularly in crime dramas. Currently these make up the vast majority of "representations" of transgender people in mainstream media, which includes very few positive images of transgender people. While some transgender people use sex work as a way of surviving (due to a lack of viable job alternatives because of the intense discrimination), there are many more transgender people who have traditional sources of employment. Likewise, the stereotype that transgender women are trying to trick straight men into gay sex is based on several false assumptions—including that transgender people's identities and medical transitions are about deceiving other people rather than reflecting the true purpose of trying to live authentic lives, that transgender people are undeserving of relationships, that transgender people are morally obligated to disclose their gender and medical history to others, and that there is such a thing as "gay" sex (rather than there being many types of sexual behaviors in which people engage).

Source: Bettcher, T. M. (2007). Evil deceivers and make-believers: On transphobic violence and the politics of illusion. *Hypatia: A Journal of Feminist Philosophy, 22*(3), 43-65.

5. **MYTH** or FACT: Elderly transgender people in need of long-term medical care are usually able to access housing placements where their gender identity is affirmed, particularly if they live in or near urban areas.

There is currently a scarcity of consistent and viable options for older and elderly transgender people to access when they are in need of long-term assisted housing or end-of-life care. Older people are less likely to be viewed as sexual beings, and this includes a person's gender identity. While LGB people may be forced to remain closeted about their sexual orientation, transgender people face different challenges due to the medical component of transgender care and requirement of physical contact and nudity. There is increasing evidence that suggests that transgender people in need of these types of support find themselves having to revert to the sex that they were assigned at birth in order to receive care. While urban areas are often assumed to be more liberal, accepting, and have better services, this is not always the case. To date, there are only a handful of LGBTQ specific eldercare facilities across the country.

Source: Addias, S., et al. (2009). The health, social care, housing needs of lesbian, gay, bisexual and transgender older people. *Health and Social Care in the Community, 17*(6), 647-658.

Source: Perrson, D. (2009). Unique challenges of transgender aging: Implications from the literature. *Journal of Gerontological Social Work, 52*, 633-646.

6. MYTH or **FACT**: Transgender People of Color face consistently higher rates of prejudice and discrimination, including discrimination from other People of Color, when compared with White transgender people.

Due to the intersections of race, class and gender, transgender People of Color consistently report facing more severe and frequent discrimination when compared with transgender people who are white. According to the Injustice at Every Turn reports, 34% of Black, 28% of Latino/a, and 18% of Asian & Pacific Islander (API) transgender people have to survive on less than $10,000 a year in income, 1 out of 2 Black transgender people face harassment at school, while 77% of Latino/as do, Black transgender people are more than 10 times more likely to be HIV-positive than other transgender people, and suicide attempts are particularly high for all people of color: 49% of Black, 47% of Latino/a, and 56% of API transgender people attempt suicide as a result of discrimination.

Sources: National Center for Transgender Equality. (2012.) Injustice at Every Turn: A Look at Latino/a Respondents in the National Transgender Discrimination Survey; Injustice at Every Turn: A Look at Asian American, South Asian, Southeast Asian and Pacific Islander (API) Respondents in the National Transgender Discrimination Survey; Injustice at Every Turn: A Look at Black Respondents in the National Transgender Discrimination Survey.

7. **MYTH** or FACT: As of 2010, there is a national law in place that protects transgender people from employment discrimination as a part of the legal protections that are provided to members of the LGBTQ communities.

There is currently no national law that protects LGBTQ people from employment discrimination (or other types of discrimination). There have been many attempts to pass various forms of legislation (both transgender inclusive, and transgender non-inclusive) at the federal level, but none has never been passed. As of 2014, the only national law that provides specific protections for transgender people is the Matthew Shepard and James Byrd Jr Hate Crimes Act, which allows for greater punishment when it can be proven that a physical attack was motivated by hate or bias, in this case, anti-transgender prejudice. While some guidelines pertaining to sex discrimination are interpreted to provide protections for transgender people, this is generally seen as a case-by-case question and does not provide proactive legal protections for transgender people.

Source: National Center for Transgender Equality. (2014). *Issues: Discrimination*. Available online at: http://transequality.org/Issues/discrimination.html

8. MYTH or **FACT**: Over 50% of transgender youth report that they are physically harassed in school, and 1 out of 4 transgender young people reports being physically attacked in school. Two-thirds of these students reported that the administration did not respond effectively or respectfully.

Research published by GLSEN in 2009 showed that young people frequently experience harassment and violence in schools¬–both from peers and from teachers and administrators. Verbal harassment was even more common, with 87% of transgender and gender non-conforming young people reporting that they were called names or threatened in school. Only 1/3 of the students felt that the teachers or administration had handled the situations effectively. Youth who experienced this verbal and physical violence were more likely to miss school because they were concerned for their safety and had GPAs that were lower than those of their peers.

Source: Greytak, E.A., Kosciw, J. & Diaz, E.M. (2009). *Harsh Realities: The Experiences of Transgender Youth in Our Nation's Schools.* New York, NY: GLSEN.

9. **MYTH** or FACT: Generally speaking, transgender people tend to experience little anti-transgender prejudice when accessing healthcare services because medical providers receive training on working with transgender people.

While we may assume that medical professionals and medical settings are less likely to engage in discrimination, this has not been shown to be true for transgender people. Nineteen percent (19%) of the 6,456 respondents to the National Transgender Discrimination Survey reported that they were refused medical care because of their identity, with 28% reporting that they were harassed by medical providers, and 2% reporting that they were victims of violence in medical settings. There have also been multiple cases in which transgender people were reported to have received inappropriate medical care in emergency settings after medical providers noted genitals that did not match the person's gender presentation, where the lack of treatment resulted in death.

Source: Grant, J., Mottet, L., Tanis, J., Harrison, J., Herman, J., & Keisling, M. (2011). *Injustice at every turn: A report of the National Transgender Discrimination Survey.* Retrieved from http://endtransdiscrimination.org/PDFs/NTDS_Report.pdf

10. **MYTH** or FACT: Most of the prejudice and discrimination faced by transgender people comes in the form of verbal and physical harassment perpetrated by people who are openly prejudiced against people who are transgender.

Typically studies report on instances of major discrimination as singular events that have a significant effect on a person's life. There has been less attention paid to smaller events of discrimination and prejudice, but it is commonly understood that transgender people, particularly those who are visibly transgender or gender non-conforming, experience consistent hostility and discrimination whenever they are engaging with other people.

Source: Nadal, K. L. (2013). *That's so gay! Microaggressions and the lesbian, gay, bisexual, and transgender community.* American Psychological Association.

PARTICIPANT HANDOUT

myth or fact

Review the 10 statements below and decide whether you believe each statement is a myth or a fact. Circle the answer you believe to be correct.

1. **MYTH or FACT:** Transgender is an extreme presentation of a homosexual sexual orientation.

2. **MYTH or FACT:** Mental health counseling can be successful in helping a transgender or questioning person change their gender identity to be consistent with the sex that they were assigned at birth.

3. **MYTH or FACT:** Anyone under the age of 18 is developmentally and psychologically too young to know who they are or what they want, and are quite likely to change their mind about their gender identity down the line.

4. **MYTH or FACT:** Many transgender women are prostitutes who are tricking straight men into having gay sex.

5. **MYTH or FACT:** Elderly transgender people in need of long-term medical care are usually able to access housing placements where their gender identity is affirmed, particularly if they live in or near urban areas.

6. **MYTH or FACT:** Transgender People of Color face consistently higher rates of prejudice and discrimination, including discrimination from other People of Color, when compared to White transgender people.

7. **MYTH or FACT:** As of 2010, there is a national law in place that protects transgender people from employment discrimination as a part of the legal protections that are provided to members of the LGBTQ communities.

8. **MYTH or FACT:** Over 50% of transgender youth report that they are physically harassed in school, and 1 out of 4 transgender young people reports being physically attacked in school. Two-thirds of these students report that the administration did not respond effectively or respectfully.

9. **MYTH or FACT:** Generally speaking, transgender people tend to experience little anti-transgender prejudice when accessing healthcare services because medical providers receive training on working with transgender people.

10. **MYTH or FACT:** Most of the prejudice and discrimination faced by transgender people comes in the form of verbal and physical harassment perpetrated by people who are openly prejudice against people who are transgender.

9
COMING OUT:
Always & Again

Overview & Rationale

While many people have a basic understanding of "coming out" as lesbian, gay, or bisexual, most people have not thought through the unique implications of coming out as transgender and how this must be navigated on a consistent basis. This empathy-based lesson helps participants to explore some of these challenges to better understand the experiences of transgender people. This lesson works particularly well when paired with **Lesson 10: Thanks for Sharing: Responses to Coming Out** on page 100.

Audience

This lesson works well with people who are relatively new to learning about transgender people and for more advanced participants who have a strong knowledge base but will benefit from further exploration of the nuances of being transgender. This lesson will work well with a range of target audiences. While ideally implemented with 30 people or less, it can be modified for up to 48 people.

Objectives

By the end of this lesson, participants will be able to:
- Identify 3 unique situations in which transgender people may have to disclose their transgender identity to others (that do not apply to cisgender people).
- Explain why these 3 situations may result in additional complexity or challenges for transgender people

Background Knowledge for Facilitators

It will be useful for facilitators to have knowledge about the emotional, logistical, and safety risks of coming out as transgender in various situations—particularly family and intimate partner reactions, as well as discrimination that may occur as a result of coming out.

Time

- Preparation: 15 minutes
- Implementation: 45 minutes

Materials

- Copies of the *Coming Out: More Than the First Time* handout (1 per participant)
- Optional: Index cards (1 per participant)

Preparation

- Make copies of the handouts
- It is recommended that facilitators complete the A-E questions for each of the 12 scenarios independently prior to implementing this lesson. This will help ensure that you have had a chance to think through each of the situations prior to leading the discussions.

Procedure

1. Explain that: When most people think of "coming out" they think of a person sitting down with a family member or friend to tell them that they are lesbian, gay, bisexual, transgender or queer, and that it is more or less a one-time event. The reality for most transgender people is that coming out is something that has to be navigated consistently throughout life, and often involves having to come out to people other than friends or family. This activity will help us to consider some of the situations in which transgender people have to come out and what the potential consequences of this might be.

2. Break participants into 4 small groups of 4-7 people per group and instruct the groups to sit together. If working with an audience of more than 28 people, divide the audience into groups of no

larger than 7 people per group and no larger than 8 groups. *(Note: This division structure mirrors the structure of Lesson 9: Thanks for Sharing: Responses to Coming Out, to ease facilitating these lessons sequentially. If not using Lesson 9, participants can be broken up into small groups of 4-5 people.)*

3. Once participants are in their small groups, pass out the **Coming Out: More Than the First Time** to participants. Assign each of the groups 2-3 of the scenarios and ask them to read through the situations and discuss their responses to each of the A-E questions. Allow about 15 minutes for the activity. Rotate through the small groups as they are working and answer questions and provide support to each of the small groups as needed.

4. Ask participants to come back to the large group. Discuss the activity using the following prompts, explaining that there are no "right" or "wrong" answers:
   - Out of all of the statements presented, which do you think was the most challenging scenario to make decisions about coming out? Why?
   - What were some of the factors that you considered when deciding the pros and cons of coming out?
   - How do you think these situations might impact individuals' decisions about how and when to come out?
   - What were some of the affirming responses you came up with? What made them affirming?

5. If using this as a standalone lesson, conclude the lesson by passing out the index cards and asking participants to write down 2 things that they learned during this activity. Based on time available, ask each participant to select 1 of their items with their small group. Alternatively, participants can be asked to turn in their index cards. (This can be a useful tool for the facilitator in assessing the success of the activity).

Evaluation Questions

✔ What are 3 situations in which transgender people may have to consider whether they will disclose their transgender identity to others?

✔ How might the repercussions of these 3 situations affect how a transgender person navigates their life?

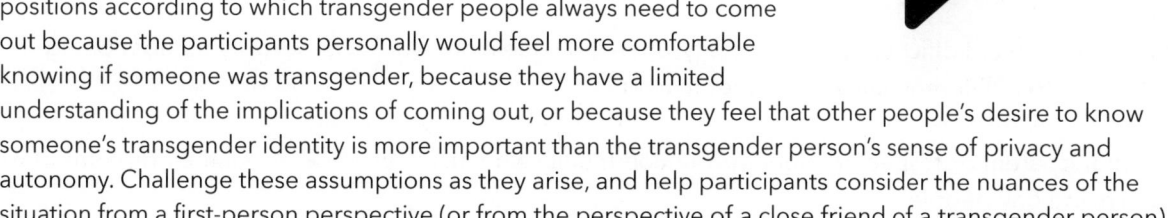

TIPS FOR FACILITATORS

If pressed for time, assign specific pairs a limited number of statements on the Coming Out handout. For example, have one half of the room work on the odd-numbered statements, and have the other half of the room work on the even-numbered statements.

• • •

During the coming out portion of the lesson, participants may default to positions according to which transgender people always need to come out because the participants personally would feel more comfortable knowing if someone was transgender, because they have a limited understanding of the implications of coming out, or because they feel that other people's desire to know someone's transgender identity is more important than the transgender person's sense of privacy and autonomy. Challenge these assumptions as they arise, and help participants consider the nuances of the situation from a first-person perspective (or from the perspective of a close friend of a transgender person).

• • •

If participants get stuck on the specifics of when a transgender person "should" or is "obligated" to come out, or seem to feel that transgender people are lying about their histories or identities, it can be useful to remind participants that social and medical transition are steps that some transgender people take to live authentic, fulfilling lives and have nothing to do with "tricking" or "deceiving" other people. It can also be useful to point out that the media has often inaccurately portrayed the latter stereotype.

PARTICIPANT HANDOUT

Coming Out: More Than the First Time

While "coming out" narratives often focus on the first time that a person communicates their identities to other people, for transgender people coming out is often a uniquely lifelong process that involves having to make decisions about when to disclose their identities and histories. Different people will experience these situations in different ways, particularly based on decisions related to medical transition, comfort in communicating affirming name and pronouns, and how gender-conforming a person is perceived to be.

Situations in which people might have to make decisions about how or when come out (or may be "outed" against their will):

1. To the EMS workers or admitting staff at the emergency room after a car accident.

2. To family you have not seen in a long time while at a funeral of an extended family member.

3. To the receptionist at a doctor's office when you have to present an insurance card that has a gender marker that is incongruent with your appearance.

4. To someone you have recently met and are interested in dating.

5. To the state patrol officer when you are pulled over for a traffic stop and you have to present identification with an old name or gender marker.

6. To someone you used to be friends with when you were growing up when they friend/follow you on social media.

7. To a home healthcare worker when you are interviewing them to provide long-term medical support services for you as a part of palliative care.

8. To the financial aid officer at your university when they question your social security number being connected to a different name or gender marker.

9. To a grandparent or respected elder in your community who has been vocal about their discomfort with lesbian and gay people.

10. To an acquaintance who asks you directly if you "used to be the other sex."

11. To the clerk at a store that you have frequented for years, when they mention that you are looking very different from how you used to look.

12. To a former partner with whom you were in a relationship several years ago.

Select one of the scenarios you were assigned and consider:

A. What might be some reasons that you would or would not come out as transgender in this situation?

_____
_____
_____
_____

B. How easy or difficult would it be to come out in this situation? Why?

_____
_____
_____
_____

C. What are some of the possible emotional, logistical, or safety implications of coming out or being outed against your will in this situation?

_____
_____
_____
_____

D. What would be the most affirming response that someone could give in this situation?

_____
_____
_____
_____

E. What steps might allies of transgender people take to help mitigate or make these situations easier?

_____
_____
_____
_____

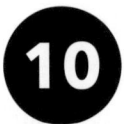

THANKS FOR SHARING:
Responses to Coming Out

Overview & Rationale

This lesson presents the Nelson Continuum as a framework for understanding the range of reactions that transgender people experience when coming out. By examining a range of quotes from popular and online media, participants will increase their understanding of how people can avoid rejecting responses and increase affirming ones. This helps participants understand the emotional, physical and economic implications of coming out as transgender, while practicing affirming responses. This lesson works particularly well when paired with **Lesson 9: Coming Out: Always & Again** on page 96.

Audience

This lesson works well with people who are relatively new to learning about transgender people and for more advanced participants who have a strong knowledge base but will benefit from further exploration of the nuances of being transgender. This lesson will work well with a range of target audiences. While ideally implemented with 30 people or less, it can be modified for up to 48 people.

Objectives

By the end of this lesson, participants will be able to:
- Name and describe the 5 stages of the Nelson Continuum as they relate to reactions to a person coming out as transgender.
- Provide 1 example from each stage of how a person might respond and explain how that type of response might affect a transgender person.
- Demonstrate at least 1 potential affirming response to a person coming out as transgender.

Background Knowledge for Facilitators

In addition to having an understanding of the coming out process for transgender people, it will be very helpful to have knowledge of each of the stories being quoted, particularly that of Leelah Alcorn.

Time

- Preparation: 20-30 minutes
- Implementation: 60 minutes

Materials

- *Nelson Continuum: Applications to Transgender Affirmation* handout (1 per participant)
- *Responses to Coming Out* handout (1 per participant)
- Blank index cards (1 per participant)

Preparation

- Make copies of the handouts
- In advance of the lesson, review the *Nelson Continuum: Applications to Transgender Affirmation* handout to make sure that you are comfortable explaining each stage. Review each of the quotes and familiarize yourself with the backstory of each, particularly that of Leelah Alcorn.

Procedure

1. Break participants into 4 small groups of 4-7 people per group and instruct the groups to sit together. (If working with an audience larger with more than 28 people, then divide the audience into groups of no larger than 7 people per group and no more than 8 groups).

2. Once participants have settled into their small groups, explain that this activity will focus on the ranges of reactions people have to someone coming out as transgender. Pass out the Nelson Continuum: Applications to Transgender Affirmation handouts, and Responses to Coming Out handouts, so that each participant has one of each.

3. Using the Facilitator's Guide to the Explaining the Nelson Continuum, read and explain each of the stages of the Nelson Continuum out loud, using the detailed examples to help participants better understand each of the stages.

4. Once you have reviewed and explained each of the stages, assign each of the small groups 2 of the quotes from the Responses to Coming Out handout and ask them to work together as a group to determine the stage and explain why the quote fits that stage. (If working with 5-7 small groups, assign each group 2 scenarios. If working with 8 small groups, assign each group 1 of the quotes).

5. Allow 10-15 minutes for the small groups to discuss the quotes they've read. Move through the room during this time, answering questions and monitoring the conversations. Once most of the groups have finished their assigned quotes, bring everyone back to the large group.

6. Ask each group in turn to read out their quote and explain to which stage of the Nelson Continuum they assigned it and why. (If there is a second group with the same quote, ask them if they had a similar answer, and provide the opportunity for the second group to add any talking points from their small group conversation that were not covered by the previous group). Using the Facilitator's Guide to the Responses to Coming Out Handout, provide the correct answers and explanations as necessary. For each of the quotes, ask the participants to consider how they think that the person felt in that situation.

7. If using this as a standalone lesson, conclude the lesson by handing out the index cards and asking participants to write down 3 examples of affirming responses that they would use themselves or recommend that someone else use. Based on time available, ask each participant to select one of their items from the group. Alternatively, participants can be asked to turn in their index cards. (This can be a useful tool for the facilitator in assessing the success of the activity).

Evaluation Questions

✔ What are 3 situations in which transgender people may have to consider whether they will disclose their transgender identity to others?

✔ How might the repercussions of these 3 situations affect how a transgender person navigates their life?

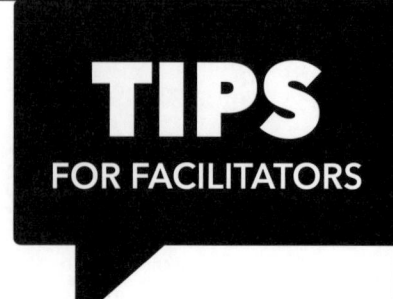

TIPS FOR FACILITATORS

The *Nelson Continuum: Applications to Transgender Affirmation* and corresponding *Facilitator's Guide* provide supporting examples from a variety of settings. When preparing to implement the lesson, it may be useful to create examples that are specific to the setting or target audience. For example, if conducting a professional development training for K–12 educators, it may be useful to refer to talking points that explain how each of the stages might present in a K–12 school setting. Or, if conducting a training for therapists, it may be useful to refer to talking points that explain how each of the types of rejections affects a person's mental health. Designing talking points that are specific to the setting/target audience will help ensure that the participants are able to connect the materials to their own experiences. Alternatively, if working with a mixed audience, it may be useful to ask participants to explore and explain potential connections or applications to their own settings (individually or in small groups).

• • •

When discussing the answers to the *Nelson Continuum: Applications to Transgender Affirmation* handout, participants may push back on why they feel that a specific quote represents a different stage of the continuum. To a certain extent, each of the quotes is open to interpretation—it is more important that participants are able to articulate and explain their response than it is for them to have the "correct" answer. Provided that the response is logical, their ability to defend their belief that a quote represents a different stage generally indicates greater depth of understanding.

• • •

Due to the "pop culture" references in some of the quotes, it will be helpful to have a basic understanding of who Cher, Chaz Bono, Drea Kelly, R. Kelly, Jay Kelly, Caitlyn Jenner and Kayne West are to aid in leading the conversation. Note that, since these figures and stories are widely known, participants may be particularly eager to talk about them and may be easily taken off track. Be sure to facilitate the group conversation in a way that keeps the dialogue focused on the activity/topic of responses to coming out as transgender.

• • •

When discussing Leelah Alcorn's quote (#6) participants may have strong emotional reactions to learning that this was written as a part of Leelah's suicide note. *Facilitators may wish to give a "trigger warning" at the start of the lesson to notify participants that this activity contains potentially triggering examples of rejection and suicide.* When facilitating, it will be helpful to be familiar with Leelah's story and the rest of her note, particularly that she used it as a call to action to help make sure that people work harder to advocate for change so that other people don't have to have the same experiences that she did. Statistics are provided in the corresponding *Facilitator's Guide* to help contextualize this information.

• • •

Some participants may have strong reactions to the mention of religion as a reason for rejection in Leelah's quote. This often evokes one of two kinds of responses: 1) wanting to distinguish between types of Christianity that are rejecting and those that are affirming, or 2) wanting to discuss religious perspectives on being transgender. In part this may be because participants feel that their faith is being misrepresented or attacked, and also in part as a reaction to feelings of discomfort. It is often useful to validate and redirect participants back toward the discussion of how these responses to coming out impact the person coming out.

SOURCES FOR QUOTES:

1. Bellino, D. (July 2, 2014). Exclusive: Drea Kelly on Her Transgender Son, Her Pending Divorce and Life After the Show. *VH1*. Retrieved from: m.vh1.com/blog/2014-07-02/drea-kelly-on-transgender-son-pending-divorce/
2. Annika. (September 13, 2012). Disowned: When Coming Out Doesn't Go As Planned. Retrieved from: www.autostraddle.com/disowned-when-coming-out-doesnt-go-as-planned-145663/
3. Keyishian, A. (September 15, 2011). Cher defends transgender son, Chaz Bono, on 'Ellen.' *The Stir*. Retrieved from: thestir.cafemom.com/entertainment/126049/cher_defends_transgender_son_chaz
4. Beam, C. (2007). *Transparent: Love, Family and Living the T with Transgender Teenagers*. Orlando, FL: Harcourt Books.
5. Written by: Anon. SOURCE: faggotboi.wordpress.com/2011/05/06/my-moms-first-post-transition-visit/
6. Alcorn L. (December 28, 2014). Untitled. Originally posted on: http://lazerprincess.tumblr.com/ Retrieved from: www.dailymail.co.uk/news/article-2891267/Transgender-teenager-leaves-heartbreaking-suicide-note-blaming-Christian-parents-walking-tractor-trailer-highway.html
7. Rolling Stone. (July 1, 2015). Kim Kardashian gets real: 11 revelations from the new cover story. Retrieved from: www.rollingstone.com/culture/news/kim-kardashian-gets-real-11-revelations-from-the-new-cover-story-20150701
8. Kellaway, M. (July 8, 2015). Two Black Trans Boys, Two NY Families and Boundless Love. *The Advocate*. Available at: www.advocate.com/families/2015/07/08/two-black-trans-boys-two-ny-families-and-boundless-love

FACILITATOR'S GUIDE
to the Explaining the Nelson Continuum

Rejecting Punitive ▶ **Rejecting Non-Punitive** ▶ **Qualified Acceptance** ▶ **Full Acceptance** ▶ **Advocacy**

Rejecting Punitive

Explicitly punishing or harming a transgender person (physically or economically) or creating a hostile environment that is emotionally abusive, because their gender identity or expression is incongruent with the sex they were assigned at birth.

> *Examples:* Firing a person for coming out as transgender; physically attacking a person who appears to be visibly transgender; parents kicking a transgender teenager out of their home because they are transgender; or intensive bullying of someone who is transgender.

> *Explaining Rejecting Punitive:*
> This is a rejection of a transgender person that comes with significant punishment or consequences. The consequences can be physical, such as violence, or economic, such as reduced income/security. In a professional setting, an example of a Rejecting Punitive response might be a supervisor firing a person for coming out as transgender, or creating a hostile workplace environment by refusing to use the person's affirming name and/or pronoun. Examples of Rejecting Punitive responses from families of origin might include a parent responding to their child's coming out by kicking them out of their home, or a grandparent removing a transgender grandchild from their will because they are transgender.

Rejecting Non-Punitive

Rejecting (verbally or emotionally) a person because their gender identity or expression is incongruent with the sex they were assigned at birth.

> *Examples:* Telling a person that their transgender partner cannot attend family events; refusing to use the affirming name and pronouns for a transgender person; socially isolating a transgender person at school or work.

> *Explaining Rejecting Non-Punitive:*
> This is a verbal or emotional rejection of a transgender person that has a significant emotional consequence for the transgender person. This often happens through messages that say a person's identity is invalid or immoral. For example, a teacher who is refusing to use affirming names and pronouns for a student is responding in a rejecting way that is not technically punitive because it is not intended to punish the student. (If the teacher failed the student because they were transgender that would be an example of Rejecting Punitive). This creates an emotionally unsafe and non-affirming environment for that student, which in a school setting, may lead to bullying from peers. Another example might be a faith leader responding to a transgender person's coming out with a "love the sinner, hate the sin" approach. While the approach may be intended to be positive, the transgender person is being told that their being who they are (transgender) is wrong/immoral.

Qualified Acceptance
Giving mixed and ambiguous messages about acceptance of a person's gender identity or expression—often presented as accepting the person, but rejecting transgender identity or transition process.

Examples: A parent telling a child that they love them for who they are but don't approve of their choice to medically transition; a social worker who intermittently misstates a transgender person's name or pronouns; asking a transgender person to change their presentation based on the context or situation.

Explaining Qualified Acceptance:
Qualified Acceptance means that a transgender person's identity is accepted only in certain spaces, settings or circumstances. While generally intended as an accepting response by the person giving it, Qualified Acceptance is often experienced by a transgender person as a form of rejection—particularly when the person is asked to change their expression/presentation, or hide their transgender identity. For example, if a person's best friend from high school is getting married, the friend might ask that the person not reveal any information that might indicate that they are transgender, or ask them to wear clothing that can be perceived as "gender neutral" so that other guests are not uncomfortable. Another example might be when a social worker tells their client who is transgender that they will have to remind them (the social worker) to use affirming pronouns.

Full Acceptance
Unequivocally affirming a transgender person's gender identity and/or expression.

Examples: A friend consistently using the affirming name and pronoun; a partner emotionally or financially supporting medical transition; a school creating affirming records for a transgender child.

Explaining Full Acceptance:
Full Acceptance is the unconditional affirmation of a transgender person's gender identity or expression. An example of a response that demonstrates Full Acceptance would be when a person comes out to their romantic partner as transgender and the partner responds by saying "I love you for who you are, and I will support you however I can." Another example might be a school working collaboratively with a parent to change the student record of a transgender young person to reflect affirming gender markers and their chosen name, and making sure that only the affirming name and pronouns are used.

Advocacy
Taking proactive steps to publically support transgender people, including advocating for overall changes that makes transgender people's experiences better.

Examples: An ally asking a medical provider to change their intake forms to include transgender-affirming options; a community member petitioning to create a local anti-discrimination ordinance; a friend asking their colleague not to make anti-transgender jokes.

Explaining Advocacy:
Advocacy can best be described as Full Acceptance plus taking actions that make things better for individual transgender people or transgender communities as a whole. This can be small increments of change such as asking friends or family members not to make anti-transgender jokes or comments, medium increments of change such as asking a medical provider to change their intake forms so that they have options that are affirming of transgender people, or large increments of change such as working on public campaigns to raise awareness or funds to support transgender causes, for example advocating for increasing protections for transgender people.

This resource is based on the work of:
Nelson, J.B. (1978). *An Approach to Sexuality and Christian Theology.* Minneapolis: Augsburg Publishing House, and subsequent works of Hall, D.M. (2009). *Allies at Work: Creating a Lesbian, Gay, Bisexual and Transgender Inclusive Work Environment.* San Francisco, CA: Out and Equal Workplace Advocates.; and; Satterly, B. A., & Dyson, D. A. (2010). Social work practice with gay, lesbian, bisexual, and transgender persons. In J. Poulin (Ed.), *Collaborative social work: Strengths-based generalist practice* (3rd ed.). Belmont, CA: Wadsworth.

FACILITATOR'S GUIDE
to Responses to Coming Out Handout

Rejecting Punitive ▶ Rejecting Non-Punitive ▶ Qualified Acceptance ▶ Full Acceptance ▶ Advocacy

1. "All I can say about Jay is he makes it so easy to be a proud mom. For parents, we need to realize, [our kids] have their own journey. Parents get it wrong when they don't support their children. They have to go out and fight every day and face this world. The first battle should not be at home. I think that a lot of children in the LGBT community don't succeed because the one thing they need the most is a foundation. I just tell Jay all the time, baby you won the war. You're gonna have a lot of battles but you won the war. Mama accepts and loves you for who you are." - Drea Kelly

   What stage of the Nelson Continuum does this represent? Why?
   Full Acceptance. Drea Kelly is communicating unconditional acceptance and support of Jay.

2. "When I came out, I didn't expect a very good reaction from my father, but I thought that my mother might be more accepting—maybe even happy to learn that the daughter she always wanted had been here all along. Things didn't turn out quite as well as I had hoped. After reading the letter, my parents quickly progressed from shock to disbelief to grief and disgust. I tried to send them resources for parents of trans* children, but when it became clear that I was serious about transitioning, they cut off all contact. I received a formal disowning letter last March, in which my father warned that my life as a trans girl would be 'bleak with much unhappiness.' He told me that he didn't want to know me as female, and that I should change my last name and only contact him if I 'decided to be a boy again.'" - Annika

   What stage of the Nelson Continuum does Annika's father response represent? Why?
   Rejecting Punitive. Annika's father responded to her medical transition by rejecting her identity, and punishing her by cutting off all contact.

3. "'My child is a wonderful child,' she says, expressing a true mom's sentiment and bypassing the pronouns that have gotten her in trouble. 'There are people,' she says, 'who'll hold their hands up and say no, but there are more who'll hear Chaz talk and say, "Oh, what a lovely person."' To the people who demand a boycott of the TV show her son will appear on, she said, 'I have no words to soothe you into not being terrified if my child dances on *Dancing With the *** Stars!*'" - Cher

   What stage of the Nelson Continuum does Cher's response represent? Why?
   Advocacy. Cher demonstrates her support of Chaz, and also advocates for him by denouncing people who are rejecting him. (Facilitator's note: Some may argue that this is Qualified Acceptance because of Cher's not using male pronouns to refer to Chaz, which would also be an accurate interpretation and speaks to the idea that affirming responses are multi-layered).

4. "Nina's mother cried and cried and said wasn't there something they could work out? Maybe Nina could just dress up on weekends and leave late at night, when the neighbors wouldn't see? Maybe they could work together to hide Nina's girl things from the mother's new live-in boyfriend, who wouldn't tolerate girlie dress-up? This new boyfriend had a decent heart, her mother said, and he paid half the rent so, Dios mio, the boyfriend had to stay. The boyfriend helped Nina's mother afford her youngest son's good Catholic school.

Everybody has to sacrifice something in this life, and wasn't there a compromise, wasn't there a way? Nina told her mother no and gently hung up the phone. For Nina, then 16, prostitution was easier." – Cris Beam, in *Transparent*

What stage of the Nelson Continuum does Nina's mother represent? Why?
Rejecting Non-punitive. While Nina's mother wants to maintain contact with her, she has placed (strict) conditions on how and when this can happen. This narrative particularly reflects the idea that there are other intersectional constraints that can affect affirming responses. In Nina's case, while her mother seems to want to support her, Nina's mother is financially dependent on the boyfriend who is rejecting. As a result, Nina's mom is forced to choose between affirming Nina and putting herself and youngest son in a more finically precarious situation.

5. "My mom came to visit, and she seems to have backtracked some from her initial, surprisingly supportive position on me being trans. She informed me that I am no longer welcome in her house, both because her husband can't stand to be near a transsexual (her exact words were that I would make him 'very uncomfortable,' because my transition was 'very hard for normal people to understand'), and because she would feel 'very uncomfortable' having to explain to friends and neighbors why I was no longer female. She has *totally* gone back on her prior *very* generous offer to talk to my Puerto Rican family about my transition in person when she visits. She now says that it is my responsibility to talk to them and to get over any initial bumps with them. She doesn't even want to be present if and when I'm first allowed to visit after discussing the transition with them. And she went to great lengths to warn me about what a difficult time they are likely to have accepting and understanding it. Therefore, what she is currently envisioning in terms of the future of our relationship is her coming to see me every two to three years. No family time whatsoever." – Anonymous

What stage of the Nelson Continuum does Anonymous' mom's response represent? Why?
Rejecting Non-Punitive or Rejecting Punitive. This person's mother appeared to offer some degree of initial support, but then reversed her decision when she had to speak about her transgender child with the boyfriend, family and peers. Previous messages of emotional support are reversed, creating a situation in which this person will see their mother only under very specific, limited circumstances. (Facilitator's Note: Depending on how one interprets the stages, this can be considered either Rejecting Non-Punitive or Rejecting Punitive. When facilitating the discussion, it is more important to focus on the severity and impact of the rejection than on which is the more accurate).

6. "When I was 14, I learned what transgender meant and cried of happiness. After 10 years of confusion I finally understood who I was. I immediately told my mom, and she reacted extremely negatively, telling me that it was a phase, that I would never truly be a girl, that God doesn't make mistakes, that I am wrong. If you are reading this, parents, please don't tell this to your kids. Even if you are Christian or are against transgender people don't ever say that to someone, especially your kid. That won't do anything but make them hate them self. That's exactly what it did to me." – Leelah Alcorn

What stage of the Nelson Continuum does Leelah's mom's response represent? Why?
Rejecting Punitive. Upon coming out to her mom the response was rejecting and created an extremely hostile situation for Leelah, particularly since it was given when Leelah was 14 and dependent on her parents for her basic needs and survival. Unfortunately, Leelah ended her life at the age of 17, and the quote used here comes from her suicide note. Contemplating and attempting suicide is a shockingly common experience for transgender people, particularly transgender youth.

Supporting statistics: In a report by the Williams Institute, 41% of transgender and gender non-conforming adults have attempted suicide compared with less than 5% of cisgender people (Herman, Haas & Rogders, 2014). Transgender People of Color, those who have not completed college, and those who live in poverty

are particularly vulnerable—as are people who report that they are visibly transgender. The overall rate of attempts by transgender people is also 4 times higher than with cisgender people who identify as lesbian, gay or bisexual.

7. "'If you can't be authentic and you can't live your life, what do you have?'" – Kayne West, in response to Caitlyn Jenner's coming out as transgender.

What stage of the Nelson Continuum does Kayne's response represent? Why?
Affirming. In this quote, Kayne expresses his acceptance of and admiration for Caitlyn Jenner living her life as her authentic self.

8. "When Jodie Patterson and Joseph Ghartey realized their 7-year-old Penel was a transgender boy, the Brooklyn couple says they never considered challenging his identity. . . . 'As a family, we embrace happiness in all forms. So everyone's championing Penel,' explained Patterson, who says she and her husband have gone to family members and their son's school community to educate them, making sure that Penel is seen as more than just 'the transgender kid.'"

What stage of the Nelson Continuum does Penel's parents' response represent? Why?
Advocacy. Penel's parents are expressing their complete and unconditional acceptance of Penel, and are making active efforts to help ensure that Penel's school and community is also affirming of him.

PARTICIPANT HANDOUT

The Nelson Continuum: Applications to Transgender Affirmation

Rejecting Punitive

Explicitly punishing or harming a transgender person (physically or economically) or creating a hostile environment that is emotionally abusive, because their gender identity or expression is incongruent with the sex they were assigned at birth.

Examples: Firing a person for coming out as transgender; physically attacking a person who appears to be visibly transgender; parents kicking a transgender teenager out of their home because they are transgender; or intensive bullying of someone who is transgender.

Rejecting Non-Punitive

Rejecting (verbally or emotionally) a person because their gender identity or expression is incongruent with the sex they were assigned at birth.

Examples: Telling a person that their transgender partner cannot attend family events; refusing to use the affirming name and pronouns for a transgender person; socially isolating a transgender person at school or work.

Qualified Acceptance

Giving mixed and ambiguous messages about acceptance of a person's gender identity or expression—often presented as accepting the person, but rejecting transgender identity or the transition process.

Examples: A parent telling a child that they love them for who they are but don't approve of their choice to medically transition; a social worker who intermittently misstates a transgender person's name or pronouns; asking a transgender person to change their presentation based on the context or situation.

Full Acceptance

Unequivocally affirming a transgender person's gender identity and/or expression.

Examples: A friend consistently using the affirming name and pronoun; a partner emotionally or financially supporting medical transition; a school creating affirming records for a transgender child.

Advocacy

Taking proactive steps to publically support transgender people, including advocating for overall changes that make transgender people's experiences better.

Examples: An ally asking a medical provider to change their intake forms to include transgender-affirming options; a community member petitioning to create a local anti-discrimination ordinance; a friend asking their colleague not to make anti-transgender jokes.

Citation: This resource is based on the work of: Nelson, J.B. (1978). *An Approach to Sexuality and Christian Theology.* Minneapolis: Augsburg Publishing House,; Hall, D.M. (2009). *Allies at Work: Creating a Lesbian, Gay, Bisexual and Transgender Inclusive Work Environment.* San Francisco, CA: Out and Equal Workplace Advocates.; and; Satterly, B. A., & Dyson, D. A. (2010). Social work practice with gay, lesbian, bisexual, and transgender persons. In J. Poulin (Ed.), *Collaborative social work: Strengths-based generalist practice* (3rd ed.). Belmont, CA: Wadsworth.

PARTICIPANT HANDOUT

Responses to Coming Out

INSTRUCTIONS: Read the quotes below, and decide which stage of the Nelson Continuum it best represents and explain why.

Rejecting Punitive ▶ Rejecting Non-Punitive ▶ Qualified Acceptance ▶ Full Acceptance ▶ Advocacy

1. "All I can say about Jay is he makes it so easy to be a proud mom. For parents, we need to realize, [our kids] have their own journey. Parents get it wrong when they don't support their children. They have to go out and fight every day and face this world. The first battle should not be at home. I think that a lot of children in the LGBT community don't succeed because the one thing they need the most is a foundation. I just tell Jay all the time, baby you won the war. You're gonna have a lot of battles but you won the war. Mama accepts and loves you for who you are." – Drea Kelly

What stage of the Nelson Continuum does this represent? Why?

_____
_____
_____
_____

2. "When I came out, I didn't expect a very good reaction from my father, but I thought that my mother might be more accepting—maybe even happy to learn that the daughter she always wanted had been here all along. Things didn't turn out quite as well as I had hoped. After reading the letter, my parents quickly progressed from shock to disbelief to grief and disgust. I tried to send them resources for parents of trans* children, but when it became clear that I was serious about transitioning, they cut off all contact. I received a formal disowning letter last March, in which my father warned that my life as a trans girl would be "bleak with much unhappiness." He told me that he didn't want to know me as female, and that I should change my last name and only contact him if I "decided to be a boy again." – Annika

What stage of the Nelson Continuum does Annika's father response represent? Why?

_____
_____
_____
_____

3. "'My child is a wonderful child,' she says, expressing a true mom's sentiment and bypassing the pronouns that have gotten her in trouble. 'There are people,' she says, 'who'll hold their hands up and say no, but there are more who'll hear Chaz talk and say, "Oh, what a lovely person."' To the people who demand a boycott of the TV show her son will appear on, she said, 'I have no words to soothe you into not being terrified if my child dances on *Dancing With the *** Stars!*'" – Cher

What stage of the Nelson Continuum does Cher's response represent? Why?

_____

_____

_____

_____

4. "Nina's mother cried and cried and said wasn't there something they could work out? Maybe Nina could just dress up on weekends and leave late at night, when the neighbors wouldn't see? Maybe they could work together to hide Nina's girl things from the mother's new live-in boyfriend, who wouldn't tolerate girlie dress-up? This new boyfriend had a decent heart, her mother said, and he paid half the rent so, Dios mio, the boyfriend had to stay. The boyfriend helped Nina's mother afford her youngest son's good Catholic school. Everybody has to sacrifice something in this life, and wasn't there a compromise, wasn't there a way? Nina told her mother no and gently hung up the phone. For Nina, then 16, prostitution was easier."
– Cris Beam, in *Transparent*

What stage of the Nelson Continuum does Nina's mother represent? Why?

_____

_____

_____

_____

5. "'My mom came to visit, and she seems to have backtracked some from her initial, surprisingly supportive position on me being trans. She informed me that I am no longer welcome in her house, both because her husband can't stand to be near a transsexual (her exact words were that I would make him 'very uncomfortable,' because my transition was 'very hard for normal people to understand'), and because she would feel 'very uncomfortable' having to explain to friends and neighbors why I was no longer female. She has *totally* gone back on her prior *very* generous offer to talk to my Puerto Rican family about my transition in person when she visits. She now says that it is my responsibility to talk to them and to get over any initial bumps with them. She doesn't even want to be present if and when I'm first allowed to visit after discussing the transition with them. And she went to great lengths to warn me about what a difficult time they are likely to have accepting and understanding it. Therefore, what she is currently envisioning in terms of the future of our relationship is her coming to see me every two to three years. No family time whatsoever." – Anonymous

What stage of the Nelson Continuum does Anonymous' mom's response represent? Why?

_____

_____

_____

_____

6. "When I was 14, I learned what transgender meant and cried of happiness. After 10 years of confusion I finally understood who I was. I immediately told my mom, and she reacted extremely negatively, telling me that it was a phase, that I would never truly be a girl, that God doesn't make mistakes, that I am wrong. If you are reading this, parents, please don't tell this to your kids. Even if you are Christian or are against transgender people don't ever say that to someone, especially your kid. That won't do anything but make them hate them self. That's exactly what it did to me." – Leelah Alcorn

What stage of the Nelson Continuum does Leelah's mom's response represent? Why?

_____
_____
_____
_____

7. "'If you can't be authentic and you can't live your life, what do you have?'" – Kayne West, in response to Caitlyn Jenner's coming out as transgender.

What stage of the Nelson Continuum does Kayne's response represent? Why?

_____
_____
_____
_____

8. "When Jodie Patterson and Joseph Ghartey realized their 7-year-old Penel was a transgender boy, the Brooklyn couple says they never considered challenging his identity. . . . 'As a family, we embrace happiness in all forms. So everyone's championing Penel,' explained Patterson, who says she and her husband have gone to family members and their son's school community to educate them, making sure that Penel is seen as more than just 'the transgender kid.'"

What stage of the Nelson Continuum does Penel's parents' response represent? Why?

_____
_____
_____
_____

11

EVERYBODY'S GOTTA GO:
The Importance of Restroom Access

...

Overview & Rationale

Many people take the availability and use of safe restrooms for granted. But for some people, deciding whether, when, and where to use a restroom is a major safety concern. It may affect their ability to work, interact in their community, travel for work or leisure, and generally participate in society. This lesson helps participants explore issues pertaining to bathrooms that may affect transgender people (and sometimes cisgender people whom others perceive might be transgender) differently, and offers suggestions for addressing them. It can help participants gain knowledge, build empathy and reduce anti-transgender prejudice.

Audience

This activity is designed for people who are new to transgender-related topics or who have not had the opportunity to learn about the importance of bathroom access as a fundamental need. This lesson works best with groups of 10–30 people, and can be used with groups of up to 50 people, if facilitated carefully.

Objectives

By the end of this lesson, participants will be able to:
- Describe 2 reasons working to insure access to restrooms is essential for equality and health
- Identify 2 groups of people (other than transgender people) who would benefit from the availability of single-user restrooms

Background Knowledge for Facilitators

It will be useful for facilitators to know about the physical, emotional, logistical, health, and safety risks transgender people face when using restrooms outside of their homes. If needed, review *Bathroom Access: Talking Points for Facilitators* to become familiar with these issues.

Time

- Preparation: 15 minutes
- Implementation: 30 minutes

Materials

- Easel paper & markers (or computer, projector & PowerPoint)

Preparation

- *Review Bathroom Access: Talking Points for Facilitators.* Use other resources in this book, or online, for further information on this topic.
- Write the 3 interview questions from Procedure step 3 on easel paper or insert them in a PowerPoint slide for easy reference, so that participants can keep them in mind during the discussion.

Procedure

1. Explain: This lesson is designed to help participants better understand the challenges transgender people face when using restrooms outside of their homes—when they are at work, school, out in their communities, etc.

2. Explain that restrooms often cause stress for transgender people because they are sex-segregated. Many people take the availability and use of safe restrooms for granted. But for transgender people, deciding whether, when, and where to use a restroom is a major safety concern. It may affect their ability to work, interact in their community, travel for work or leisure, and generally participate in society. This can also affect anyone who expresses their gender differently from what

others expect. Sometimes gender non-conforming cisgender people are also affected by the lack of restrooms that are safe for transgender people.

3. Ask participants to turn to a neighboring participant and "interview" them using 3 questions (below). Explain that each pair will have about 3 minutes for one to ask the other the questions. When the facilitator calls time, the pairs will switch roles. Explain that after each person has had a chance to interview their neighbor, the facilitator will call the large group back to order and invite participants to share their experiences. While the pairs are interviewing each other, circulate among the pairs and offer support to each pair as needed.

   INTERVIEW QUESTIONS:
   - Can you think of a time when you (or a loved one) needed to access a safe restroom and were unable to do so? What happened in that situation?
   - What is the importance of consistent access to restrooms for all people (cisgender and transgender) where they are confident they will be safe?
   - What are some possible concerns people may have about transgender people and restrooms? Are any of these concerns potentially stereotyped or based on false information? If not, what information have we used to determine that these concerns are legitimate risks (as opposed to expressions of discomfort)?

4. Once each pair has completed their interview and time has been called, bring the pairs back into the large group. Ask for someone who is willing to start, and invite several participants to share some of the themes that arose for each question.

5. Lead a short discussion using the following questions, and use *Bathroom Access: Talking Points for Facilitators* to guide the discussion.

   DISCUSSION QUESTIONS
   - In what ways might access to restrooms affect transgender people's job and school performance?
   - How does access to restrooms affect transgender people outside of work and school?
   - Would people who are non-binary (or cisgender people who are gender non-conforming) be affected similarly, or differently?
   - How might some cisgender people be affected by anti-transgender prejudice regarding restrooms?
   - What are the impacts of the availability of individual, single-person unisex or gender-neutral restrooms on people who are transgender?
   - What are the potential impacts of the availability of individual, single-person unisex or gender-neutral restrooms on people who are not transgender?

6. If using this as a standalone lesson, conclude the activity by giving participants about 5 minutes to return to their pairs, brainstorm slogans for gender-neutral restroom campaigns and report back to their peers. For example, Single Stall Restrooms: The Best Cure for Pee Shyness, or Private Restrooms: So You Don't Have to Hear Anyone Fart, or [A picture of a toilet] Everyone Deserves Access to a Safe Restroom.

Evaluation Questions

✔ What are 2 reasons working to insure access to restrooms is essential for equality and health?

✔ What are 2 groups of people (other than transgender people) who would benefit from the availability of single-user restrooms?

TIPS FOR FACILITATORS

Some participants may resist the idea of allowing transgender people to use the restroom that corresponds with their gender identity. Often this resistance is based on a fear that transgender people are predators, or that people who are not transgender will pretend to be transgender to access bathrooms for sexual or nefarious purposes. It is important to stress that when violence or sexual assault occurs in bathrooms, transgender and gender non-conforming people are much more likely than cisgender people to be victims and are very, very rarely perpetrators. It can be helpful to refocus the discussion on why access to restrooms is important for all people, how laws are already in place to prevent harassment in restrooms, or how policing restrooms is unnecessary, unrealistic and an invasion of privacy for everyone.

• • •

Participants may have detailed questions about the legalities of bathroom use; they may, for example, ask specific questions about local or state regulations in their area. Be sure to include the discussion points on these topics listed under Background Knowledge for Facilitators under the discussion section of the lesson, and *Bathroom Access: Talking Points for Facilitators* as a guide.

• • •

Participants may be surprised to learn about proposed bathroom bills, or simply not understand why some people have so much focus on how, whether, where, and when others should be allowed to use the restroom. Or, they may have a difficult time believing that this could happen. Refer to the discussion points and Background Knowledge for Facilitators, and encourage participants to seek out additional information about this issue. Remind participants that because this issue is rooted largely in anti-transgender prejudice, myth, and misinformation, it's important to know the facts and work toward providing safe restrooms for everyone.

Bathroom Access: Talking Points for FACILITATORS

Impacts

- Transgender people frequently experience discrimination, such as being questioned or challenged about whether they are in the "correct" bathroom, being verbally or physically harassed or threatened, or fearing for their physical safety. So do people who are not transgender, but whom others believe don't look masculine or feminine enough for the bathroom they're in.

- Many transgender people report avoiding using public bathrooms. Or they may restrict their fluid intake. This can have a significant negative impact on physical health, (including extensive dehydration or urinary tract infections) and mental health (including anxiety, depression and isolation).

- Some transgender people avoid situations in which they will be away from safe or private bathrooms for extended periods of time, try to create a "buddy system" to ensure their safety, or go out of their way to find restrooms that are gender-neutral or private.

- Many transgender people, people with non-binary genders, and people who are perceived as gender non-conforming must think every day about whether they have access to a safe restroom at work, in school, in restaurants and coffee shops, at bus and train terminals, at airports, when they are out the community or traveling elsewhere, and generally wherever they are outside of their homes.

- Transgender people may use a lot of time and energy trying to structure their work or school day to avoid having to use the bathroom. This may also affect their work or school performance, if they need to leave early, arrive late, or try to take breaks to travel back home or to another safe location in order to use the restroom.

Risk, Harassment, and Discrimination

- Transgender people are at risk when using restrooms outside the home. It is common for transgender people to be harassed by cisgender people in restrooms. In one survey, fifty percent of transgender respondents reported having experienced harassment or assault in a public restroom (San Francisco Human Rights Commission, 2002). When this happens, the person may be verbally or physically harassed, asked to leave the restroom, removed by the establishment in which the restroom is located, or arrested by the authorities.

- There are no recorded instances of cisgender people being harassed by transgender people in restrooms. And, a recent report found no instances of harassment or inappropriate behavior in 17 of the largest school districts in the country in which transgender students are allowed to use the restrooms and locker rooms that match their gender identity (Media Matters, 2015).

- Most people, whether transgender, cisgender, or another gender, simply wish to use the restroom in peace, and leave.

- Sometimes cisgender people find themselves affected by anti-transgender prejudice in restrooms when someone else perceives them as transgender. If this happens, the cisgender person might suffer the same difficulty as a transgender person. They may be verbally or physically harassed, asked to leave the restroom, removed by the establishment in which the restroom is located, or arrested by the authorities.

Myth, Misinformation, and More Discrimination

- There is a great deal of myth and misinformation about transgender people and restroom use. Because of this, some people are fearful or angry when they think about transgender people's access to restrooms, or if they believe a transgender person may have access to a restroom they might use—or to any restroom at all.

- In 2015, several states introduced laws that would jail people whose chromosomes or birth sex do not match the restrooms they are using. Some of these bills also proposed a "bounty" of up to $4,000 be paid to anyone who turns in someone they believe is using the "wrong" restroom to the authorities. Other laws have proposed fines or criminal charges for schools or business owners if they allow a transgender person to use the restroom.

- There are already laws in place that make harassment in restrooms (or anywhere) illegal, which makes additional legislation unnecessary and shows that the abovementioned laws exist solely to penalize transgender people.

- Multiple-person restrooms don't prevent people from entering who seek to harass others. Bathrooms with multiple stalls don't have a "force field" or other magical powers to keep such individuals out.

- Requiring transgender people to use only a specific restroom (for instance, requiring a person to use only a single-person, gender-neutral restroom, or requiring a person to use a restroom that is not open to all other members of the public/employees/students) is disrespectful, an invasion of privacy, and could reveal someone's transgender status to others and thereby place them at risk for violence. In some places it is against the law.

Strategies and Solutions

- There are strategies that can assist transgender people in finding access to safe restrooms. These include websites and apps that provide listings of single-person, gender-neutral restrooms in some communities, making plans in advance to visit the restroom accompanied by a trusted friend, seeking out only single-user restrooms (those with "unisex" or gender-neutral signage that have facilities inside for one person, and a locking door).

- At its root, much of the fear and anger others harbor about transgender people and restrooms is a reflection of anti-transgender prejudice, and assumptions that people with penises (cisgender or transgender) will use them to harm women, if given the opportunity.

- Reducing anti-transgender prejudice so that transgender people could simply use any restroom that corresponds to their gender identity would eliminate the need for many of these strategies.

- Providing some single-user restrooms is one way to provide more options not only for transgender people and people whose gender expression differs from what others might expect, but for many other people as well. Single-user restrooms may also meet the needs of people in a variety of situations, including:
  o parents assisting a small child or a person of another gender,
  o people accompanying an elderly relative of another gender who requires assistance,
  o people who have personal care attendants of another gender than themselves
  o people who are very shy and find it difficult to use a public restroom if others are present
  o anyone seeking additional privacy or security while using a restroom.

UNDERSTANDING & ADDRESSING Anti-Transgender Prejudice

POWER, PRIVILEGE, AND PRONOUNS:
Transforming Education Beyond Transgender 101

By Jaymie Campbell, MA, MEd
Professional Development Manager, Mazzoni Center

• • •

As a mixed-race child, I didn't have to go far to experience racism because I experienced it frequently within my own family. Although I received conflicting messages about what it meant to be White and what it meant to be Black, both sides of my family were in agreement about what it meant to be a boy or a girl; namely, a child is born either a boy or a girl and certain gender roles and expressions should follow from the sex assigned at birth. With its abstinence focus, sexuality education in grade school was of no help for learning about the breadth and complexity of human sexuality. Everywhere I turned I was faced not only with a racial binary—White people versus People of Color—but also gender and sex binaries. As a mixed-race transgender adult, I am constantly tasked with teaching beyond binaries, but I can't do it alone.

How can others respectfully and accurately teach about marginalization, discrimination, and oppression they have not experienced? While many shy away from the call out of fear of making a mistake, no social movement was forwarded without the help of allies, and allies are essential to the Transgender Rights Movement. An educator does not have to have had personal experience to create options for students and lead them beyond the confines of previously limited curricula. Regardless of identity, the best educational work begins with the basics—learning terminology, exploring attitudes and beliefs, and then applying this new knowledge in the classroom. Transgender 101 is an essential building block of social change, but it cannot stop there. It is essential that we tackle anti-transgender prejudice head-on and work to build allies in change. This requires more than just an intellectual understanding of transgender identities, pronoun options, and why this information is important—it requires interrogation of unconscious cultural conditioning that makes transgender lives precarious.

In order to teach about anti-transgender prejudice, it is essential that we as educators also do the work to address our own biases. We must hold ourselves accountable to ensure that our good intentions as educators don't end up being a breeding ground for microaggressions. This starts with expanding our knowledge of transgender people's experiences—particularly from an intersectional perspective, examining our choices in language, reconsidering what we include or exclude from our trainings, and being mindful of the impact of our actions. While this work can feel overwhelming, the goal is not to accomplish perfection; the goal is to recognize when we have made a mistake, commit to using it as an opportunity for growth, and continuing to do better as we move forward.

According to a Buddhist saying, "When the student is ready, the teacher will appear," but it is also important for the teacher to be ready for the student. The lessons included in this section will help participants explore how their worldviews inform the lives of transgender people and related social change efforts both positively and negatively. These lessons help participants understand the systematic, institutional, and individual biases that cause harm for transgender and gender non-conforming people, and provide a framework for contributing to a world that affirms transgender and gender non-conforming people. As teachers, educators, and facilitators we have incredible opportunities to powerfully transform society. This book offers tools for social change—use them to prepare yourselves as teachers for students who are ready to join you in changing the world.

A THOUSAND CUTS:
Understanding Anti-Transgender Microaggressions

•••

Overview & Rationale

This powerful lesson asks participants to vocalize some of the common microaggressions that transgender people (particularly those who are visibly transgender or gender non-conforming) may face, as a way of understanding the impact that small acts of prejudice and discrimination can have on a person's experience. Following the activity, participants are provided with the opportunity to process the experience and discuss the emotions they feel during the activity. This lesson is designed to elicit empathy and increase basic awareness of the systematic oppression and prejudice that transgender people face in their daily lives. The lesson helps participants see that one person's negativity can have a significant impact on a transgender person's experiences, and better understand the interactions that transgender and gender non-conforming people may face on a daily basis.

Audience

This lesson works particularly well with college audiences and social service providers in medical, mental health and community-based settings. Works best with 25 participants or less.

Objectives

By the end of this lesson, participants will be able to:
- Define "microaggression" and provide examples of 2 transgender-specific microaggressions
- Name 3 common situations in which transgender people regularly endure microaggressions
- Explain the impact of microaggressions on the mental health and well-being of transgender and gender non-conforming people

Background Knowledge for Facilitators

It is important that facilitators have a high level of comfort facilitating lessons that evoke strong emotions in participants. It will also be very useful for facilitators to be familiar with the frequency and context of the microaggressions used in the activity.

Time

- Preparation: 10 minutes
- Implementation: 35–45 minutes

Materials

- 5x8 Index Cards
- Markers
- *Overview of Microaggressions & Discriminations Terms* handout (1 per participant)

Preparation
- Make copies of the handouts
- Print out Microaggression Activity Cards from www.teachingtransgender.com/printables (PW: TTTprep15) or label the index cards with the microaggression statements on the *Microaggression Statements Facilitator Resource*.

Procedure
Hand out index cards to each of the participants as they arrive.

1. Explain that: This session focuses specifically on various types of prejudice that are faced on a regular basis by transgender people. [If using, pass out the Microaggressions handout].

2. Explain that: Microaggressions are most often *individual* acts of subtle prejudice or hostility that can be unintentional or conscious (Nadal, 2013), generally committed against another individual. "Micro" does not mean that the action is insignificant—in fact, microaggressions can have a profound impact on a person's experience. All people engage in microaggressions, usually without knowledge or the intention of offending or hurting the other person. It is important that we understand the impact of our microaggressions on others, particularly transgender and gender non-conforming people.

3. Explain that: There are 3 types of microaggressions:

   Microassaults – small behaviors that are intentional and purposefully hurtful (e.g., using the wrong name or pronouns, name-calling, or making derogatory statements or threatening gestures).

   Microinsults – rude statements that are usually unintentional or unconscious that indicate ignorance or bias (e.g., asking inappropriate questions about genitals or surgical status, redirecting someone to another bathroom, or making facial expressions that reveal confusion or disgust).

   Microinvalidations – statements or actions that are usually unintentional or unconscious that ignore, minimize, or nullify a person's identity (e.g., having only two options for sex/gender on forms, telling gender non-conforming people that they should not be upset if people are confused by their gender, or saying "I am sure they didn't mean it that way" in response to a report of anti-transgender prejudice).

4. Explain that: You will be participating in an activity that shows how microaggressions affect transgender people's experiences and the struggles that transgender people have to navigate when engaging with people who are not knowledgeable about transgender issues. This activity is meant to be challenging and you may experience emotional discomfort during this activity.

5. Ask participants to create a circle in the center of the room, so that everyone is standing shoulder to shoulder.

6. Once participants have settled, physically move to the center of the circle, and ask for 2-3 participants to volunteer to join you in the center, explaining that volunteers will be playing a scripted role. (Ask for 2 volunteers with groups smaller than 16, and 3 volunteers with groups larger than 15). [Alternatively, if there are no volunteers, or there is concern about undue burden on the volunteers, the facilitator can serve as the volunteer].

7. Distribute the prepared index cards to each of the participants standing in the circle, asking them to keep their cards to themselves.

8. Instruct the volunteers in the center of the circle that they will be going to individuals in the circle one at a time and each person will read aloud what is written on their card. Instruct the participants in the circle that when they are approached, they should say only what it is on their card, and lower their card back to their side when they are done.

9. Have the participants start the activity by having one of the volunteers approach a participant, and then have the next volunteer approach a different participant. (The goal here is that there is constant reading of the participants' cards).

10. Have the volunteers approach the participants until each participant has read their card aloud. Thank everyone for participating in the activity, and ask everyone to return to their seats.

11. Process the activity using the following questions, explaining that the volunteers who were going from person to person will be asked to respond first, and those asked for help will be asked to respond next:
    - For the volunteers who faced the microaggressions from the other participants, how was this experience for you?

- How did it feel to have these negative statements read to you?
- Did you want to be able to respond at any point? What would you have said?
- How were you feeling at the end of the activity?
- For the participants who were being asked for help, what was this experience like for you?
- How did it feel to be read the card aloud?
- How did it feel to hear all of the other cards read aloud?
- Were there any statements in particular that were especially upsetting?
- How were you left feeling at the end of the activity?
- All of these microaggressions were verbal. Can you suggest some microaggressions that are non-verbal, and how would their impact be similar or different?
- What do you think the impact of experiencing these microaggressions might be on a person's mental health and well-being?
- How might your life and your general well-being change if you knew that you were likely to encounter microaggressions every time you went out?

12. Explain: While this is a dramatization, it represents the types of prejudice that transgender people face on a regular basis as well as the types of remarks that transgender people face when interacting with people. It is one of the goals of this session to better understand the experiences of transgender people.

13. Provide an opportunity for people to share any further thoughts

Talking Points

- Cisgender participants may experience disbelief or shock that these microaggressions are common occurrences for transgender people. This is an expected response, and facilitators should be prepared to explain that these microaggressions are common, particularly towards those who are visibly transgender or gender non-conforming—regardless of how rude, shocking, or distasteful the statements seem to be.
- Participants often assume that prejudice occurs only at the hands of people who are intentionally discriminating against a group. It is important that participants understand that the majority of microaggressions are committed unintentionally, and that this lack of intent does not diminish the impact.
- It is important to help participants understand the difference between impact and intention. Particularly when discussing microaggressions, folks may get hung up on the "but I didn't mean it that way" or "I am sure that person didn't intend to be hurtful" as a strategy for minimizing discomfort about having said something hurtful or offensive. (This can also emerge in arguments that people don't really make such statements or that they are not really microaggressions.) As a talking point, it is helpful to reframe the conversation to focus on the *impact* the statements have, rather than on the intention of the person committing the microaggression.

Evaluation Questions

✔ What is a microaggression?
✔ Please describe 3 common situations in which transgender people are likely to encounter microaggressions.
✔ What are 2 examples of transgender-specific microaggressions?
✔ What is the potential impact of microaggressions on the mental health and well-being of transgender and gender non-conforming people?

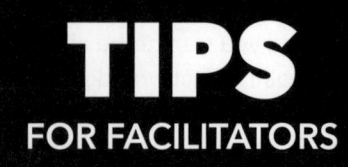

TIPS FOR FACILITATORS

This activity works best in a group with some pre-existing degree of cohesion, and may not be as effective in groups where there is a low level of trust among participants. Minimally, using ice breakers prior to this activity will be helpful.

• • •

This activity can be very powerful, and may upset some participants. It is essential that participants be given ample time to process their feelings, and that their feelings are validated. It is also essential that the facilitator leverage the empathy created and help participants connect their experience in the circle activity to the impact that they have on transgender and gender non-conforming people. This lesson is most powerful when followed by one of the other lessons in this section designed to help participants actively support transgender people and/or a lesson on intervening when witnessing anti-transgender prejudice.

• • •

If there are transgender participants, they may experience discomfort that their cisgender peers do not. Some people who are "out" as transgender may wish to share their personal experience, while others may remain silent, participate minimally, or withdraw. It is recommended that during the discussion facilitators remind participants that we never know anyone's personal history, and that there may be transgender people in the room.

• • •

If there is concern that the circle portion of the activity will be too intense for participants, facilitators can modify the activity by distributing a list of microaggressions as a handout, and ask the participants to gather in small groups to discuss the microaggressions and determine which type of microaggression is involved in each case. The discussion questions can then be used to discuss how the participants would feel if these statements were said to them.

• • •

Participants may push back about whether or not the aggressions named are *micro* or *macro*. Often this reflects the belief among participants that "micro" equates to minimal impact. It is important to clarify that the *micro* in microaggression does not imply that transgressions are insignificant; rather, it refers to the phenomenon of oppression that is perpetuated by individuals on a daily basis. It can be helpful to remind participants that their strong reaction is similar to what transgender and gender non-conforming people experience, and that being subject to these microaggressions on a consistent basis often amplifies their impact.

• • •

Participants may exhibit frustration or resistance to the topics being presented, particularly if they have a hard time acknowledging that their actions may contribute to causing harm—even when it is not intended. It is important to stress the difference between impact and intent, and help participants see that their actions can have significant ramifications even when not intended.

SOURCE:
Nadal, K. L. (2013). *That's so gay! Microaggressions and the lesbian, gay, bisexual, and transgender community.* American Psychological Association.

Microaggression Statements:
FACILITATOR'S RESOURCE

STATEMENTS TO BE WRITTEN ON INDEX CARDS & READ DURING THE ACTIVITY:

1. As soon as I saw you, I knew you were transgender.
2. But you are not really a woman, because you haven't had the surgery yet.
3. Did you see that transgender person in the coffee shop? He is clearly never going to pass as a real woman.
4. Excuse me, I think that you are in the wrong bathroom.
5. Faggot.
6. God made men and women, and meant for them to stay that way.
7. Have you had the surgery yet?
8. Hiring you would negatively affect business.
9. I don't care what you call yourself, if you have a penis, you are a man.
10. I don't think that we can provide transgender services here. Have you tried the LGBT Center?
11. I want to see your (post-operative) results!
12. If you dressed more appropriately, you wouldn't get treated badly.
13. Mommy, is that a man or a woman?
14. Our other clients wouldn't be comfortable with your being here.
15. So, you want to cut off your penis?
16. This location does not have any gender-neutral bathrooms.
17. This position is not going to be a good fit for you.
18. We don't have any safe housing for homeless transgender people.
19. We don't hire trannies.
20. We have a dress code here and you cannot wear that here.
21. We need a transgender person on this committee to help us diversify.
22. What do your genitals look like?
23. What do your parents think of you doing this?
24. Which direction are you going, male or female?
25. You are sick! Trying to fool people into thinking you are the opposite sex.
26. You look like a real man. If you hadn't told me, I never would have known.
27. You need to see a psychiatrist to fix your gender issues before we can treat you.
28. You will have to remind me to use the right pronoun. It's hard for me.
29. You're violating God's laws.
30. Your record has a different gender marker.

PARTICIPANT HANDOUT

Overview of... Microaggressions & Discrimination Terms

Individual Microaggressions:
Small acts of subtle prejudice or hostility that can be unintentional or conscious, generally committed by one individual toward another individual.

- **Microassaults** – small behaviors that are intentional and purposefully hurtful (e.g., using the wrong name or pronouns, name-calling, making derogatory statements or threatening gestures).

- **Microinsults** – rude statements that are usually unintentional or unconscious that indicate ignorance or bias (e.g., asking inappropriate questions, redirecting someone to another bathroom, or facial expressions that reveal confusion or disgust)

- **Microinvalidations** – statements or actions that are usually unintentional or unconscious that ignore, minimize, or nullify a person's identity (e.g., having only two options for sex/gender on forms, telling gender non-conforming people that they should not be upset if people are confused by their gender, or saying "I am sure they didn't mean it that way" in response to a report of anti-transgender prejudice).

Intersectional Microaggressions
Microaggressions (of all types) that are connected to multiple parts of a person's identity (such as race and gender or religion and ethnicity).

Prejudice
Negative attitudes or feelings towards an individual or group because of their identity. These negative attitudes can include discomfort, derision, or hostility.

Discrimination
Actions based on prejudice that treat a person differently because of, or punish them for, their identity (e.g., not hiring someone because the gender marker on their identity documents does not match their gender expression, physically assaulting or harming someone because they are gender non-conforming, or preventing someone from accessing a space because they are transgender).

Systematic Microaggressions & Discrimination
Institutionally based microaggressions that cannot be attributed to one specific person, but that affect many or most members of a group (e.g., lack of gender-neutral bathrooms, sex designations on identification, or gender-segregated facilities).

For more information about microaggressions against LGBT people, check out our source:

Nadal, K. L. (2013). *That's so gay! Microaggressions and the lesbian, gay, bisexual, and transgender community.* American Psychological Association

AT THE CRUX:
Intersecting Identities

Overview & Rationale

It is important that participants understand that being transgender is just one aspect of a person's experience and that other components of their identities will have a significant impact on their experiences in this world. Utilizing a multi-layered activity, this lesson will help demonstrate how oppressions intersect and encourage participants to act as agents of change.

Audience

This lesson works well with a variety of audiences. It works best with 30 or fewer people, and will not work with fewer than 15 people. Can work with up to 50, when facilitated carefully.

Objectives

By the end of this lesson, participants will be able to:
- Summarize the definition of "intersecting oppression."
- Name 3 ways in which transgender people are uniquely affected by intersecting oppressions.

Background Knowledge for Facilitators

In addition to being familiar with the teaching strategies included in the **Understanding Intersecting Identities & Oppressions** section on page 20, it will be necessary for facilitators to have a strong foundational knowledge of Intersectional Analysis. (See: www.whiteprivilegeconference.com/pdf/intersectionality_primer.pdf).

Time

- Preparation: 15 minutes
- Implementation: 45 minutes

Materials

- Identity Cards & Oppression Cards (on differently colored paper)
- *Understanding Intersecting Oppressions* handout (1 per participant)
- Ball of string
- Several pairs of scissors
- Masking tape

Preparation

- Make copies of the handouts
- Print out the Identity Cards and the Oppression Cards from www.teachingtransgender.com/printables (PW: TTTprep15) so that the Identity Cards and Oppression Cards are colored differently.
- Alternatively, create the sheets by labeling three sheets of one color paper (1) Individual (2) Organizational and (3) Systematic, so that they are each on their own sheet of paper. Repeat the process with the other color paper and label them: (1) Ableism, (2) Ageism, (3) Citizenship, (4) Classism, (5) Ethnicity & Cultural Heritage, (6) Heterosexism, (7) Racism, (8) Religion, and (9) Sexism.
- Manipulate the physical space so that it can accommodate a circle of 9 people.
- Read through all of the *Understanding Intersecting Oppressions* handouts, and become familiar with the circumstances in which intersecting oppressions occur and with their impact on transgender people.

Procedure

1. Explain that there are 3 types of oppression:

    Individual: In which one person directly discriminates against another person, usually with intent. For example, not hiring someone because they are transgender, or physically attacking someone because they are gender non-conforming.

    Organizational: In which a particular organization intentionally or unintentionally creates an environment that is unwelcoming or hostile. For example, a middle school requiring students to wear uniforms based on gender, or a social service organization requiring state-issued identification to enter the location.

    Systematic: In which an established system intentionally or unintentionally creates additional barriers and burdens for marginalized groups. This cannot be tied to one specific office or policy. For example, all identity documents being tied to the sex marked on someone's birth certificate and the difficulty of the process involved in changing these documents.

2. Divide participants into 9 groups, and give each of the groups 1 of the Identity Cards. (If there are not enough people to create 9 groups, assign each group 2 Identity Cards). Pass out the *Understanding Intersecting Oppressions* handout.

3. Explain: During this lesson we will be examining several ways in which intersecting oppressions affect transgender people's lives and experiences. Ask each of the groups to spend about 15 minutes reviewing the section of the handout that corresponds to their Identity Card(s). For each of the bulleted statements, the groups should identify whether the statement represents **Individual, Organizational** or **Systematic** oppression, and note that on the *Understanding Intersecting Oppressions* handout. Rotate through the small groups as they are working and provide additional support as needed.

4. After the 15 minutes, direct participants back to the large group, and ask for 1 volunteer from each group, and for 3 additional volunteers from any group. These volunteers should be able to toss and catch a ball. Ask the 3 volunteers to stand in the middle of the circle with their backs facing each other. Ask the other 9 participants to create a circle around the center 3. It should look like the image to the right. (Optional: Tape the Oppression Cards to the shirts of the 3 people standing in the center triangle. Tape the Identity Cards to the 9 people who are standing in the outside circle.)

5. One at a time, ask each of the participants who are standing in the outer circle to read 1 of the bullet statements aloud (or have someone from their small group read it on their behalf) and then share which of the 3 types of oppression the group decided it represented. The person standing should then toss the ball of string (while holding on to one end of it) to the person in the center triangle who represents that type of oppression. The person in the triangle should toss the ball of string to another person in the outside circle. This should be repeated until at least 3 statements from each of the types of oppression have been called out. The end result should be a relatively tangled web of strings.

6. Explain that this web represents the ways in which oppressions intersect for transgender people. There is no "easy" way of disconnecting the distinct strings of oppression. Then ask the people who are holding the "individual" strings to drop their strings. Ask the participants to observe how even though the individual acts of oppression have been dropped, much of the web still remains. Ask the participants to share their thoughts on how hard it might be to disentangle this web. (Answer: It would be quite hard because everything has become so entangled).

7. Distribute the pairs of scissors to a few participants who are not in the circle, and ask them to see if they can find the strings that are holding up most of the web and cut them. (It should take the cutting of several strings in order for the web to collapse). Explain to the participants that while many forms of prejudice and discrimination are systematic, with enough people working to make even small changes in those systems, it is possible to make a significant difference. (Optional: You may wish to cut the string into smaller pieces and give a small piece to each of the participants as a reminder of their ability to contribute to change.)

Evaluation Questions

✔ Write 2-3 sentences summarizing what "intersecting oppression" means.
✔ List 3 ways in which transgender people are uniquely impacted by intersecting oppressions.

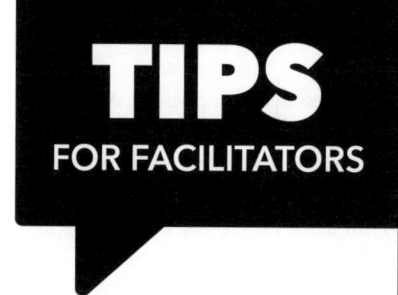

Participants may struggle to determine whether a given form of oppression is individual, organizational or systematic. There are many arguments for each, and there are not necessarily "right" answers—it is more important that participants have the dialogue and consider the various perspectives. It can be helpful to reassure participants that there are many right answers.

...

This activity is a particularly dense one that can bring up a lot of feelings and reactions to what is being presented—reactions of defensiveness, frustration, and being overwhelmed or triggered are common. How participants react will also depend on the demographics of the group and their current degree of understanding of intersecting oppressions. It is particularly useful for facilitators to demonstrate patience and empathy for participants by validating their reactions while encouraging them to continue with the activity.

...

It will be very important to make sure that participants who experience intersectionality, particularly those who are highly marginalized by intersectionality, have a strong voice in the conversations (if they so choose), and that as a facilitator you work to support their sharing and manage any pushback from other participants to help make sure that the person sharing does not feel that they are being attacked or targeted by other participants.

...

Participants may exhibit frustration or resistance to the topics being presented, particularly if they have a hard time acknowledging that their actions may contribute to causing harm—even when it is not intended. It is important to stress the difference between impact and intent, and help participants see that their actions can have significant ramifications even when not intended.

PARTICIPANT HANDOUT

Understanding Intersecting Oppressions

"If you add together separate oppressions, you are left with a grand oppression greater than the sum of its parts."
—Patricia Hill-Collins, 1993, p. 26

All people have experiences of gender, orientation, race, ethnicity, class, religion, ability, and age that are intersecting and complex. To truly contribute to social change for transgender people, we must pay particular attention to how intersecting identities and oppressions affect the lives of transgender people. Just as each cisgender person and their constellation of experiences and background are unique, the same is true for transgender people. Different backgrounds may yield different levels of societal privilege. Each transgender person will have a unique experience of the world, based on the combination of their gender identity and expression with their ability, age, citizenship, class, ethnic & cultural heritage, race, religion, and sexual orientation.

Here are some examples of the ways in which being transgender intersects with other aspects of a person's identity:

ABLEISM:
Prejudice against people who are perceived as physically, mentally, or intellectually atypical. Examples of how being transgender intersects with ableism:
- Will medical providers doubt my gender identity because I have also been diagnosed with Bipolar Disorder?
- Once I find one of the few affirming medical and mental health providers in my area, how accessible is the public transportation I need to use to get to their office?
- Due to my chronic illness, will my body physically be able to handle hormonal or surgical interventions?
- As a transgender person with Down Syndrome, how will my intellectual abilities affect whether people will validate my gender identity?
- What are the American Sign Language signs for transgender-related terms, and will people understand them?

AGEISM & ADULTISM:
Prejudice against older people, and prejudice against young people. Examples of how being transgender intersects with ageism and adultism:
- Will people believe me because I am a child?
- Will malpractice laws prevent me from surgical interventions before I turn 18?
- If I am a minor in foster care, will my foster parents respect and affirm my identity?
- How will being older affect my ability to medically transition?
- If I develop age-related dementia, how will the people in my life affirm my gender?
- Will I be able to find a long-term care facility that will respect and affirm my identity?

CITIZENSHIP:
Rights and privileges afforded to being a documented citizen or lack thereof if one is undocumented or not a citizen. Examples of how being transgender intersects with citizenship:
- Does my country of origin or country of immigration allow me to change my identity documents, (e.g. passport, driver's license)?
- As a genderqueer person, how will I navigate not being able to have identity documents that validate my gender identity?
- Can I return to my country of origin if I have medically transitioned?
- Is it illegal for me to be transgender in my country of origin? To visit certain countries?
- If I am undocumented, how will I have access to affirming identity documents?
- Do I have to delay social or medical transition in order to obtain citizenship?
- If I am detained for deportation due to a lack of documentation, which sex will I be housed with and will I be safe from violence from peers and guards?
- What will the impact be of my not being able to change my name or gender markers once I have applied to become a US citizen?
- Since the US does not have legal protections for transgender people, will I be able to seek and receive asylum from my own country based on persecution there due to my gender identity?

→

CLASSISM:
Lack of access to social and economic power based on socioeconomic status. Examples of how being transgender intersects with class:
» Access to sexual and reproductive services (e.g., egg harvesting, freezing sperm, fertility)
» Can my family afford pubertal suppression drugs?
» How will I pay for medical transition, if my insurance doesn't cover it?
» Can I afford to buy a gender-affirming wardrobe?
» Will my access to jobs be restricted because of my gender identity or expression?
» How will I be able to find the information I need online if I can't afford Internet access?

ETHNICITY & CULTURAL HERITAGE: **One's ethnic and cultural backgrounds and experiences. Examples of how being transgender intersects with ethnicity and cultural heritage:**
» Does my cultural background acknowledge that transgender and genderqueer people exist?
» How will I handle the lack of gender-neutral words and affirming terms in my native language?
» How will I navigate the traditional dress and roles of my culture?
» Is gender non-conformity forbidden by law or custom?

HETEROSEXISM:
The assumption that all people are, or should be, heterosexual and that heterosexual people must be gender conforming (based on sex assigned at birth). Examples of how being transgender intersects with heterosexism:
» Will people assume that, because I am transgender, I must be attracted to the opposite sex?
» Might my marriage or my custody of my children be subjected to heightened scrutiny because I am a transgender person?
» If people know that I am a transgender woman, will my heterosexual male partner be subjected to gay bashing?

RACISM:
One's racial background or perceived racial background. Examples of how being transgender intersects with race:
» How will being targeted by the police as a transgender or genderqueer person of color affect my safety?
» Since people of color are more likely to be targeted as potential shoplifters, will I be able to shop for affirming clothing without additional scrutiny or harassment?
» How will historical stereotypes of Native Americans influence how people perceive my gender identity?
» How will I be able to succeed in school, given that gender non-conforming students face high rates of bullying, and teachers are less likely to intervene on behalf of students of color?
» If I experience rejection from my family, friends and community because I am transgender, who will I turn to, to process and cope with the racism that I experience as a person of color?

RELIGION:
One's faith, agnosticism or atheism. Examples of how being transgender intersects with religion:
» Does my religion condemn transgender people?
» Does my faith tradition require that men and women be separated during worship or life?
» Will I have to choose between affirming my gender and my faith?
» How will I handle my faith's requirements to cover my head (e.g. hijab, yarmulke, wigs, apostolnik) or sit in a certain part of a worship space?
» Does my religion prohibit me from modifying my body?
» Will I be allowed to be a faith leader? Will my faith leaders support me?
» Will I be allowed to participate in the traditions and rites of passage that are gendered?

SEXISM:
The ways in which people are treated differently based on whether they are perceived as men or women. Examples of how sexism intersects with being transgender:
» Will my income change after I transition medically because of the pay disparities between men and women?
» As a transgender man, how will I handle other men's sexist comments or treatment of women?
» As a transgender woman, will I experience extra scrutiny about whether my fashion choices are considered to be "trying too hard" or "too sexual"?
» As a transgender woman, will people in LGBQ communities expect me to be "femme"? Will people invalidate my gender identity if I want to express masculinity?
» As a gay transgender man, will other gay men reject me because I don't have traditional male genitals?
» As a genderqueer person, how will other people's discomfort with my non-binary identity impact me?

What other examples of intersecting identities can you think of?

1. _____
2. _____
3. _____
4. _____
5. _____

CHECK YOUR PRIVILEGE:
Understanding and Building Awareness

By Maureen Kelly

• • •

Overview & Rationale

This lesson gives participants an opportunity to learn about and discuss cisgender privilege through a mini-lecture, a brief video clip, small- and large-group activities, and scenario brainstorming. Through this lesson, participants will learn the definition and origins of the term "cisgender" and understand cisgender privilege. Exploring how unquestioned privilege means not having to think about things that those without cisgender privilege face on a daily basis will help cisgender people develop empathy, awareness, and skills as more effective collaborators in social justice and social change work. This lesson works particularly well when paired with **Lesson 15: In Solidarity With: Allies as Agents of Social Change** on page 137.

Audience

This lesson works particularly well with cisgender participants who are likely to have professional or social interactions with transgender people. Works best with 30 participants or less.

Objectives

By the end of this lesson, participants will be able to:
- Define cisgender and cisgender privilege.
- Explain 2 examples of cisgender privilege.

Background Knowledge for Facilitators

It will be useful for facilitators to know about and understand systems of privilege, particularly regarding the ways in which our culture favors cisgender people. It will also be useful for facilitators to be familiar with Janet Mock's book *Redefining Realness: My Path to Womanhood, Identity, Love & So Much More,* and/or her coming out story published in 2011 by *Marie Claire* magazine.

Time

- Preparation: 10 minutes
- Implementation: 90 minutes

Materials

- *Putting Ourselves in Transgender People's Shoes* handout (1 per participant)
- Computer, projector and PowerPoint
- Large easel paper and markers (if not using PowerPoint)
- Technology system that allows trainer to show video clip with sound on the Internet
- Video clip: "Activist Janet Mock Flips the Script on Reporter: Asks Her to Prove Her Womanhood." Clip available at: http://youtu.be/ISsdSvJhniQ

Preparation

- Make copies of the handouts
- Read through the procedure and choose your best method (easel paper or PowerPoint) for communicating definitions to your participants. If using PowerPoint, download the slides from www.teachingtransgender.com/printables PW: TTTprep15). If using easel paper, write the definitions on the paper.
- Review video clip in advance.
- Familiarize yourself with the talking points for the discussion questions.

Procedure

1. Introduce the lesson by explaining that, to better understand the role of transgender allies, it is important to understand the terms "cisgender" and "cisgender privilege." Use the talking points below to explain the definitions for each.
    - The term "cisgender" refers to someone whose gender identity matches the sex they were assigned at birth.
    - The term "cisgender" helps name the unstated assumption that everyone's sex assigned at birth is congruent with their gender identity.
    - "Cisgender" is preferred to "normal" because "normal" implies that transgender people are "abnormal."
    - The prefix "cis" means "on the same side as" (that is, the opposite of *trans*).
    - While "cisgender" refers to the alignment of someone's sex and gender, cisgender privilege denotes how perceived gender/sex alignment is often a quiet, internal, unquestioned experience. This frequently means not having to think about or address challenges transgender people have to deal with, often on a daily basis. This is referred to as "cisgender privilege."

2. Explain: One example of cisgender privilege is not having to answer deeply personal questions about one's identity or body. This is beautifully illustrated by author Janet Mock's satirical interview with a reporter. In the video clip we are about to watch, Ms. Mock shows how inhumanely journalists treat transgender women when they ask inappropriate questions. Ms. Mock "flips the script" and interrogates a journalist on what it's like to be a cisgender woman.

3. Show the 3-minute video clip "Activist Janet Mock Flips the Script on Reporter: Asks Her to Prove Her Womanhood" Available at: http://youtu.be/ISsdSvJhniQ

4. Facilitate a brief conversation with the large group about their reflections and reactions to the clip using the following questions:
    - What did you see in this clip? Can you summarize the key points?
    - What are your personal reactions to this clip? What stands out to you?
    - Has it ever occurred to you that someone might question the legitimacy of your gender identity? How do you think you would respond if they did?
    - What might it feel like to have someone ask such personal questions? What might someone's motivations be for asking such questions?

TIPS FOR FACILITATORS

If participants resist the idea that they have privilege, it is important to gently challenge them. This resistance is often rooted in the idea that they are not intending to cause harm to others, or did not ask to be bestowed with additional privilege. Challenge participants to action by helping them identify strategies for being an ally to transgender people.

• • •

It may be useful to view other clips by Janet Mock to use as a reference point during the post-video discussion. You may find it useful to be familiar with various interviews in which Janet has been asked these types of questions. However, it is not recommended that you show clips of other interviews to audiences unless they already have a strong understanding of why/how those types of questions and comments are problematic. (Otherwise they will be more likely to focus on Janet's personal story, rather that the problematic and invasive nature of the questions).

• • •

Participants may exhibit frustration or resistance to the topics being presented, particularly if they have a hard time acknowledging that their actions may contribute to causing harm—even when it is not intended. It is important to stress the difference between impact and intent, and help participants see that their actions can have significant ramifications even when not intended.

5. Explain: For the next part of the session, you will be pairing up with a peer to further explore some of the challenges that transgender people experience on a daily basis. Ask participants to find a peer that they do not know particularly well and sit with that person to work on this activity together. Pass out copies of the *Putting Ourselves in Transgender People's Shoes* handout and instruct the pairs that they will have about 15 minutes to work through the scenarios and questions. (Optional: If short on time, assign each of the pairs one of the 4 scenarios to discuss). Rotate through the small groups while they are working on this task and provide additional support as needed.

6. Once pairs have completed the activity, bring everyone's attention back to the large group to discuss their answers. Use the talking points on the *Putting Ourselves in Transgender People's Shoes: Facilitator's Guide* to guide your discussion.

7. If using as a standalone lesson, conclude the activity by asking participants to return to the peer with whom they partnered and spend 5 minutes discussing possible steps that they could have taken as an ally in these situations to support the transgender person in the scenario. Have participants share these steps with the larger group and record these steps on easel paper to create a list of potential ally steps.

Evaluation Questions

✔ How are "cisgender" and "cisgender privilege" defined?

✔ What are 2 examples of cisgender privilege?

Putting Ourselves in Transgender People's Shoes:
FACILITATOR'S GUIDE

1. **You plan to attend a football game at your high school. You'll be going with friends. You know that with the halftime show the event will last for several hours and you will likely need to use the restroom.**

   ### TALKING POINTS:
   - Bathrooms are often a source of stress for transgender and gender non-conforming people because they are sex-segregated.
   - Transgender and gender non-conforming people frequently report microaggressions and discrimination such as being questioned or challenged about whether they are in the "correct" bathroom, being verbally harassed or threatened, or being put in fear for their physical safety.
   - As a result, many transgender and gender non-conforming people report avoiding using public bathrooms. This can have a significant negative impact on physical health, (including extensive dehydration or urinary tract infections) and mental health (including anxiety, depression and isolation).
   - Some transgender and gender non-conforming people may avoid situations in which they will be away from safe or private bathrooms for extended periods of time, have to create a "buddy system" to ensure safety, or go out of their way to find bathrooms that are gender neutral or private.

2. **You have plans to go on a trip! This will require air travel, navigating TSA screening, showing identification and using restrooms.**

   ### TALKING POINTS:
   - In order to travel by air, it is necessary to have identity documents, which are required to include a legal name and gender marker (e.g., a driver's license or passport). Depending on a person's present location or where they were born, it may be logistically, legally or financially difficult or impossible to obtain identity documents that have a name and/or gender marker that accurately reflects a person's gender identity. This can lead to increased scrutiny by security officials and the person may be prohibited from traveling.
   - Screening procedures often involve backscatter scanning technology. Security agents are required to select a gender for the person in the machine based on visual appearance. The machine scans the person's body for anomalies, which can reveal genitals that are non-congruent (such as a penile prosthesis, chest-binding materials, breast forms, wigs, etc.). Anything that is considered an anomaly will result in an invasive pat down, body search, or interview—often conducted in public and escalating to private areas with increased risk of harassment or discrimination.
   - This affects how transgender and gender non-conforming people approach travel. Some avoid air travel altogether, which means not being able to travel for work, school or pleasure. Others experience high levels of stress and anxiety related to concerns around safety and harassment.

3. **You are a part of group that has decided to do something fun to get to know one another better. Everyone has been invited to bring in a baby picture to share to see if the group can guess who is who.**

   ### TALKING POINTS:
   - For transgender people, showing pictures from one's youth can be embarrassing or humiliating. Making excuses to avoid such activities may result in being perceived as unfriendly or standoffish.
   - For people who have medically transitioned, being asked to show pictures from their youth forces a person to reveal themselves as transgender.

- If a person does choose to share a picture, peers may make a "fuss" over the person's previous gendered presentation, express disbelief at their previous gender expression, or make other inappropriate or offensive remarks about how "beautiful" or "handsome" a person was before they transitioned.

4. **You are applying for a new job. You have been asked for the names and contact information for three previous employers so that your prior employment can be verified.**

   ## TALKING POINTS:

   - If a person has changed their name, socially transitioned, or medically transitioned since a previous job, the prior employer may not recognize the new name or gender marker. Even if a person supports another person's transition, they may still unintentionally slip and use an old name or wrong pronoun for that person. The incongruence in name or gender markers may out the person as transgender, which can lead to discrimination, often including not being considered or hired for a position.
   - A person may have left a job to transition, or because they were being harassed or discriminated against. They will then have to explain why they were terminated or explain the gap in their employment. Alternatively, due to hiring discrimination, a person may not have three previous jobs to record.
   - As a result of these factors, transgender people may feel limited in their job options. Some transgender people have to change careers, or remove previous degrees, awards, or publications from their résumés to avoid being "outed."

PARTICIPANT HANDOUT

Putting Ourselves In Transgender People's Shoes

While "cisgender" refers to the apparent alignment of someone's sex and gender, "cisgender privilege" reflects how perceived gender/sex alignment is often a quiet, internal, unquestioned experience. This frequently means not having to think about or address challenges transgender people have to deal with, often on a daily basis. The following four scenarios describe situations in which transgender people may experience aggression, discrimination, injustice, or violence. Read through the scenarios and answer the accompanying questions.

1. You plan to attend a football game at your high school. You'll be going with friends. You know that with the halftime show the event will last for several hours and you will likely need to use the restroom.

   - What might a transgender or gender non-conforming person need to think about or do to be able to use the restroom?

     _____
     _____
     _____

   - What might make this uniquely challenging, frightening or distressing for a transgender or gender non-conforming person?

     _____
     _____
     _____

2. You plan to go on a trip! This will require air travel, navigating TSA screening, showing identification and using restrooms.

   - What might a transgender or gender non-conforming person need to think about or do to be ready for travel?

     _____
     _____
     _____

   - What might make this uniquely challenging, frightening or distressing for a transgender or gender non-conforming person?

     _____
     _____
     _____

3. You are a part of group that has decided to do something fun to get to know one another better. Everyone has been invited to bring in a baby picture to share to see if the group can guess who is who.

   - What might a transgender or gender non-conforming person need to think about or do when this group activity is announced?

   _____
   _____
   _____

   - What might make this uniquely challenging, frightening or distressing for a transgender or gender non-conforming person?

   _____
   _____
   _____

4. You are applying for a new job. You have been asked for the names and contact information for three previous employers so that your prior employment can be verified.

   - What might a transgender or gender non-conforming person need to think about when giving this information?

   _____
   _____
   _____

   - What might make this uniquely challenging, frightening or distressing for a transgender or gender non-conforming person?

   _____
   _____
   _____

15

IN SOLIDARITY WITH:
Allies as Agents of Social Change

By Maureen Kelly and Calvin Kasulke

Overview & Rationale

This lesson gives participants an opportunity to learn about and discuss being an ally* to transgender people through a mini-lecture, small- and large-group activities and a self-assessment activity. Allies that develop empathy, awareness, and skills are more effective collaborators in social justice and social change work. This lesson works particularly well when paired with **Lesson 14: Check Your Privilege: Understanding and Building Awareness** on page 130 **and Lesson 12: A Thousand Cuts: Understanding Anti-Transgender Microaggressions** on page 119.

Audience

This lesson works particularly well with people who identify as allies or would like to expand their skills. This lesson works best with 10–30 participants, but can be modified for larger audiences.

Objectives

By the end of this lesson, participants will be able to:
- Identify 2 of the 10 components of being an effective ally
- Identify 1 situation in which an inappropriate comment or question may occur, and explain why the comment or question would be problematic

Background Knowledge for Facilitators

It will be helpful for facilitators to understand a range of strategies that people can utilize to be better allies. It will also be very helpful to know personal narratives from allies that indicate why being an ally is important to them and narratives from transgender people that describe being positively affected by allies.

Time

- Preparation: 10 minutes
- Implementation: 90 minutes

---

*The word **"ally"** can be contentious. Some people identify with it and use it with conviction. Others view it more negatively and use "in solidarity with" instead. This is often based on the idea that "ally" is a problematic label because it takes focus away from the people being marginalized. There are also some who challenge the idea that someone can identify as an ally, or has the right to do so. We choose to use the word "ally" here because it remains the best word we can find to assign to people with privilege who stand in solidarity with marginalized people, in this case, transgender people. We realize language matters and changes, and we expect to learn new words to add to the conversation.

Materials
- *Ten Components of Being an Effective Ally* handout (1 per participant)
- *Ally Role Play* handout (1 per pair)

Preparation
- Make copies of the handouts
- Review the *Ally Role Play Activity: Facilitator's Guide* to ensure clarity of the situations and talking points

Procedure
1. Explain: We will be exploring what it means to be an ally to and advocate for transgender people. There are many components of being an ally and it is important to understand how to be the best possible ally.

2. Pass out copies of the *Ten Components of Being an Effective Ally* handout, and ask for volunteers to read one of the statements aloud.

3. Ask participants to find a peer they do not know particularly well and sit with that person to work on this activity together. Direct the pairs to pick out which of the 10 components stands out the most to them and discuss why they believe it is an important part of being an ally. After 10 minutes, ask all of the pairs to come back to the large group, and ask for 3-5 volunteers to share which component they chose and why.

4. Once participants have shared their statements and rationales, conclude the activity by emphasizing the following talking points:
   - Because anti-transgender prejudice is so prevalent, there are ample opportunities to engage or advocate as an ally.
   - Ally work can take on a variety of approaches, styles and actions.
   - Ally work changes based on time, places, and situation.
   - There are situations in which allies have unique opportunities to act as advocates when transgender people do not have access to or are not welcome or safe in a venue or space.

5. Explain: Being an ally is more than declaring a lack of prejudice toward transgender people or having a desire to be supportive of transgender people. There are a variety of ways to approach being an ally, but one of the most important and prevalent opportunities available to potential allies is calling out instances of ignorance, bias or discrimination.
   - Explain that the following activity will involve a volunteer being presented with a brief scenario that addresses one of the ways in which transgender people are asked questions or talked about in ways that are inappropriate and require interruption, correction, and education. Distribute the *Ally Role Play* handouts to the participants.
   - For the first 2 scenarios, ask for 2 volunteers, and ask 1 volunteer to read the scenario with the problematic statement. Ask the large group to identify a few reasons why the statement is problematic. Then ask the other volunteer to read the possible responses aloud and explain which one they would select and why.
   - For the remaining 3 scenarios, ask people to return to their previous pairs. Direct participants that 1 person will read a statement that is ignorant, biased or prejudiced, and the other person in the pair will practice how they would respond. Allow 5 minutes for each of the scenarios, stopping to discuss the following questions briefly after each scenario:
     - Why was the statement problematic?
     - What was it like for you to try to respond to this statement? How easy or hard was it to do?
     - How did you respond? What were the statements you made?
     - How comfortable would you feel in responding this way in real life?

Talking Points

- Stress that the most effective strategy for calling someone out is to provide useful content in a warm and non-shaming tone. It is also helpful to provide context and clarity about why a statement is problematic, and offer a simple correction.
- Validate that it can be stressful, or that it can be hard, to find the words to call someone out at the exact moment that a hurtful remark occurs. It is often better to try to intervene in that moment because it helps raise awareness and communicates solidarity with and support of transgender people.
- There are situations in which an intervention may be more effective when done privately or at a later time. (For example, if you are addressing your supervisor, or if you are concerned about a defensive response). When it is not possible or advantageous to call someone out at a particular moment, it may be possible to re-approach the person later in a more private location.

Concluding Discussion Questions

After the group has completed all 5 scenarios, lead the whole group in a culminating discussion using the following questions:

- Why is it important that allies intervene in situations in which there is bias or prejudice?
- Where do you think that you might encounter some of these situations?
- How likely do you think it is that you would speak up in an instance in which someone makes a statement that is ignorant, biased, or prejudiced?
- What additional steps could you take to become more confident as an ally or advocate in such situations?

Evaluation Questions

✔ There are 10 components of being an effective ally. Name 2.

✔ What are 2 situations in which an inappropriate comment such as "What was your name before?" might occur, and why would this be a problematic comment?

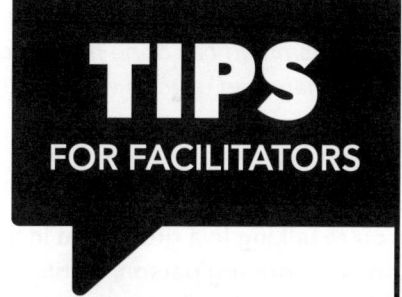

TIPS FOR FACILITATORS

For groups larger than 30 or if there are time constraints, assign each pair a scenario rather than having each pair do all scenarios. This will shorten the time required to process the role-play

• • •

Role-play activities often raise participants' anxiety. Validate that these practices can be stressful but are an essential part of acquiring the skill of successfully advocating for transgender people and communities.

• • •

Participants may exhibit frustration or resist the topics being presented, particularly if they have a hard time acknowledging that their actions may contribute to causing harm—even when it is not intended. It is important to stress the difference between impact and intent, and help participants see that their actions can have significant ramifications even when not intended.

• • •

Ally work is hard and can be thankless. Allies often receive conflicting messages about their role in advocating for and supporting transgender people—including whether or not it is even okay to call themselves an ally. Transgender communities will include multiple perspectives on this question. In the end, it is more important that allies advocate for transgender people than worry about what they call themselves. As a facilitator, if participants raise these concerns, it will be helpful to validate that it can be difficult to navigate and redirect them back to their initial goal of wanting to be an ally. Allies do play an essential role in creating social change.

Ally Role Play Activity:
FACILITATOR'S GUIDE

ROLE PLAY 1

You're having a conversation with a co-worker. The co-worker is referring to a staff member who is an out transgender man named Mohammad, and says "Oh, you know her, when she started working here she worked in facilities, now she's the one you need to talk to in the IT department to get your new email login."

Why this is problematic:
- The co-worker used the wrong pronoun.
- This is a common microaggression against transgender people.

Suggested Reponses:
- "Hey, just so you know, Mohammad uses male pronouns."
- "I get that it can feel confusing to talk about Mohammad's past work, before he transitioned, but it's really important that we all use his name, Mohammad, and male pronouns when we talk about him in the past, present, or future."
- "If you actually need to talk about other work Mohammad has done here, you can just say, 'Mohammad used to work in facilities.'"

ROLE PLAY 2

You're talking in a group that includes a gender non-conforming person, Terrill. A friend turns to this individual and with compassion and heartfelt emotions exclaims "Oh my gosh, you're so brave being who you are like that!"

Why this is problematic:
- Even though the person's intentions may be positive and affirming, the statements call attention to Terrill's gender expression in a way that may be embarrassing or demeaning.
- Telling Terrill that they are brave implies that their gender expression is a choice or decision.
- This can be perceived as patronizing.
- This is a common microaggression against transgender people.

Suggested Responses:
- "I think it's less about Terrill being brave and more about working to get the rest of the world to discriminate and stigmatize transgender people less."
- "Yes, I think there are unique challenges and discrimination that transgender and gender non-conforming people face, but calling it 'brave' might be seen as unintentionally patronizing."
- "Sometimes when 'bravery' is used it sets transgender people apart or 'others' them. It further stigmatizes transgender or gender non-conforming people."

ROLE PLAY 3

You're talking with a small group of friends that includes an out transgender woman, Sylvia. She is sharing a story of frustration and stress caused by rejection and lack of understanding of her family of origin. One friend chimes in and says, "Oh don't worry, they'll come around someday, you're so great."

Why this is problematic:
- While this may be well intentioned, this can be perceived as dismissive, minimizing or invalidating.
- The transgender woman may have been looking for support, and may feel further rejected or misunderstood.
- This implies that the transgender woman's impression of her family is inaccurate, and denies the reality that many people are rejected by their families.
- This is a common microaggression against transgender people.

Suggested Responses:
To the friend and transgender woman:
- "I'm sure she knows her family best."
- "Families can be really complicated; I don't think it's right for us to try to oversimplify a really personal issue like this."

To the transgender woman:
- *"I can't speak for your family, but we're here if you need support."*
- *"I'm sorry they're creating difficulties for you."*

ROLE PLAY 4

A co-worker asks to talk with you privately. She says she knows that you are close with an out transgender co-worker, Marsha, and she was curious about whether you know if Marsha had had "the surgery" yet.

Why this is problematic:
- Asking about a person's surgical status is invasive, inappropriate and rude.
- Decisions about whether to disclose private medical information should be Marsha's.
- Asking a co-worker behind Marsha's back is gossipy and inconsiderate.

Suggested Responses:
- "Marsha's medical history is private, just like the medical history of the rest of our co-workers."
- "That's really private information."
- "Regardless of what operations Marsha may or may not have had, she has the right to have her privacy respected. Especially privacy about her personal medical history, that's not at all a workplace discussion."
- "I don't think Marsha feels comfortable sharing that information with people, and it doesn't affect your ability to do your job effectively."

ROLE PLAY 5

In the course of a small meeting, Yasmin mentions that she is a transgender woman. Another person in the meeting turns and says, "I never would have known, you look so much like a real woman!"

Why is this problematic?
- This implies that Yasmin is not a "real" woman, and that she is really a man.
- While potentially intended as affirming, the statement undermines Yasmin's validity as a woman.
- This is a common microaggression against transgender people.

Suggested Responses:
- "That's because Yasmin is a real woman."
- "Wow, if I were Yasmin, I might find that really offensive."
- "I understand you meant that as a compliment, but Yasmin's appearance doesn't dictate the reality of her womanhood."

PARTICIPANT HANDOUT

Ally Role Play Activity

ROLE PLAY 1

You're having a conversation with a co-worker. The co-worker is referring to a staff member who is an out transgender man named Mohammad, and says "Oh, you know her, when she started working here she worked in facilities; now she's the one you need to talk to in the IT department to get your new e-mail login."

ROLE PLAY 2

You're talking in a group that includes a gender non-conforming person, Terrill. A friend turns to this individual and with compassion and heartfelt emotions exclaims "Oh my gosh, you're so brave being who you are like that!"

ROLE PLAY 3

You're talking with a small group of friends that includes an out transgender woman, Sylvia. She is sharing a story of frustration and stress caused by rejection and lack of understanding of her family of origin. One friend chimes in and says, "Oh don't worry, they'll come around someday, you're so great."

ROLE PLAY 4

A co-worker asks to talk with you privately. She says she knows that you are close with an out transgender co-worker, Marsha, and she was curious about whether you know if Marsha had had "the surgery" yet.

ROLE PLAY 5

In the course of a small meeting, Yasmin mentions that she is a transgender woman. Another person in the meeting turns and says, "I never would have known, you look so much like a real woman!"

PARTICIPANT HANDOUT

10 Components of Being an Effective Ally

1. Allies proactively seek understanding and awareness of the marginalization that transgender people face, and advocate for a safer and more affirming world.

2. Allies actively cultivate transgender people's leadership as a contribution toward creating social change.

3. Allies take primary responsibility for learning about how oppression affects the lives of transgender people.

4. Allies seek out transgender people's perspectives as experts on transgender identities, experiences, and needs. Allies amplify the experiences of transgender people to a broader audience.

5. Allies acknowledge their own cisgender privilege and leverage it for the benefit of transgender people.

6. Allies seek to understand the connections between all forms of injustice, and understand how oppressions intersect.

7. Being a cisgender ally to transgender people means seeking understanding and awareness of transgender lives and experiences, and speaking out against injustice directed at transgender people.

8. Allies take pride in their work without being self-congratulatory.

9. Allies seek out and are receptive to feedback from transgender communities and hold themselves accountable to this feedback.

10. Allies call out and raise awareness about ignorance, bias and discrimination toward transgender people, in both individual instances and broader systems of oppression.

*Note: This is not an exhaustive list.

K-12 Professionals

K-12 PROFESSIONALS
Why Affirming Schools Matter

By Emily A. Greytak, PhD
Director of Research, GLSEN

• • •

"Being transgender in high school is almost impossible because of how much harassment we receive."

— Transgender student from GLSEN's 2013 National School ClimateSurvey

Despite great strides in visibility that transgender people have made over the past few years, such as increased media representation and frequent mention in popular culture, safety and equity for transgender youth in schools lags behind. Transgender and gender non-conforming students continue to face high levels of violence and bias in their schools (Grant et al., 2011; McGuire et al., 2010; Greytak et al., 2013; Veale et al., 2015). Over the past fifteen years, our research at GLSEN has routinely documented that transgender and other gender non-conforming youth experience more hostile school climates than their peers. For example, in our National School Climate Survey we found that approximately three-quarters of transgender students experienced regular harassment at school and two-thirds of genderqueer students have felt unsafe at school because of their gender expression (Kosciw et al., 2014). Not only are transgender and gender non-conforming youth more likely to be victimized by other students (Mitchell et al., 2014; Reisner et al., 2014), but they also regularly face discrimination and, at times, hostility from school officials. In fact, the majority of transgender students report being required to use the bathrooms or locker rooms of their sex assigned at birth and 40% were prevented from using their preferred names in school (Kosciw et al., 2014).

In response to increased awareness and advocacy, we are seeing growing attention to transgender rights at the federal, state, and local levels. Recently, the U.S. Department of Education's Office of Civil Rights explicitly affirmed that transgender students are protected under Title IX, the provision of the Civil Rights Act that explicitly prohibits sex discrimination in schools (Title IX, 1972). Furthermore, states and districts are increasingly enacting measures to ensure that schools are safe and supportive for transgender youth. For example, in 2013, California passed the School Success and Opportunities Act, enshrining into state law the obligation on the part of schools to allow transgender students to participate in all school activities and facilities based on gender identity. In 2014, the New York City Department of Education joined several other districts (e.g., Boulder Valley, Colorado and Los Angeles) to enact official guidelines related to transgender students. And although we see positive gains for transgender students in these locales, we have also seen inaction and even active opposition to addressing these issues in schools in many other locales. Legislatures in some states, such as Nevada, Florida, and Arizona, have proposed anti-transgender bills that apply to schools, most commonly by prohibiting transgender students from using bathrooms that correspond to their gender identities. Although these efforts have predominantly failed, they demonstrate the difficult challenges transgender youth often face in their schools and communities. Of course, transgender and gender non-conforming students are not the only ones who may face a hostile school climate. Transgender parents, teachers, and other school staff may be subject to mistreatment as well. Therefore, schools need to be affirming for all members of the school community.

As concerns about the educational environment for transgender and other gender non-conforming people come to the forefront and schools are increasingly obligated to address these issues, increased interest in professional development and training related to transgender people has arisen. Educators must be provided with the critical knowledge, skills, and dispositions not only to effectively address incidents of bias but to also proactively create school environments that support transgender and gender non-conforming youth of all ages. It is crucial that professional development efforts explicitly address transgender topics. Proficiency around issues of sexual orientation is not sufficient, and in fact professional development that professes to be "LGBT" often lacks transgender-specific content, potentially rendering transgender people invisible or further stigmatized. Unfortunately, most educators are not provided with professional development opportunities that address transgender topics (GLSEN & Harris Interactive, 2012; Kull, 2014). For example, only 14% of public school principals indicated that their school provided professional development related to bullying or harassment based on gender identity or expression (GLSEN & Harris Interactive, 2008).

Clearly there is an urgent need for action to ensure that transgender and gender non-conforming people are afforded safe, supported, and affirming school environments. And yet, there are few opportunities for educators or other members of school communities to develop the capacity to ensure effective transgender inclusion in schools. The activities provided in this section provide an accessible way for educators at all levels to begin to engage in critical exploration of their role in supporting transgender and gender non-conforming members of the school community and to develop concrete strategies to ensure their school environments are welcoming and affirming of transgender and gender nonconforming students, parents, and educators. Particularly in K–12 settings, it is imperative not only to ensure that transgender people are valued and supported, but also to deconstruct the gender binary and challenge traditional gender stereotypes that can limit all children, particularly those who challenge traditional notions of gender, especially in elementary grades. Therefore, the activities described in this section, in addition to increasing educators' capacity to create affirming schools for transgender individuals, provide opportunities for educators to consider a more expansive view of gender that can allow for more authentic expression for all children. The activities in this section can be a critical tool in a broader professional development effort to ensure that educators have the skills and competencies to respond appropriately to transgender students and proactively ensure an environment that allows transgender and all gender non-conforming youth to fully participate in school and achieve their full potential.

16

STORY TIME:
Gender Messages in Children's Books

...

Overview & Rationale

This lesson helps participants look deeply at the everyday messages that we convey to children about gender roles, stereotypes and conformity, and asks participants to view these messages through a gender-affirming lens. While this lesson was written specifically so that it can be used for people preparing to become elementary school educators as well as current elementary school teachers, it can also be modified for use with a variety of audiences, including families.

Audience

This lesson is designed for people who will be interacting with elementary-aged children in professional or social settings, and can be adapted for use with families. It can also be beneficial in college courses that include child development or gender themes. This lesson works best with 10–30 participants, but can be modified for larger audiences.

Objectives

By the end of this lesson, participants will be able to:
- Identify 3 common gender-related messages in children's books that reinforce gender roles, stereotypes, or conformity.
- Determine 2 strategies that can be used to create affirming classroom environments.

Background Knowledge for Facilitators

It will be useful for facilitators to have background knowledge of gender messages in children's books, toys and other media. When facilitating with K–12 educators, it will be useful to have read and reviewed Chapters 4 & 6 of Jennifer Bryan's book: *From the dress-up corner to the senior prom: Navigating gender and sexuality diversity* in pre K–12 schools.

Time

- Preparation: 10 minutes (plus acquiring the books)
- Implementation: 90 minutes

Materials

- 10–12 General themed children's books (See Tips for Selecting Books in Preparation below)
- 1–5+ Transgender-specific children's books (see **Resources & Recommended Reading** section on page 251)
- Copies of the *Mapping Gender Messages* handout (1 per participant)
- Easel paper & markers

Preparation

- Make copies of the handouts.
- Pre-select 10–12 children's books for use in this activity.
- Review each of the children's books that you will be using during this session and chart out the gender-related themes using the handout provided. (If you are comfortable doing so, create this as a handout to share with participants after they have completed the activity.)

Tips for selecting books:

- Books may be easy to preview and obtain from a local library or school library.
- Some children's books are also available online. A

search of titles may yield versions of the books in PDF form, Google Books, other free e-formats, or even YouTube versions.
- Select short books intended for younger children.
- Select a sampling that includes characters who are boys and men as well as girls and women.

Procedure

1. Explain that this lesson is designed to help us better understand the intensity and frequency of the gender messages that young children receive on a daily basis.

2. Break participants up into 5 small groups, give each of the groups 1 or 2 of the "general" children's books, and pass out the handout. Direct participants to read the book(s) aloud within their small groups and then complete the handout for each book. Explain that they will have about 20 minutes to complete the exercise and then they will be sharing their responses with the large group. For a shorter lesson, have each group read, review, and report on one book. For a longer lesson, invite groups to read, review and report on more than one book. During the small-group time, circulate through each of the small groups and offer support as needed.

3. Once the participants have completed both of their books and the corresponding handout for each one, bring the small groups back to the large-group format. Ask for a group who is willing to start, and have them share their responses to their book(s). Rotate among each of the small groups until each has shared its responses.

4. After each of the groups has reported back, lead a short discussion using the following questions:
   - What was this process like for you?
   - Were you surprised by any of your findings?
   - Did you notice anything about these books that you had not noticed before?
   - What do you think the impact of these messages might be, particularly on children who are gender non-conforming or transgender? On cisgender children? On children with non-binary gender identities?

5. Explain that you will now look at children's books that specifically convey messages of role-modeling affirmation to children who are gender non-conforming or transgender. (If you only have 1 transgender-specific book, ask for a volunteer to read the book aloud to the whole group. If you have enough books for each of the small groups, distribute the books to the groups and ask them to read them aloud to each other within the small group).

6. Lead a group discussion using the questions and talking points in the *Transgender Book Discussion: Facilitator's Guide*. If facilitating the lesson with Elementary School educators, extend the conversation by including the additional questions on the *Facilitator's Guide*.

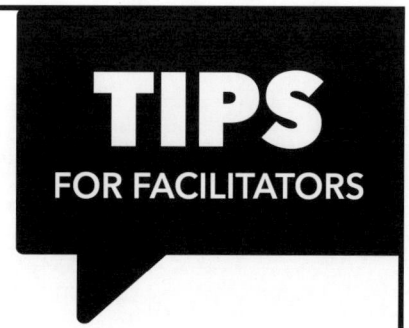

If leading this activity with educators, you may experience some resistance to the idea of talking about gender specifically, particularly when it comes to reading books that are transgender specific. Often this resistance is based in a fear of backlash from parents or administrators. It can be helpful to walk educators through the talking points pertaining to the books, (e.g. general themes of respect, empathy, self-care, etc.), and map those to their required core curriculum standards.

• • •

Participants may have questions about gender expression and children. For instance, they may wonder whether children who express their gender in ways that are gender non-conforming are always transgender. Or if children who express their gender in expected or even stereotypical ways are not transgender. Gender expression and gender identity are distinct. Be sure to include the discussion points on these topics listed under Background Knowledge for Facilitators, and under the discussion section of the lesson.

7. If using this as a standalone activity, ask participants to turn to the person next to them and briefly discuss 1 thing that they can do to incorporate something that is affirming of all children that allows all to express gender in the way that feels most comfortable to them. (For example, not teasing children about their gender expressions, using more gender-neutral language, not limiting play options or toys based on gender, etc.).

Evaluation Questions

✔ What were 3 common gender-related messages you observed in the children's books that reinforce gender roles, stereotypes, or conformity?

✔ What are 2 strategies that teachers can use to create affirming classroom environments for students of all genders?

ADDITIONAL RESOURCES:
Bryan, J. (2012). *From the dress-up corner to the senior prom: Navigating gender and sexuality diversity in preK–12 schools.* New York: R&L Education.

Transgender Book Discussion:
FACILITATOR'S GUIDE

DISCUSSION QUESTIONS

- What did you notice that was different about this book compared with the others you mapped?
- What are the overall messages and themes of this book?
- What do you think the impact of these messages might be, particularly on children who are gender non-conforming or transgender? On cisgender children? On children with non-binary gender identities?
- Did you find the books more gendered than you expected? Did the types or number of gender stereotypes they contained surprise you? If so, in what ways?
- Are stereotypes inherently bad? Why or why not?
- What do you think are some reasons that children's books place such an emphasis on gender?
- What are the possible impacts of this book (and the other books) on people of all genders?

DISCUSSION TALKING POINTS

- Gender stereotypes in children's books can reinforce binary and rigid ways of viewing what is considered acceptable or appropriate for people based on their gender. This can limit or restrict the ideas, interests, goals, and expression of children of all genders.
- Sometimes transgender children express their gender in ways that are perceived as gender non-conforming.
- Gender expression and gender identity are distinct. Just because a child may not fit gender expression norms does not mean they are transgender. Some children who don't fit gender norms are/will be transgender, while others aren't/won't be.

ADDITIONAL DISCUSSION QUESTIONS FOR ELEMENTARY SCHOOL EDUCATORS:

Note: It will be useful to record responses on easel paper as they are shared with the group.

- What are some of the ways in which we impart gender messages to children in our classrooms (for example, using the phrase "boys and girls" or asking children to line up by gender)?
- What are some alternative language/strategies that could be used?
- What are some other possible ways to create a classroom environment that is affirming to students of all genders (for example, making sure to include images of gender diversity in classroom artwork, leading discussions about gender messages when reading books, using examples in classroom activities that represent gender diversity)?

PARTICIPANT HANDOUT

Mapping Gender Messages

DIRECTIONS: For (each of) the book(s) that you read aloud in your small group, discuss the answers to the questions below and provide examples to support your responses.

Title of the Book: _____

Author: _____ Year Published: _____

1. What was the overall theme of this book (e.g., respect, empathy)?

   _____
   _____
   _____

2. How was gender portrayed through the characters' attire (e.g., the boy character wore a collared shirt and tie)?

   _____
   _____
   _____

3. What gender roles are portrayed in this book (e.g., the girl character plays pretend tea party)?

   _____
   _____
   _____

4. What could have been changed in this book to make it more inclusive of diverse gender expressions and genders?

   _____
   _____
   _____

17

KIDS IN THE HALL:
Transgender Kids in School

Overview & Rationale

This lesson gives participants an opportunity to consider the unique experiences of transgender and gender-diverse students in middle and high school, and strategize ways in which to provide personal support and act as allies. Using information about transgender students drawn from two national research resources as a tool for facilitated discussion, participants will learn more about the experiences of transgender students. Through this process, participants will develop a better understanding of issues that many transgender and gender-diverse students face in middle and high school. Participants will be better prepared to act as allies to transgender students, and will identify ways in which they can act as advocates and allies in terms of personal support as well as institutional change.

Audience

This lesson is designed for people who will be interacting with middle and high school youth in professional settings. It can also be beneficial in college courses that include child development or gender themes. This lesson works best with 10–30 participants, but can be modified for larger audiences.

Objectives

By the end of this lesson, participants will be able to:
- Identify 3 challenges that middle school and high school transgender students face.
- Identify 2 ways to be supportive of transgender students at school.
- Discuss 2 ways to make a school more sensitive and friendly to transgender students.

Background Knowledge for Facilitators

Facilitators are encouraged to familiarize themselves with the findings and implications of the two GLSEN publications used in this lesson, both available for free on GLSEN.org: *Harsh Realities: The Experiences of Transgender Youth in Our Nation's Schools* and *The 2013 National School Climate Survey*, both of which can be found at http://glsen.org/students/tsr/resources GLSEN conducts a biennial survey of LGBT youth, the National School Climate Survey, and the most recent results of this survey are always available at www.glsen.org.

Time

- Preparation: 15 minutes
- Implementation: 60 minutes

Materials

- *Statistics Signs Set 1 & Set 2,* with each set printed on a different color paper from www.teachingtransgender.com/printables (PW: TTTprep15)
- Blank paper
- Easel paper & markers
- Tape

Preparation

- Download two sets of *Statistics Signs* from www.teachingtransgender.com/printables (PW: TTTprep15). Alternatively, use easel paper to create posters, using differently colored markers for the two sets.
- Hang the first set of sheets of paper around one half of the room so that there is enough room for a small group of people to stand in front of that sign. Hang a blank piece of easel paper below each of the statistics signs, so that participants can write on the easel paper.

- Hang the second set of sheets of paper around the other half of the room—but for the second set, tape a sheet of paper over each of the posters so they are all covered. In this way, participants will not be able to see what is written on them until the facilitator removes the covering sheet. (If using easel paper, tape the bottom part of the sheet so that it folds over and covers the top part of the sheet.)

Procedure

1. Break participants into small groups. Direct the participants to stand in front of the first set of papers on the wall. Pass out 1-2 markers to each group.

2. Tell participants that each poster contains a statistic reflecting the challenges that transgender students face in schools, based on GLSEN's research on transgender students and its biennial survey of LGBT youth, the National School Climate Survey. Explain that they will have 3 minutes to write down as many ideas as they can think of that might help reduce this specific challenge, and that they will then move to the next poster and repeat the process until they have provided strategies on all of the posters. Time each group and, after about 3 minutes, instruct them to move clockwise to the next poster.

3. After all posters have been completed, participants may return to their seats. Lead participants in a discussion based on the questions provided in the *Discussion Questions* facilitator resource.

4. Next, call participants' attention to the second set of posters. One by one, remove the cover sheets so that the text can be seen. Read each one aloud (or ask participants to volunteer to read them aloud). Explain that this set of posters describes some of the things that can address or support the transgender students in the challenges that that can face in school. Tell participants that these facts are also from GLSEN's research on transgender students.

5. After reviewing all of these posters, lead participants in a discussion based on the questions and talking points provided in the *Discussion Questions* facilitator resource.

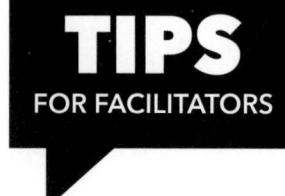

Familiarize yourself in advance with the research findings used in this lesson by visiting glsen.org. This will assist you in addressing questions participants may raise about how the research was conducted, who the respondents were, and what the most current data demonstrate.

...

This lesson focuses on the experiences of transgender students. The 2013 National School Climate Survey also included respondents who identified as genderqueer (about 10% of the sample) or in other non-cisgender and usually non-binary ways, for example as pangender, bigender, and other identities (about 4% of the sample). Students who identified in those ways also experienced an unwelcoming and hostile school climate much as those who identified as transgender did. However, their school experiences were slightly less negative than were those of students who identified as transgender.

6. If using as a standalone lesson, conclude the activity by asking each of the participants to select one of the strategies from the second set that they can commit to implementing and ask them to name 1 specific thing that they will do to make that happen

Evaluation Questions

✔ What are 3 challenges that middle school and high school transgender students face?

✔ What are 2 ways educational professionals can be more supportive of transgender students at school?

DISCUSSION QUESTIONS: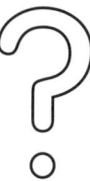

FIRST SET OF POSTERS:

- What are your initial reactions to reading the posters of challenges faced by transgender students (e.g., shocked, overwhelmed, surprised, felt they were accurate, etc.)?
- Did you have a particularly strong reaction to any of the posters? Why?
- Which of the research findings on the posters do you think might indicate a condition or circumstance that is particularly damaging or harmful to transgender students?
- How might these realities affect transgender students in school? How might they affect students at any time during the school day (e.g., they might affect their sense of self-worth or self-esteem, they might cause them to limit their school and work goals because of academic, social, and safety challenges at school, etc.)?
- How do you think these realities might affect students who are not transgender?
- What strategies did you come up with to address the information on the posters?

SECOND SET OF POSTERS:

- What are your initial reactions to reading the posters that describe ways to support transgender students in school?
- Did you have a particularly strong reaction to any of the posters? Why?
- Which of the research findings on the posters indicate a condition or circumstance that might be particularly helpful for transgender students?
- How might these helpful support strategies affect transgender students?
- How do you think that these helpful support strategies might affect students who are not transgender?
- What other strategies can you think of whereby you can act as advocates for or allies to transgender students in terms of personal support or institutional change?

CONCLUDING TALKING POINTS:

- Most transgender youth attend schools with hostile school climates.
- The majority of students surveyed in this research did not have access to supportive resources, such as GSAs (Gay Straight Alliances or other supportive LGBTQ clubs), inclusive curricula, or comprehensive anti-harassment policies.
- Many transgender students could identify at least one supportive educator.
- Having access to a GSA in their school, supportive school staff, comprehensive anti-harassment policies, and inclusive curricula helped support transgender students in schools.
- There are many ways in which school personnel can act as advocates for and allies to transgender students in terms of personal support as well as institutional change.

FACILITATOR RESOURCE
Statistics Signs Set 1: Challenges Faced by Transgender Students

- Most transgender students reported that they felt unsafe at school because of their gender expression (75%). (2)

- Almost all transgender students heard negative remarks about someone's gender expression sometimes, often, or frequently in school (90%). (1)

- Almost all transgender students had been verbally harassed (e.g., called names or threatened) in the past year at school because of their gender expression (87%). (1)

- Over half of all transgender students had been physically harassed (e.g., pushed or shoved) in school in the past year because of their gender expression (53%). (1)

- Nearly half of all transgender students had been personally prevented from using their preferred names in school (42%). (2)

- More than half of all transgender students had been required to use the bathroom or locker room of their legal sex at school (59%). (2)

- Nearly a third of all transgender students had been prevented from wearing clothes at school because they were considered inappropriate based on their legal sex (32%). (2)

- Transgender students were more likely to have experienced school disciplinary actions (such as receiving detention, being suspended or being expelled) than cisgender LGB students.

- Transgender students had somewhat higher rates of overall contact with the criminal/juvenile justice system as a result of school disciplinary actions than their cisgender LGB peers.

- Less than half of all transgender students reported that they could find information about LGBT people, history, or events in their school library (46%) while nearly a third were able to access this information using the school Internet portal (31%). (1)

- Less than a fifth of transgender students reported that LGBT-related topics were included in their textbooks or other assigned readings (16%), and only a tenth were exposed to an inclusive curriculum that included positive representations of LGBT people, history, or events in their classes (11%). (1)

- A third of all LGBT students heard negative remarks about transgender people (i.e. "tranny," "he/she") frequently or often at school (33%). (2)

- Over half of LGBT students heard negative remarks about gender expression (not acting "masculine enough" or "feminine enough") frequently or often at school (56%). (2)

- LGBT students who experienced higher levels of victimization because of their gender expression were more than three times as likely to have missed school in the past month than those who experienced lower levels (59% vs. 17%). (2)

- LGBT students who were more frequently harassed because of their gender expression had lower grade point averages than students who were harassed less often. (2)

- LGBT students who experienced higher levels of victimization in school because of their gender expression were twice as likely to report that they did not plan to pursue any post-secondary education (e.g., college or trade school) than those who experienced lower levels (8% vs. 4%). (2)

REFERENCES

(1) Greytak, E. A., Kosciw, J. G., and Diaz, E. M. (2009). *Harsh Realities: The Experiences of Transgender Youth in Our Nation's Schools*. New York: GLSEN.

(2) Kosciw, J. G., Greytak, E. A., Palmer, N.A. & Boesen, M. J. (2014). *The 2013 National School Climate Survey: The experiences of lesbian, gay, bisexual and transgender youth in our nation's schools*. New York: GLSEN.

FACILITATOR RESOURCE
Statistics Signs Set 2: Addressing or Reducing Challenges

- LGBT students with a GSA (Gay Straight Alliance or other supportive LGBT student club) were more likely to report that school personnel intervened when hearing homophobic remarks or negative remarks about someone's gender expression (compared with students without a GSA). (2)

- LGBT students with a GSA had a greater sense of connectedness to their school community than students without a GSA. (2)

- LGBT students with many supportive staff reported higher grade point averages than other students (3.2 vs. 2.9). (2)

- LGBT students with a greater number of supportive staff also had higher educational aspirations—students with many supportive staff were about a third more likely to say they were not planning on attending college compared to students with no supportive facilitators (2)

- Transgender students who attended a school with a GSA experienced lower levels of peer victimization. (3)

- Transgender students who were exposed to an LGBT-inclusive curriculum in at least one of their classes experienced lower levels of peer victimization. (3)

- Transgender students with LGBT-supportive educators experienced lower levels of peer victimization. (3)

- Transgender students who attended a school with a GSA were less likely to miss school because they felt unsafe or uncomfortable. (3)

- Transgender students who were exposed to an LGBT-inclusive curriculum in at least one of their classes were less likely to miss school because they felt unsafe or uncomfortable. (3)

- Transgender students with LGBT-supportive educators were less likely to miss school because they felt unsafe or uncomfortable. (3)

- Transgender students in schools with comprehensive anti-bullying policies (i.e., enumerated sexual orientation and gender identity/expression) were less likely to miss school because they felt unsafe or uncomfortable. (3)

- The more transgender students discussed LGBT issues in school, the more likely they were to feel like a part of their school communities. (1)

- Transgender students who were out to most or all other students and school staff reported a greater sense of belonging to their school communities than those who were not out or only out to a few other students or staff. (1)

- LGBT students in schools with comprehensive anti-bullying policies (i.e., including sexual orientation and gender identity/expression) were more likely than students in schools with a generic policy or no policy to report that staff intervened when hearing negative remarks about gender expression. (2)

REFERENCES

(1) Greytak, E. A., Kosciw, J. G., and Diaz, E. M. (2009). *Harsh Realities: The Experiences of Transgender Youth in Our Nation's Schools.* New York: GLSEN.

(2) Kosciw, J. G., Greytak, E. A., Palmer, N.A. & Boesen, M. J. (2014). *The 2013 National School Climate Survey: The experiences of lesbian, gay, bisexual and transgender youth in our nation's schools.* New York: GLSEN.

(3) Greytak, E. A., Kosciw, J. G., & Boesen, M. J. (2013). Putting the "T" in "resource": The benefits of LGBT-related school resources for transgender youth. *Journal of LGBT Youth, 10*(1-2), 45–63.

SUPPORTIVE SERVICES:
Creating Safe Havens of Affirmation In Schools

Overview & Rationale

In many schools, the nurse's office, school counselor or social worker's office, or the guidance office are among the few spaces where students can find safe spaces and adults who support them. It is essential that these support professionals understand how to be supportive of transgender and gender non-conforming students and students who identify their gender in non-binary ways.

Audience

This lesson is designed for professional support staff (such as school nurses, social workers, and guidance counselors) who work with middle and high school youth. This lesson works best with 10–30 participants, but can be modified for larger audiences.

Objectives

By the end of this lesson, participants will be able to:
- Identify 2 reasons why transgender, non-binary, or gender non-conforming students may seek support from a nurse, school counselor, or guidance counselor.
- Practice 2 strategies that can be used to affirm transgender, non-binary, or gender non-conforming students and provide them with support.

Background Knowledge for Facilitators

When facilitating with professionals working in K–12 settings, it may be useful to have them read Jennifer Bryan's book: *From the dress-up corner to the senior prom: Navigating gender and sexuality diversity in pre-K–12 schools,* and review the transgender-related resources at GLSEN.org *(http://glsen.org/students/tsr/resources)*.

Time

- Preparation: 10 minutes
- Implementation: 45 minutes

Materials

- *Role Play Scenario* handout (1 per pair)
- *Strategies for Affirming Transgender Students* handout (1 per person)

Preparation

- Make copies of the handouts

Procedure

1. Explain: According to GLSEN's *Harsh Realities* report, guidance counselors and nurses are often reported as sources of support for transgender and gender non-conforming students. Over 50% of transgender youth report that they are physically harassed in school, and 1 out of 4 transgender young people report being physically attacked in school (Greytak, Kosciw & Diaz, 2009). More than one-fifth of transgender students said they were not out at school specifically about being transgender (Kosciw, Greytak, Palmer & Boesen, 2014). Students who identify as genderqueer or in other non-cisgender and non-binary ways (such as pangender, bigender, etc.) also experience an unwelcoming and hostile school climate (Greytak, Kosciw & Diaz, 2009).

2. Because there are increasing numbers of youth becoming aware of their transgender identities at younger ages (and also making decisions about how, whether, and when to come out to family, friends, or at school), it is essential that schools understand how to proactively support transgender students. Students who many not identify as transgender but identify in other non-cisgender ways also need supportive schools to increase their safety and well-being.

3. Explain that many of the same methods and skills that are used to support cisgender students also apply to transgender, gender non-conforming and non-binary students. These include:
   - Providing a space where students can share their experiences and tell their stories
   - Validating students' feelings
   - Helping students identify sources of support and connect them with others
   - Taking steps to make sure that students threatened with harm are protected
   - Understanding school policies on bullying and non-discrimination, in particular who they protect and how to file a complaint

4. Divide participants into pairs by asking them to partner with someone they don't know very well (the goal is to try to separate people who already have strong relationships so that all participants are on equal footing). Ask participants in the pairs to decide which person will be Person A, and which will be Person B.

5. Distribute a *Role Play Scenario* handout to each pair, and a *Strategies for Affirming Transgender Students* handout to each person.

6. Asking person A to play the role of the nurse/school counselor and person B to play the role of the student, present the first role-play scenario. Give the participants about 5-7 minutes to complete the role-play, and then ask the participants to share their experiences of completing the role-play (e.g., what they felt worked well, what they struggled with, what questions they have).

7. Repeat, alternating which person in each pair plays each role, until each of the scenarios has been completed. Invite the participants to reflect on how they might manage these situations in their jobs.

Assessment Questions

✔ What are 2 reasons that transgender, non-binary or gender non-conforming students may seek support from a school nurse or school counselor?

✔ What are 2 strategies that you can use to affirm transgender, non-binary or gender non-conforming students and provide them with support?

TIPS FOR FACILITATORS

Many participants experience anxiety about role-plays. They are often concerned that they are going to be put on the spot in front of their peers, will "mess up" or feel uncomfortable about participating in general. It can be helpful to reassure participants that this anxiety is normal, and explain that role-plays are important because they offer the opportunity for participants to practice how they might respond if presented with these scenarios, so that they are better prepared when they happen.

• • •

Participants may have concerns about whether they will be able to provide support for transgender students—e.g., whether administrators, families, or peers will support their efforts. It is important to help participants focus on why it is so essential that transgender students receive as much support as possible.

• • •

Depending on time allotted and the willingness of the participants, facilitators may modify this lesson in several ways. Pairs may be instructed to role-play 1 or 2 of the scenarios first for practice, and then several volunteer pairs may be invited to role-play a scenario in front of the large group. The facilitator may also serve as one of the role players for the first scenario along with a volunteer, to demonstrate the exercise before having participants pair off to role-play additional scenarios.

PARTICIPANT HANDOUT

Role Play Scenarios

1. A transgender student comes to you and tells you they are being harassed every time they try to use the bathroom.

2. A gender non-conforming student makes up an excuse to come see you every time they are supposed to be in gym class.

3. A teacher of a student who identifies as having a non-binary gender has mentioned to you that the student is being verbally harassed by peers, and is concerned that it might escalate to physical harassment. They have reported it to the Assistant Principal but are including you in the loop because they are concerned for the student's emotional well-being.

4. A student has recently revealed to you that their parent has just come out as transgender and is in the process of transitioning medically. They are concerned about other students finding out and harassing them for it.

5. A teacher has mentioned to you that one of their students has been electing to write all of their class assignments about transgender people, and the teacher is wondering if it is something the student might be thinking about.

6. A transgender student mentions to you that their father has been hitting them when they are wearing clothes that match their gender identity, so they have been changing clothes in the bathroom as soon as they get to school in the morning.

7. A transgender student mentions to you that they are experiencing a lot of gender dysphoria, and they are wondering if you could help them to research and access medical transition, specifically hormones.

8. A student comes to you and tells you that their best friend (also a student at the school) has been really struggling with depression and thinks that they might be transgender. The student is nervous that their friend might be considering suicide.

9. A student applying for college asks for your assistance in finding out about whether there are any transgender-affirming colleges to which they might apply.

PARTICIPANT HANDOUT

Strategies for Affirming Transgender Students

1. Believe them
When a young person shares that they are transgender or non-binary, it is critical that they feel that the person receiving the information understands what they are saying and believes them. Similarly, when students report bullying, harassment, discrimination, or isolation at the hands of peers, staff/faculty, at home, or in the community, it is essential that they know that the adult they are reporting to believes them.

2. Validate & Empathize
Just as you would with any young person who is navigating something potentially difficult, it is important to show that their feelings are valid and demonstrate empathy. Many transgender and non-binary young people suffer because they do not have people in their lives who listen to them and support them.

3. Use Affirming Name & Pronouns
One of the most effective ways of demonstrating affirmation is to consistently use the name and pronouns that the young person has said that they would like to be used. If you make a mistake, apologize, correct it, and move on.

4. Help Connect to Support & Resources
Transgender and non-binary young people often have limited allies who are willing to advocate for them. Helping students identify and connect with additional affirming, supportive resources (in person or online), can reduce their sense of isolation.

5. Advocate
Whether one is advocating for a specific student in a specific situation or working towards creating a transgender-affirming school, advocacy is essential to ensuring that students are safe, respected and affirmed while they are in school.

6. Be Proactive
Being proactively prepared to support a young person will help you provide quality services and support when they are needed. For example, researching local supportive organizations, online resources, and connecting with school leadership about how to best support transgender and non-binary students will allow you to be ready when a student walks into your office. Do some research to figure out who your allies are and how they can support you in this work.

COLLEGE & UNIVERSITY
Professionals

The Journey to Becoming a Trans-Affirming University

By Nancy Jean Tubbs, Director
LGBT Resource Center, University of California, Riverside

• • •

Fifteen years ago when I began my career as a director of LGBT resources on a college campus, I knew just enough about gender identity to differentiate it from sexual orientation on educational materials and during trainings. Transgender folks remained a hidden population on my campus for several years, with the exception of gender non-conforming students and a visiting professor who happened to be a transgender woman.

We reached a turning point as a campus when students system-wide began organizing for gender-inclusive restrooms, trans-identified staff joined our center, and more and more students embraced "genderqueer" as a self-identity. As a community, we learned to respect people's chosen names and not assume the pronouns used by folks. I discovered that my students were much more adaptive than me regarding the use of "ze," but I stumbled my way through the learning curve.

Then, as a campus, we chose a path that many other colleges are embracing: create the resources and the education regardless of the number of "out" transgender students, staff, and faculty. Our center developed a Trans Allies training program for students, faculty and staff. A student proposal led to a Gender Inclusive Housing option for any resident, including first-year students. The first action we asked of a new Chancellor was to finally change signage on single-occupancy restrooms. After three hard-fought years of student and staff activism, our campus negotiated transgender-inclusive student health insurance. A Trans Task Force recently implemented the first steps to a Preferred Name Policy as our campus transitions to a new student information system.

All of these gains in resources and policies do not tell the most profound story for our campus: our center finally hosts a visible transgender student population that provides peer support, challenges cisgender people (both queer and straight) to embrace transgender inclusion, and actively educates others inside and outside the classroom.

The year more students applied from my campus to attend T*Camp (an intercampus retreat for trans* college students) than we had spots available for signaled another milestone in community development. And yet, at the intersections of identity, other struggles carry on. Students of color who were invited to T*Camp were forced to drop out because of pressure from their families. We know that our transfeminine and transgender students of color are more likely to attend peer-based support groups than formal educational programs. These students rely more on peer-to-peer support. For example, I witnessed a moment in which two transgender women were sitting in my office, with one encouraging the other to attend one of our social events so that she could connect with other students with similar experiences. These moments become powerful turning powerful turning points in engaging our most vulnerable students.

I speculate that most college and university campuses do not yet serve a visible transgender population. Transphobia and the gender binary workings of a bureaucracy are too powerful. Yet college campuses also provide the academic elixir of new language and theory, the critical study of social norms, and the fierce exchange of experiences and ideas. Faculty and staff do invest in creating safe learning environments and courageous spaces for students, many of whom are young adults exploring their gender identities for the first time.

Where else but on a college campus would organizers of a trans* conference share a mission that "affirms all people who transcend gender norms, including transgender, genderqueer, genderfluid, non-binary, transsexual, agender, third gender, two-spirit, bigender, trans man, trans woman, gender non-conforming, masculine of center, gender questioning, and many other gender-awesome identities and experiences"?

Yes, most college campuses are starting with the basics of understanding gender identity, transphobia, and gender oppression. Yet this also means that you can choose to provide support, education, and advocacy and make an immediate difference for your campus. Maybe your efforts will lay the foundation for future policy change. Maybe it will mean the difference in one student's life. Maybe it will begin the conversation for a campus community transformed by gender awesomeness.

In the past 15 years of work toward becoming an affirming campus, professional training has been a cornerstone of our work. In combination with the lessons provided in the "Transgender 101" section, the lessons in this section will help you to start conversations among key stakeholders on your campus, which will contribute to a campus that is welcoming and affirming of transgender and gender non-conforming students.

RESIDENCE LIFE:
Working Towards Safe & Affirming Residence Halls

...

Overview & Rationale

This lesson gives participants the opportunity to consider the unique experiences of transgender and gender-diverse students in residence halls on college campuses, and to strategize how to provide personal and professional support in their roles as RAs, Residential Life staff, and peers. Safe and affirming housing on campus allows transgender students to gain key interpersonal skills and participate in experiences that support their academic development (outcomes noted by Robison, 1998) as well as contribute to the vibrancy of a residence hall environment and experience a sense of belongingness and community. Housing can firmly establish (or detract from) transgender students' feelings of safety and having their needs met (Rankin, 2007, Beemyn, 2005). Vignettes and case studies provide the opportunity to assist participants in making connections between informational content and lived experiences.

Audience

This lesson works best with college and university residential life staff. It is also appropriate for college and university faculty, staff, and administrators; and may be adapted for use with participants who work in other residential settings with teens or young adults. It may also be appropriate for some college student audiences in disciplines such as education, higher education administration, sociology, psychology, and other fields. This lesson works best with 10-30 participants, and can be modified for larger audiences.

Objectives

By the end of this lesson, participants will be able to:
- Identify 1 thing they personally can do to help make their campus affirming for transgender students.
- Identify 2 things their college or university could do, or do differently, to make their campus more affirming for transgender students.

Background Knowledge for Facilitators

Facilitators will benefit from knowledge of the issues that uniquely affect college students, with a particular focus on housing concerns and strategies that can be implemented by Residence Life staff to indicate that they are affirming. It will be very helpful for the facilitator to be familiar with the specific policies of a particular campus, or to have a professional staff member in the training who is familiar with the policies and can explain them during the training.

Time

- Preparation: 15 minutes
- Implementation: 75-90 minutes, (plus 30 minutes for professional staff)

Materials

- *Residence Life Vignettes* handout (1 per participant)
- *Proactive Planning for Professional Residence Life Staff* handout (1 per participant, if using)
- 4 differently colored index cards (1 of each color per participant)
- Assorted stickers
- Easel chart paper and markers

Preparation

- Make copies of the handouts
- Place stickers on the *Residence Life Vignettes* handout so that participants will end up in small groups of the desired size (for example, use 4 types of fruit to break participants into 4 smaller groups, or 8 stars of different colors to break them into 8 small groups). To save time during the activity, you may wish to distribute the handouts as people walk in, or place them on the seats in advance.
- On the easel paper (or in a PowerPoint slide), write out the 4 closing prompts from Procedure step 5.

Procedure

1. Explain that this activity is designed to help us think about how we might mitigate some of the challenges faced by transgender students who live on campus in gender-segregated housing.

2. Instruct participants to break into small groups by finding the other participants with the same stickers as them and sitting together. Once the participants have settled into their groups, assign each group 1 vignette to work on. (Depending on the number of groups, there may be multiple groups working on the same vignette, or groups working on multiple vignettes). Direct participants to read their assigned vignettes and then work together for about 10-15 minutes to answer the questions. Rotate among of the small groups as they are working and provide additional support as needed.

3. After about 15 minutes, bring all of the participants back to the large group. Using the *Residence Life Vignettes: Facilitator's Guide,* lead a large-group discussion about each of these vignettes. Start by asking group 1 to read their vignette out loud (or summarize the key points) and provide their answers. Repeat with each group. Depending on the time available, it may not be possible to review all answers for all questions—select those that seem the most relevant and least redundant based on the flow and pace of the discussion.

4. If conducting this lesson exclusively with professional Residence Life staff (i.e. not student staff), pass out the *Proactive Planning for Professional Residence Life Staff* handout, and ask the staff to return to their small groups to discuss the questions listed. After about 15-20 minutes of discussion, ask the small groups to return to the large group to identify and assign action steps.

5. If using as a standalone lesson, conclude the activity by handing out 4 differently colored index cards (for example: pink, green, blue, yellow) to participants, so that each participant has 1 of each color. Allow 10 minutes for participants to provide their answers to the prompts below. They should not write their names on the cards. Once the participants have completed their responses, collect the cards by color, shuffle them and return them to participants, so that each person has 4 new cards—1 of each color. Have each participant read off the responses written on their card in turn. (For a shorter version, ask for a few volunteers to read off responses that they really like.)
   - On the pink card, write 1 thing that you learned during the session.
   - On the green card, write 1 thing that you personally can do to help make your campus more affirming for transgender students.
   - On the blue card, write 1 thing that your college or university could do, or do differently, to make their campus more affirming for transgender students.
   - On the yellow card, write 1 question that they still have about working with transgender students.

6. *Optional:* The cards can be collected and turned into a bulletin board as an ongoing reminder of the commitments made to create a more affirming campus. Prior to displaying, answers should be provided for the question cards.

Evaluation Questions

✔ What is 1 thing you can personally do to help make your campus more affirming for transgender and gender non-conforming students?

✔ What are 2 things your college or university could do, or do differently, to make your campus more affirming for transgender students?

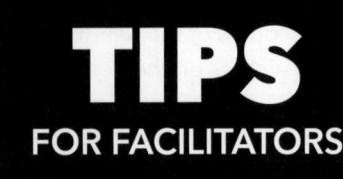

TIPS FOR FACILITATORS

When conducting this lesson with resident assistants or other student staff, it is ideal to have the professional residence life staff complete this training as a staff professional development training in advance of student training. Student staff will likely have questions and need support from the professional staff, and this will help to ensure that staff are prepared to do this work.

• • •

If you are conducting this training as an outside facilitator (who does not work on campus), it will be very helpful to have a professional staff member in the training who is familiar with the policies (or lack thereof) and discuss them during the training. When booking the training, be sure to ask who this person might be and if you can speak to them in advance. This will help ensure that the person knows what questions are coming and can review the policy in advance.

• • •

When discussing the various scenarios, it is likely that there will be concern or discomfort regarding the potential implications of having a person with a different sex assigned at birth from that of their roommate or floormates (particularly if the campus does not have the option for mixed-gender rooms or floors). Often these concerns are vocalized in terms of the potential for harm or trauma (e.g., concern that a transgender person will sexually assault a cisgender roommate, or that a roommate with a history of trauma may be triggered by seeing a person's genitals) and related liability, or the notion that there must be disclosure of someone's transgender identity to get informed consent on the part of a cisgender roommate or floormates. Both of these concerns are generally rooted in false stereotypes depicting transgender people as physically or sexually violent, and implying that a cisgender person's desire to know that someone is transgender is more important than the transgender person's privacy or safety concerns. These concerns can be redirected by pointing out that these stereotypes are false and reminding participants that in all cases the risks are more significant and more likely to be realized for the transgender person than for cisgender people in such a situation.

• • •

Not all transgender people wish to serve in an advocacy or educational role. There are people who are professional facilitators who are able to provide training and education. Find out who these people are on your campus and in your community. Consulting with the campus-based LGBTQ Center or LGBTQ-themed campus group, if there is one, is a good first step. Many places also have a local LGBTQ community group or community center that can provide resources, referrals, and consultation. A student should never be required to educate their roommates, hallmates, other students, or staff about their identity.

Residence Life Vignettes:
FACILITATOR'S GUIDE

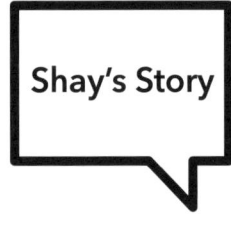

Shay's Story

You are a resident assistant in the all-female first-year residence hall. Shay is one of your residents. Shay seems to be a loner and you have not had the opportunity to interact much with this student yet. You overhear a few of your residents talking about Shay's appearance and speculating about whether or not Shay might be a lesbian. A few days later, Shay requests a meeting with you and your residence hall director. During the meeting, Shay explains that he is transgender and requests that you and your RD help with coming out to the floor and having people use male pronouns. Shay thinks that he might be more comfortable in the co-ed dorm, on a male-only floor, but is not sure yet. He is adamant that his parents not be told about any of this, out of fear that they might disown him and he would not be able to afford college without their support.

REPORT BACK FROM SMALL GROUPS:

1. **What are some positive aspects of this situation?**
   Shay sees the RA and RD as approachable and has asked them for their help. Shay is proactive about contacting you. Although your residents are already discussing Shay's appearance, there may be an opportunity for some education regarding themes of sexual orientation and gender identity, and the fact that these are distinct dimensions of a person's identity.

2. **What are some negative or concerning aspects of this situation?**
   Your residents are already talking about Shay's appearance and speculating about Shay's sexual orientation.

3. **What would you say to Shay during that meeting?**
   Responses will vary. (Note: This question should not be reported back to the large group so that participants do not have to share potentially non-affirming responses).

4. **What are some things that you would consider doing to be supportive of Shay?**
   Possible affirming responses: Asking Shay what would make him feel most safe and affirmed; asking Shay what support he needs; making sure that all staff and RAs are trained; providing a training for residents to learn about transgender identities, experiences and people; passing out affirming information about transgender and gender non-conforming people; putting up a bulletin board about gender diversity; letting Shay know about other support services for and about transgender people on and off campus (for example, campus policies and services for transgender students, local transgender support groups, LGBTQ+ student organizations, a campus or community LGBTQ Center, affirmative counseling and health services that may be available on or off campus, etc.); and contacting the campus or community LGBTQ Center or group to request additional consultation and guidance.

5. **What are some affirming things that you could say to other residents who are confused or not affirming of Shay?**
   Possible affirming responses: Transgender people are people too and deserve our respect; here are some resources to learn more about transgender people; please don't say negative things about Shay's identity (or anyone's identity) around me because I find it offensive; your room and your residence hall are your home and mine—please tell me anytime something happens here that is derogatory or disrespectful to yourself or another resident because we want to build and maintain a safe and respectful community here.

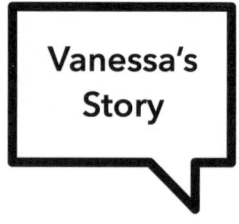

You are a resident assistant with a floor of male students in the sophomore residence hall that has a reputation for being a "party" dorm. Just before winter break, Jason asks if he can talk to you about something. You are really busy with finals, and do not have a chance to meet with Jason before you leave. When you return from break, you pass Jason in the hall. He is wearing a dress, make-up and has his long hair styled in a feminine manner. You are naturally quite surprised by this. You wave hello and continue walking to your room. When you check your voicemail, you have a message from the director of residence life saying that one of your residents is transgender and will be coming back as a woman, and would like people to start using female pronouns and calling her Vanessa. Your director wants to schedule a meeting with you to talk about how you can be supportive of Vanessa.

REPORT BACK FROM SMALL GROUPS:

1. **What are some positive aspects of this situation?**
   - Although the RA is surprised, the RA remains calm, waves hello and continues on.
   - The director wants to schedule a meeting with the RA and RD to talk about how you can be supportive of Vanessa.

2. **What are some negative or concerning aspects of this situation?**
   - The RA did not have a chance to meet with the student before the winter break.
   - You are unsure how, or if, the floor's reputation as a "party dorm" may come into play in this situation. You want to avoid stereotyping the residents of this community based on this reputation, but are also concerned others (residents, staff, or administrators) may use this as an excuse for inappropriate behavior.

3. **What do you think that your initial reactions to Vanessa might be?**
   Responses will vary. (Note: This question should not be reported back to the large group so that participants do not have to share potentially non-affirming responses).

4. **What do you think that some of the challenges might be for Vanessa?**
   Possible challenges: Being concerned about how people will react to her transition; whether her peers, professors and university staff will be supportive of her; whether her physical safety will be at risk; whether she will be socially isolated from peers because of her transition; whether the stress of navigating this will affect her academic success; finding out about support services or campus policies that might offer additional assistance or support for her needs.

5. **What might be some affirming things that you could say to other residents who are confused or not affirming of Vanessa?**
   Possible affirming responses: Transgender people are people too and deserve our respect; here are some resources to learn more about transgender people; please don't say negative things about Vanessa's identity around me because I find it offensive; your room and your residence hall are your home and mine–please tell me anytime something happens here that is derogatory or disrespectful to yourself or another resident because we want to build and maintain a safe and respectful living community here.

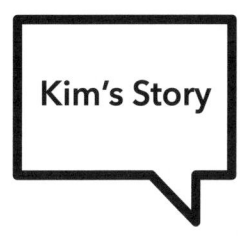

Kim's Story

You are a resident assistant on a women's floor in the co-ed sophomore residence hall. Your resident director has informed you that you will be having a new resident who is a transfer student. The resident director tells you that Kim is a transgender woman. Kim does not want anyone to know that she is transgender, and she is transferring to the school to get a new start as Kim. She is currently taking female hormones and has been for about a year now, but has not been able to have surgery yet and does not expect to for several years. Since there are no single rooms available, Kim will be living with one of your residents whose roommate left the school last semester. You and your resident director plan to meet in order to come up with a plan for how to be supportive of Kim.

REPORT BACK FROM SMALL GROUPS:

1. What are some positive aspects of this situation?
   The RA and RD plan to meet proactively to come up with a plan for how to be supportive of Kim.

2. What are some negative or concerning aspects of this situation?
   - Kim does not want anyone to know that she is transgender and so she may already have concerns or anxiety about how Residence Life staff will safeguard her privacy and keep confidentiality.
   - Kim may also arrive with the expectation/worry that she will not be treated with respect at her new institution. Residence life staff will need to address her feelings (she may be fearful, angry, stressed, or experience other feelings) and demonstrate their commitment and cultural competency to meet her needs.

3. What challenges do you expect Kim to face?
   Possible challenges: Being worried about how other people might react if they find out about her being transgender; having to navigate keeping her identity and body private; worrying about being accidentally outed; wondering how she will receive affirming medical care while on campus; wondering how she will pay the extra costs of a single room when one becomes available.

4. How do you think that her roommate might react if she finds out about Kim?
   Possible reactions: positive and affirming, supportive, curious, unconcerned, confused, feeling deceived, being upset, wanting Kim to be removed from the room.

5. How might her floor-mates react to her using the bathroom and showers?
   Possible reactions: positive and affirming, supportive, curious, unconcerned, unconcerned, feeling deceived, being upset, wanting Kim to be denied access to the bathroom and showers.

6. What are some things that you would suggest to the director of residence life as ways to be supportive of Kim?
   Possible affirming steps: Asking Kim what would make her feel most safe and affirmed; asking Kim what support she needs; making sure that all staff and RAs are trained; providing a training for residents to learn about transgender identities, experiences and people; using passive programming to help raise awareness and understanding about transgender people; engaging the campus LGBTQ group to support these efforts; making sure Kim knows about support services for and about transgender people on and off campus (for example, campus policies and services for transgender students, local transgender support groups, LGBTQ+ student organizations, a campus or community LGBTQ Center, affirmative counseling and health services that may be available on or off campus, etc.); contacting the campus or community LGBTQ Center or group to request additional consultation and guidance.

7. What are some possible affirming things that you could say to other residents who are confused or not affirming of Kim?
   Possible affirming: Transgender people are people too and deserve our respect; here are some resources to learn more about transgender people; please don't say negative things about Kim's identity around me because I find it offensive; your room and your residence hall are your home and mine—please tell me anytime something happens here that is derogatory or disrespectful to yourself or another resident because we want to build and maintain a safe and respectful living community here.

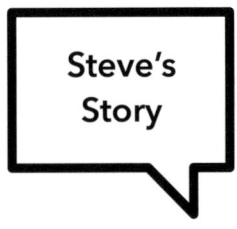

You are a resident assistant in the co-ed sophomore residence hall that has a reputation for being a "party" dorm. One of your residents, Steve, is rather androgynous. Steve tends to be a loner, rarely interacts with the other residents, and spends weekends off-campus. You have frequently overheard remarks from your other residents talking about how "weird" Steve is, and that "there is something that is not just right about Steve." One weekend, someone writes: "~~Steve~~ It is f***n' tranny!!!!" on Steve's marker board. Steve comes back to campus, sees this and reports it to the RA on duty. The RA on duty reports this to you, and you and your residence director plan a meeting to discuss the incident and figure out what to do next.

REPORT BACK FROM SMALL GROUPS:

1. **What are some positive aspects of this situation?**
   You and the residence director have planned a meeting to discuss the incident and figure out what to do next.

2. **What are some negative or concerning aspects of this situation?**
   Frequent remarks from other residents talking about how "weird" Steve is. Someone has written a slur on Steve's marker board. You are unsure how, or if, the floor's reputation as a "party dorm" may come into play in this situation. You want to try to avoid stereotyping the residents of this community based on this reputation, but are also concerned others (residents, staff, or administrators) may use this as an excuse for inappropriate behavior.

3. **What do you think Steve's reaction to the marker board message will be?**
   Possible reactions: anger, frustration, disappointment, concern for physical safety, wanting to ignore it, not wanting to cause problems, dismissing it as a prank.

4. **What are some steps that you could take to address the incident with your residents?**
   Possible affirming steps: Holding a floor meeting, passing out affirming information about transgender and gender non-conforming people, putting up a bulletin board about gender diversity, contacting the campus or community LGBTQ Center or group to ask to request consultation and guidance.

5. **What would might you would do to make Steve feel more comfortable on the floor?**
   Possible affirming responses: Asking Steve if there is anything that you can do to be of support; explaining how the incident will be handled and what will be expected of him in that process–including how his privacy will be protected; telling Steve that your room and your residence hall are your home and mine–please tell me anytime something happens here that is derogatory or disrespectful to yourself or another resident because we want to build and maintain a safe and respectful living community here.

6. **What are some affirming things that you could say to other residents who are not affirming of Steve?**
   Possible affirming responses: Transgender people are people too and deserve our respect; here are some resources to learn more about transgender people; please don't say negative things about Steve's identity around me because I find it offensive.

PARTICIPANT HANDOUT

Residence Life Vignettes

Shay's Story

You are a resident assistant in the all-female first-year residence hall. Shay is one of your residents. Shay seems to be a loner and you have not had the opportunity to interact much with this student yet. You overhear a few of your residents talking about Shay's appearance and speculating about whether or not Shay might be a lesbian. A few days later, Shay requests a meeting with you and your residence hall director. During the meeting, Shay explains that he is transgender and requests that you and your RD help with coming out to the floor and having people use male pronouns. Shay thinks that he might be more comfortable in the co-ed dorm, on a male-only floor, but is not sure yet. He is adamant that his parents not be told about any of this, out of fear that they might disown him and he would not be able to afford college without their support.

SMALL-GROUP DISCUSSION QUESTIONS:
1. What are some positive aspects of this situation?
2. What are some negative or concerning aspects of this situation?
3. What would you say to Shay during that meeting?
4. What are some things that you would consider doing to be supportive of Shay?
5. What might be some affirming things that you could say to other residents who are confused or not affirming of Shay?

Vanessa's Story

You are a resident assistant with a floor of male students in the sophomore residence hall that has a reputation for being a "party" dorm. Just before winter break, Jason asks if he can talk to you about something. You are really busy with finals, and do not have a chance to meet with Jason before you leave. When you return from break, you pass Jason in the hall. He is wearing a dress, make-up and has his long hair styled in a feminine manner. You are naturally quite surprised by this. You wave hello and continue walking to your room. When you check your voicemail, you have a message from the Director of Residence Life saying that one of your residents is transgender and will be coming back as woman, and would like people to start using female pronouns and calling her Vanessa. Your director wants to schedule a meeting with you to talk about how you can be supportive of Vanessa.

SMALL-GROUP DISCUSSION QUESTIONS:
1. What are some positive aspects of this situation?
2. What are some negative or concerning aspects of this situation?
3. What do you think your initial reactions to Vanessa might be?
4. What are some of the challenges Vanessa might face?
5. What are some affirming things that you could say to other residents who are confused or not affirming of Vanessa?
6. What are some things that you would suggest to the director of residence life as ways of supporting of Vanessa?

Kim's Story

You are a resident assistant on a women's floor in the co-ed sophomore residence hall. Your resident director has informed you that you will be having a new resident who is a transfer student. The resident director tells you that Kim is a transgender woman. Kim does not want anyone to know that she is transgender, and she is transferring to the school to get a new start as Kim. She is currently taking female hormones and has been for about a year now, but has not been able to have surgery yet and does not expect to for several years. Since there are no single rooms available, Kim will be living with one of your residents whose roommate left the school last semester. You and your resident director plan to meet in order to come up with a plan for how to be supportive of Kim.

SMALL-GROUP DISCUSSION QUESTIONS:
1. What are some positive aspects of this situation?
2. What are some negative or concerning aspects of this situation?
3. What do you think that some of the challenges might be for Kim?
4. How do you think that her roommate might react if she finds out about Kim?
5. How might her floor-mates react to her using the bathroom and showers?
6. What are some things that you would suggest to the director of residence life as ways to be supportive of Kim?
7. What are some affirming things you could say to other residents who are confused or not affirming of Kim?

Steve's Story

You are a resident assistant in the co-ed sophomore residence hall that has a reputation for being a "party" dorm. One of your residents, Steve, is rather androgynous. Steve tends to be a loner, rarely interacts with the other residents, and spends weekends off-campus. You have frequently overheard remarks from your other residents talking about how "weird" Steve is, and that "there is something that is not just right about Steve." One weekend, someone writes: "Steve It is f***n' tranny!!!!" on Steve's marker board. Steve comes back to campus, sees this and reports it to the RA on duty. The RA on duty reports this to you, and you and your residence director plan a meeting to discuss the incident and figure out what to do next.

SMALL-GROUP DISCUSSION QUESTIONS:
1. What are some positive aspects of this situation?
2. What are some negative or concerning aspects of this situation?
3. What do you think Steve's reaction to the marker board message will be?
4. What are some steps you could take to address the incident with your residents?
5. What are some things that you could do to make Steve feel more comfortable on the floor?
6. What are some affirming things you could say to other residents who are not affirming of Steve?

PARTICIPANT HANDOUT

Proactive Planning for Professional Residence Life Staff

Creating affirming spaces for transgender students requires proactive work to identify policies, procedures and resources. Consider the answers to the following questions:

1. Are there any residence life or campus policies or practices that may assist transgender students in terms of housing, academics, chosen name, access to campus services? Are there any policies or practices that may be barriers to transgender students?

2. How would a transgender student find out about these policies (e.g., are they available on the website, student handbook, or can they ask a residence life staff member)?

3. How will a transgender student's privacy be protected? How will this happen if the student contacts residence life as an incoming student? As a returning student?

4. What policies or procedures are in place that can support the RA and the resident in the scenarios outlined in the previous activity? Are the staff or RAs trained in these policies?

5. What are some additional policies or procedures that could be developed to proactively support transgender students and the RAs and staff who work with them?

6. What campus or community resources are available to support transgender students (e.g., an LGBTQ Center, affirming and supportive counseling, transgender-specific support groups, social groups)?

7. What campus or community resources are available to support cisgender students who are struggling with being affirming?

ACTION STEPS:
Identify the next steps necessary in answering these questions and addressing any related concerns. Who will be responsible for taking these steps?

_____
_____
_____
_____
_____
_____
_____
_____

SAFE AND INCLUSIVE TEAMS:
Lessons for Athletics Staff in Higher Ed

...

Overview & Rationale

This lesson gives participants an opportunity to consider the unique experiences of transgender and gender-diverse student athletes and issues of transgender inclusion in sports on college campuses, and strategize ways to provide personal and professional support in their roles as athletics and recreation staff. Vignettes and case studies are used to assist participants in making connections between informational content and lived experiences.

Audience

This lesson works best with college and university athletics and recreation staff, coaches, fitness trainers, and with some groups of student athletes. It is also appropriate for college and university faculty, staff, and administrators, and may be appropriate for some college student audiences in disciplines such as higher education administration, athletic training, sports management, and other fields. In addition, it may be of interest to others who work or volunteer in sports, recreation, and fitness settings. This lesson works best with 10–40 participants, and can be modified for larger audiences.

Objectives

By the end of this lesson, participants will be able to:
- Identify 1 thing they can do to make their campus athletics program friendlier for transgender and gender non-conforming students.
- Identify 2 things their college or university could do, or do differently, to make their campus athletics more welcoming to transgender and gender non-conforming students.

Background Knowledge for Facilitators

It will be helpful for facilitators to have foundational knowledge of sports teams and player dynamics, and also to have specific knowledge of how transgender athletes have navigated college sports (including the challenges faced). Even if not facilitating with a participating NCAA school or team, it can be useful to be familiar with NCAA guidelines on supporting transgender athletes as a point of reference to explain how other schools are creating affirming teams for transgender athletes.

Time

- Preparation: 15 minutes
- Implementation: 60 minutes

Materials

- *Transgender in Sports Vignettes* handout (1 per participant)
- Index Cards (1 of each color per participant)
- Assorted stickers
- Easel chart paper and markers

Preparation

- Make copies of the handouts
- Place stickers on the *Transgender In Sports Vignettes* handout so that participants will end up in small groups of the desired size. For example, use balls from 6 sports to create 6 small groups). To save time during the activity, you may wish to distribute the handouts as people walk in, or place them on the seats in advance.
- On the easel chart paper (or in a PowerPoint slide), write the 2 closing prompts from Procedure step 4.

Procedure

1. Explain that this activity is designed to help us think about some of the challenges that transgender athletes have to navigate and how we can make sure that every team is safe and affirming.

2. Instruct participants to break into small groups by finding the other participants with the same sticker as them and sitting together. Once the participants have settled into their groups, assign each group 1 vignette to work on. (Depending on the number of groups, there may be multiple groups working on the same vignette, or groups working on multiple vignettes). Direct participants to read their assigned vignette and then work together for about 10–15 minutes to answer the questions.

3. After about 15 minutes, bring all of the participants back to the large group. Using the *Transgender In Sports Vignettes: Facilitator's Guide,* lead a large-group discussion about each of these vignettes. Start by asking group 1 to read their vignette out loud (or summarize the key points) and provide their answers. Repeat with each group. Depending on the time available, it may not be possible to review all answers for all questions—select those that seem the most relevant and least redundant based on the flow and pace of the discussion.

4. If using as a standalone lesson, conclude the activity by handing out an index card for each participant. Allow 5 minutes for participants to provide their answers to the prompt below. They should not put their names on the cards. Once the participants have completed their responses, collect the cards and shuffle them and return them to participants, so that each person has a new card. Have each participants read off the responses written on their cards in turn.

   – *On the front:* Write 1 thing you can do to make your campus athletics programs more affirming of transgender athletes.

   – *On the back:* Write 1 thing that coaches or athletic directors can do to make every team more affirming for transgender athletes.

5. *Optional:* The cards can be collected and turned into a bulletin board as an ongoing reminder of the commitments made to create a more affirming athletic environment.

Evaluation Questions

✔ What is 1 thing that you can do to help make your campus athletics program friendlier for transgender students?

✔ What are 2 things that your college or university could do, or do differently, to make your campus athletics more welcoming to transgender students?

RELATED RESOURCES

NCAA Inclusion of Transgender Student-Athletes. NCAA Office of Inclusion
   www.uh.edu/lgbt/docs/Transgender_Handbook_2011_Final.pdf

Champions of Respect: Inclusion of LGBTQ Student-Athletes and Staff in NCAA Programs
   www.ncaapublications.com/p-4305-champions-of-respect-inclusion-of-lgbtq-student-athletes-and-staff-in-ncaa-programs.aspx

The Transgender Athlete: www.genderspectrum.org/images/stories/The_Transgender_Athlete.pdf

On the Team: Equal Opportunity for Transgender Student Athletes, online at: www.genderspectrum.org/images/stories/On_The_Team.pdf

By Dr. Pat Griffin, Former Director, It Takes A Team! Education Campaign for Lesbian, Gay, Bisexual and Transgender Issues in Sport, Women's Sports Foundation

And Helen J. Carroll, Sports Project Director, National Center for Lesbian Rights

Guidelines for Creating Policies for Transgender Children in Recreational Sports by the Transgender Law & Policy Institute. Available at:https://www.genderspectrum.org/images/stories/trans_children_in_sports.pdf

Athlete Ally: www.athleteally.org

When conducting this lesson with athletic training, recreation, sports medicine, fitness, or other student staff or student athletes, it is ideal to have the professional athletics and recreation staff complete this training as a staff professional development training in advance of student training. Student staff will likely have questions and need support from the professional staff, and this will help to ensure that staff are prepared to do this work.

• • •

If you are conducting this training as an outside facilitator (who does not work on campus), it will be very helpful to have a professional staff member in the training who is familiar with the institution's policies (or lack thereof) and can discuss them during the training. When booking the training, be sure to ask who this person might be and find out if you can speak to them in advance. This will help ensure that the person knows what questions are coming and give you a chance to review the policy in advance.

• • •

When discussing the various scenarios, it is likely that there will be concern or discomfort about the potential implications of having a person with a different sex assigned at birth from that of their teammates in the locker rooms or other changing or treatment areas that are sex-segregated. This can also apply to practice or athletic meet or game locations that can be entered only through sex-segregated locker rooms (e.g., pools, sports medicine treatment areas, some fitness center and workout equipment rooms, etc.). Often these concerns are vocalized in terms of the potential for harm or trauma (e.g., a transgender person might sexually assault a cisgender teammate, or a teammate with a history of trauma may be triggered by seeing a person's genitals) or a related liability, or the idea that there must be disclosure of someone's transgender identity to get informed consent on the part of a cisgender teammates, coaches, or opposing teams' players. Both of these concerns are generally rooted in false stereotypes about transgender people being physically or sexually violent, and the assumption that a cisgender person's desire to know that someone is transgender is more important than the transgender person's privacy or safety concerns. There are several ways to afford greater privacy to people who desire it. Lightweight portable privacy screens may be used in changing areas by cisgender athletes who have high privacy needs. They can also be offered to transgender athletes (or any athlete desiring increased privacy for any reason), but transgender athletes should never be required to use them.

• • •

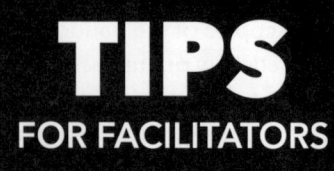

TIPS FOR FACILITATORS

Not all transgender people wish to serve in an advocacy or educational role. There are people who are professional facilitators who are able to help provide training and education. Find out who these people are on your campus and in your community. Consulting with the campus-based LGBTQ Center or LGBTQ-themed campus group, if there is one, is a good first step. Many places also have a local LGBTQ community group or community center that can provide resources, referral, and consultation. A student should never be required to educate their coaches or other school's teams and staff about their identity.

• • •

Some colleges and universities already have sport-specific participation policies and practices in place, and/or a non-discrimination policy. If your institution does not, resources exist for you and your institution to create these policies and practices. Recent Title IX interpretation guidance documents may also assist you and your university in addressing inclusion of transgender student athletes in accordance with the law.

Transgender in Sports Vignettes:
FACILITATOR'S GUIDE

Jack's Story

You are a coach of the men's track team. Jack is new on your coaching staff. He's a great addition to your staff—he has coached at another highly respected athletic program for a few years, and he's an alumnus of your university and eager to be back on campus, this time in a staff role. Jack started using hormones to medically transition (from female to male) after graduation, and has let you know he will be having top surgery within the year. He knows some people on campus will remember him from when he was a student, while for most of the current student athletes he'll be a new acquaintance. He requests a meeting with you to discuss whether and how he will come out to the team, because he wants to have clear, open lines of communication and answer any questions the students and the rest of the coaching staff may have. In particular, he's thinking ahead to whether issues in the locker room or athletic treatment or training areas like the pool or sports medicine clinic may arise. Maintaining a well-run and winning team, and succeeding in his new position are his main goals, and he is seeking your support.

SMALL GROUP REPORT BACK:

1. **What are some positive aspects to this situation?**
   Jack comes to you ahead of time so you can work together. As an alumnus, Jack is already familiar with the institution and the campus culture, so you have much common ground.

2. **What are some challenging or concerning aspects of this situation?**
   Some staff will remember Jack from his time as a student, while new students on campus will not know him, or his history, at all; which may be difficult for all involved to manage.

3. **What do you think your initial reactions to Jack might be?**
   Responses will vary. (Note: This question should not be reported back to the large group so that participants do not have to share potentially non-affirming responses).

4. **What would you say to Jack during that meeting?**
   Responses will vary. (Note: This question should not be reported back to the large group so that participants do not have to share potentially non-affirming responses; instead ask "what are some possible responses to Jack?").

5. **What challenges do you think Jack will face?**
   Possible challenges: Jack may be worried how he will navigate the varying levels of awareness about his being transgender, whether the information will be a distraction to the team, or how other coaches may respond.

6. **How do you think students might react to Jack's coming out?**
   Possible responses: positive and affirming, supportive, curious, confused, unconcerned, feeling deceived, being upset, not wanting to be on the team, not wanting to be in the locker room with Jack.

7. **What are some things that you would consider doing to be supportive of Jack?**
   Possible affirming responses: Asking Jack if there is anything you can do to be of support; asking Jack how he would like you to respond when people ask if he is transgender; checking into the university's and city/state's protections around gender identity/expression to determine if Jack is legally protected from being fired because he is transgender; asking Jack if you should arrange for student/staff training on transgender topics in sports.

Talking Points:

– There are resources to support you in your role, to support your athletes, and to support Jack in his decision to come out to the team and at his workplace in general. Consult the resources listed in this lesson to find some of them.

– Jack will probably have to negotiate his coming out on multiple levels on a college campus—with some people he has never met, and with others who knew him as a student. It is important that you have the information and resources to support him, and are familiar with policies in place at your institution regarding nondiscrimination and support for transgender employees.

> **Andrea's Story**

You coordinate the recreational sports intramural program on campus. A student, Andrea, e-mails you to ask if she can meet with you to discuss her interest in club volleyball. It's immediately prior to fall break, and you are really busy planning the upcoming winter leagues as well as some special events including the all-campus 5K run and the annual benefit golf tournament that are all scheduled for alumni weekend in a couple of weeks. You look up from your desk when Andrea comes into your office for her appointment, and you are a bit surprised because Andrea's appearance is not what you had expected. Andrea has long hair and is wearing a big sweater, skirt and tights, but speaks in a deep voice and has what looks to you like a little bit of five o'clock shadow. Andrea explains that she is very interested in joining the women's intramural volleyball team, but is worried she'll not be accepted by the team because she is a transgender woman. She also has questions about her participation—will college policy allow her to play on the women's team? Or will she be required to be on a men's team? Will she be allowed to participate at all?

SMALL GROUP REPORT BACK:

1. **What are some positive aspects to this situation?**
   Andrea proactively approaches you. You have time to consider the situation and look into the relevant policies and procedures, whether they already exist or you need to work with Andrea and the institution to develop such policies and procedures if needed.

2. **What are some challenging or concerning aspects of this situation?**
   Although you oversee the recreational sports program, you are unsure if such policies and procedures are already in place. You are busy and distracted by the other major events and leagues you are facilitating.

3. **What do you think your initial reactions to Andrea might be?**
   Responses will vary. (Note: This question should not be reported back to the large group so that participants do not have to share potentially non-affirming responses).

4. **How can you find answers to Andrea's questions, and is there other information that might be helpful to her that you can provide as well?**
   Possible responses: Consulting recreation or athletic department policies; consulting the college/university's policies and practices regarding inclusion; reviewing the institution's non-discrimination policy; reviewing the policies and practices of the specific sport's governing body; consulting the institution's legal counsel for additional assistance in identifying and acting in accordance with all institutional, local, and statewide policies and laws on this issue; utilizing outside resources including NCAA inclusion and Title IX interpretation documents for additional guidance.

5. **How do you think other students might react to Andrea if she joins the team?**
   Possible reactions: positive and affirming, supportive, curious, confused, unconcerned, feeling deceived, being upset, not wanting to be on the team, not wanting to be in the locker room with Andrea.

6. **What are some challenges that Andrea might face?**
   Possible challenges: People talking about her behind her back, people isolating her because she is transgender, people bothering or harassing her in the locker room, people on other teams being upset about someone who was assigned male at birth playing on a women's team because of a perceived unfair advantage.

7. **How can you be supportive of Andrea?**
   Possible supportive responses: Ask Andrea if there is anything that you can do to be of support; ask her how she would like you to respond when people ask if she is transgender; check into the Title IX and university's protections around gender identity/expression to make sure that Andrea is legally protected from being denied access to club sports; ask Andrea if she would like you to arrange for student/staff training on transgender people.

Talking Points:

– Some colleges and universities already have sport-specific participation policies and practices in place, and/or a non-discrimination policy. These may assist you in providing Andrea with the answers she's seeking, and assist you in supporting her full participation. If your institution does not, resources exist for you and your institution to create these policies and practices. Recent Title IX interpretation guidance documents may also assist you and your university in addressing inclusion of transgender student athletes in accordance with the law.

- Not all transgender people wish to serve in an advocacy or educational role. There are people who are professional facilitators who are able to help provide training and education. Find out who these people are on your campus and in your community. Consulting with the campus-based LGBTQ Center or an LGBTQ-themed campus group, if there is one, is a good first step. Many places also have a local LGBTQ community group or community center that can provide resources, referral, and consultation. A student should never be required to educate teammates or staff overseeing the program about their identity.

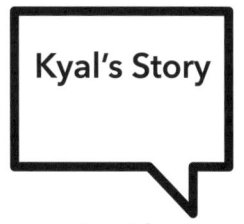

Kyal's Story

You are traveling with your team to an away game. One of your student athletes, Kyal, is friendly and outgoing, although sometimes a bit loud and rambunctious. Kyal also presents in a rather genderfluid manner, seeming sometimes quite feminine but at other times very masculine. Kyal's teammates are drawn to Kyal's easy-going manner and sense of fun, and find Kyal's genderfluidity interesting and even endearing. They are fierce allies of Kyal. When you reach your destination city, your team and an opposing team arrive at the hotel front desk at the same time. As you are trying to get all the logistics settled and rooms assigned with the desk clerk, you overhear remarks from a few of the opposing team members as they are waiting in the hotel lobby for their room keys. They are pointing and staring at Kyal and making unkind remarks. Kyal looks surprised and hurt. Just as you notice one of the opposing team's coaches beginning to laugh along with the players, a few of your own athletes walk directly toward them. Their faces are angry, and you know you have to intervene.

SMALL GROUP REPORT BACK:

1. **What are some positive aspects to this situation?**
   Kyal is easy-going, and Kyal's teammates like Kyal and are very loyal. You are present to observe the events leading up to this moment, which may be helpful to you as you consider how to act.

2. **What are some challenging or concerning aspects of this situation?**
   Opposing team members and coaches make disparaging remarks and point, stare, and laugh at Kyal. Kyal's teammates are loyal to the point of risking a confrontation with the opposing team in the hotel lobby.

3. **What do you think Kyal's reaction to this incident will be?**
   Possible reactions: Being grateful to teammates for their support, embarrassed that the incident happened, distracted from the game, angry about the unkind statements, upset that it was not stopped by the other team's coach.

4. **In this moment, what steps could you take to address the incident with your athletes? With the opposing team's coaches and athletes?**
   Possible affirming steps: Pulling the other coach aside and expressing your concerns about his team's remarks; asking your athletes to immediately reconvene with you in another place in or outside the hotel so you can re-group, talk about what happened, and have a chance for everyone to cool down; helping the team stay focused so that the incident doesn't disrupt the game; informing the team that you'll review university policy and the policies and guidelines of the NCAA or another governing body (as appropriate) to determine what reporting requirements are in place for you to report this incident so that official investigations or actions can take place.

5. **What could you would do to make Kyal feel more comfortable at this game?**
   Possible affirming actions: Asking Kyal what would be helpful or supportive in that moment; validating that the situation was upsetting/not okay; helping the team stay focused so that the incident doesn't disrupt the game; informing Kyal that you'll review university policy and the policies and guidelines of the NCAA or another governing body (as appropriate) to determine what reporting requirements are in place for you to report this incident so that official investigations or actions can take place.

6. **What steps could you take once you've returned to your home campus?**
   Possible affirming steps: Touching base with Kyal to see what would be supportive moving forward; contacting the other coach to discuss the situation; consulting with supervisor and colleagues in athletics department for support and guidance; consulting with college counsel if necessary; filing a complaint with the appropriate governing body; seeking out training for the entire team about effective bystander responses.

   Talking Points:
   - Not all people who are gender non-conforming are transgender (nor are all people who are gender-conforming cisgender). It is important not to make assumptions about gender identity or sexual orientation.
   - Not all transgender people wish to serve in an advocacy or educational role. There are people who are professional facilitators who are able to provide training and education. Find out who these people are on your campus and in your community. Consulting with the campus-based LGBTQ Center or an LGBTQ-themed campus group, if there is one, is a good first step. Many places also have a local LGBTQ community group or community center that can provide resources, referrals, and consultation. A student should never be required to educate their coaches or other school's teams and staff about their identity.

PARTICIPANT HANDOUT

Transgender in Sports Vignettes

Jack's Story

You are a coach of the men's track team. Jack is new on your coaching staff. He's a great addition to your staff—he has coached at another highly respected athletic program for a few years, and he's an alumnus of your university and eager to be back on campus, this time in a staff role. Jack started using hormones to medically transition (from female to male) after graduation, and has let you know he will be having top surgery within the year. He knows some people on campus will remember him from when he was a student, while for most of the current student athletes he'll be a new acquaintance. He requests a meeting with you to discuss whether and how he will come out to the team, because he wants to have clear, open lines of communication and answer any questions the students and the rest of the coaching staff may have. In particular, he's thinking ahead to whether issues in the locker room or athletic treatment or training areas like the pool or sports medicine clinic may arise. Maintaining a well-run and winning team, and succeeding in his new position are his main goals, and he is seeking your support.

SMALL GROUP DISCUSSION QUESTIONS:
1. What are some positive aspects to this situation?
2. What are some challenging or concerning aspects of this situation?
3. What would your initial reactions to Jack be?
4. What would you say to Jack during that meeting?
5. What are some of the challenges Jack might face?
6. How might students react to Jack's coming out?
7. What are some things you would consider doing to be supportive of Jack?

Andrea's Story

You coordinate the recreational sports intramural program on campus. A student, Andrea, e-mails you to ask if she can meet with you to discuss her interest in club volleyball. It's immediately prior to fall break, and you are really busy planning the upcoming winter leagues as well as some special events including the all-campus 5K run and the annual benefit golf tournament that are all coming up for alumni weekend in a couple of weeks. You look up from your desk when Andrea comes into your office for her appointment, and you are a bit surprised because Andrea's appearance is not what you had expected. Andrea has long hair and is wearing a big sweater, skirt and tights, but speaks in a deep voice and has what looks to you like a little bit of five o'clock shadow. Andrea explains that she is very interested in joining the women's intramural volleyball team, but is worried she'll not be accepted by the team because she is a transgender woman. She also has questions about her participation—will college policy allow her to play on the women's team? Or will she be required to be on a men's team? Will she be allowed to participate at all?

SMALL GROUP DISCUSSION QUESTIONS:
1. What are some positive aspects to this situation?
2. What are some challenging or concerning aspects of this situation?
3. What would your initial reaction to Andrea be?
4. How can you find answers to Andrea's questions, and is there other information that might be helpful to her that you can provide as well?
5. How do you think other students might react to Andrea if she joins the team?
6. What are some of the challenges Andrea might face?
7. What are some of the ways you can be supportive of Andrea?

www.TeachingTransgender.com • THE TEACHING TRANSGENDER TOOLKIT • 183

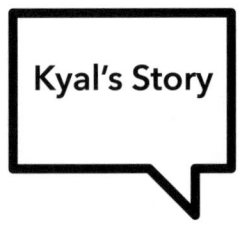

Kyal's Story

You are traveling with your team to an away game. One of your student athletes, Kyal, is friendly and outgoing, although sometimes a bit loud and rambunctious. Kyal also presents in a rather genderfluid manner, seeming sometimes quite feminine but at other times very masculine. Kyal's teammates are drawn to Kyal's easy-going manner and sense of fun, and find Kyal's genderfluidity interesting and even endearing. They are fierce allies of Kyal. When you reach your destination city, your team and an opposing team arrive at the hotel front desk at the same time. As you are trying to get all the logistics settled and rooms assigned with the desk clerk, you overhear remarks from a few of the opposing team members as they are waiting in the hotel lobby for their room keys. They are pointing and staring at Kyal, and making unkind remarks. Kyal looks surprised and hurt. Just as you notice one of the opposing team's coaches beginning to laugh along with the players too, a few of your own athletes walk stridently toward them. Their faces are angry, and you know you have to intervene.

SMALL GROUP DISCUSSION QUESTIONS:
1. What are some positive aspects to this situation?
2. What are some challenging or concerning aspects of this situation?
3. How will Kyal react to this incident?
4. In this moment, what steps could you take to address the incident with your athletes? With the opposing team's coaches and athletes?
5. What could you do to make Kyal feel more comfortable at this game?
6. What are some steps you could take once you've returned to your home campus

NOTES

CREATING
Transgender-Affirming College Health Centers

Overview & Rationale

In greater numbers than ever before, transgender students are coming out in college, or transitioning before they arrive at college. The health of transgender students is important not just to their physical well-being but also to their academic success and personal growth, and transgender college students have some unique and, too often, unmet needs. This lesson explores ways in which college and university health center professionals can offer culturally competent services and support to meet the needs of this growing population, and improve the campus climate to better meet the distinct needs of transgender students.

Audience

This lesson is designed for college and university health center staff but can also be modified to work with college and university faculty, staff, and administrators. This lesson works best with groups of 10–40.

Objectives

By the end of this lesson, participants will be able to:
- Identify 3 common needs of transgender college students in college and university healthcare settings.
- Provide 3 examples of barriers that transgender college students may face in seeking to have their needs met by college and university health centers.
- Provide examples of 3 specific strategies for making college and university health services welcoming to transgender people.

Background Knowledge for Facilitators

It will be useful for facilitators to understand the policies of the campus hosting the training regarding transgender students and health center processes, procedures and practices (e.g., non-discrimination policies, student insurance coverage for transgender healthcare services [hormones/surgeries], any established medical protocols for transgender students).

Time

- Preparation: 15–30, depending on knowledge of campus policies
- Implementation: 70 minutes

Materials

- Easel paper
- Markers
- Copies of *Health Center Check-Up* Handout (1 per participant)

Preparation

- Make copies of handouts.
- Review each of the items on the handout to make sure that you are comfortable explaining each of these items and how they might affect a transgender students' experience, particularly as it relates to being a potential risk to their emotional or physical well-being or safety.
- If possible, research the policies, practices, and procedures of the participants' campus(es) ahead of the training.

Procedure

1. Explain that this lesson focuses specifically on exploring the medical needs of transgender college students as well as the covering the potential barriers they may face, and what professionals in college and university health centers may encounter in their work regarding transgender students. This lesson is not about how to change campus policy—it is about how to raise cultural competency in meeting the health needs of transgender students, regardless of current campus policies.

2. Break participants into 5 separate groups, and explain that each group will be focusing on 1 specific area of needs, barriers, and opportunities with regard to transgender students and the college health center.

3. Distribute the *Health Center Check-Up* handout. Assign 1 section of the handout to each group, by number. Explain that each small group will review the items in their assigned section and discuss whether or not their Student Health Center has those items in place. Based on the in-group discussion, select "yes," "no," or "maybe" for each item. Ask each group to discuss the specific needs, barriers, and opportunities that transgender college students may face regarding the main theme in their section of the handout, in a college health center setting.

    For example: a student who wants to transition but not tell their parents—how does this affect health insurance?—may be one challenge facing transgender college students listed under the "health insurance" heading. Another example is the inclusiveness of intake forms or medical software—listed under "documentation."

4. During the small-group session, rotate around to each of the small groups and offer support as needed. Allow participants to ask questions or seek clarification about the reasons for, or importance of, various items on the checklist. Explain to participants that they may not know some of the answers on the checklist but that it is important for them to go back to their campuses and find out the answers.

5. After about 15 minutes, call the group back to order and ask each group to report. Use these discussion questions to frame responses:
    - Based on your small-group discussion, what needs might transgender students have when they seek healthcare services through their college health centers?
    - Based on your discussion, what barriers might transgender students face when accessing their college health centers?
    - On which questions did you find you're already doing a good job?
    - On which questions might there still be room for change?
    - Were there questions to which you were unsure of the answers? How could you find out?

6. Ask the 5 small groups to reconvene, this time with the task of discussing and describing 3 ideas or strategies that participants will take back to their campus or their role on campus to make their college or university health services more welcoming to transgender people. Provide easel paper and markers for each group to write down responses. Provide 10 minutes for small-group discussion.

7. Reconvene the large group and invite participants to share what they discussed. Small groups may also hold up or post their easel papers to display their work. Use these discussion questions to frame responses:
    - What ideas did you have?
    - Which can you implement right away?
    - Which will take more time to implement?
    - Which will require the help of other colleagues, departments, or administrators?

8. Explain that all students benefit from healthcare staff who model active and respectful listening, use inclusive language, combat stereotypes, and advocate for meeting student needs within the current environment of practices and policies or advocate for change that will be more effective.

9. If using as a standalone lesson, conclude the session by asking each participant to report back to the large group 1 thing that they are committed to investigating or doing when they return to their campus/health center to make it more affirming for transgender students.

Evaluation Questions

✔ What are 3 common needs that transgender college students seek to access at their college health centers?

✔ Describe 3 examples of barriers that transgender college students may face when accessing services at their college health centers.

✔ What are 3 specific strategies that can be implemented that would make college and university health services more welcoming to transgender students?

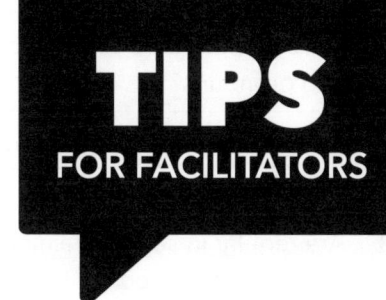

Some participants may display concern or resistance to the idea of supporting transgender students in fulfilling their transition goals. Sometimes this resistance is based in a fear that the medical transition process is dangerous. Some healthcare providers are concerned a student may not fully understand the risks or understand which physical changes involved in medical transition may be permanent. Still other providers may harbor myths or misinformation about this topic, or they may have not had the opportunity to have had professional development updates on this topic in the past.

• • •

Participants may have questions about the physical or emotional changes involved in medical transition, or be curious about surgical options and outcomes. Remind participants that there are excellent sources of information for professionals as well as first-person stories of transgender people online and in books and other publications.

• • •

Participants may express surprise when asked to consider that they may already be serving transgender students. Students may have transitioned before entering college, and/or may be receiving transgender-related health care from off-campus providers. These students may choose to disclose this information, or choose not to, for a variety of reasons. Remind participants that the most important thing is that any student—transgender or not—with health questions or maintenance needs should be monitored by a healthcare provider. College health centers that provide knowledgeable, culturally competent care are best positioned to meet students' needs.

REFERENCE

The *Health Center Check-Up* handout is based on the work of: Beemyn, B. G. (2005). Making campuses more inclusive of transgender students. *Journal of Gay & Lesbian Issues in Education,* 3(1), 77–87.

PARTICIPANT HANDOUT

Health Center Check-Up:

ACHIEVING AND MAINTAINING EXCELLENCE FOR TRANSGENDER STUDENTS

Basic Cultural Competency	Yes	No	Maybe
1. Are all staff members trained in basic cultural competency (e.g., Transgender 101, confidentiality, safe environment)?			
2. Are staff members up-to-date on current terminology and language?			
3. Are staff members comfortable asking students about preferred name and pronouns?			
2. Are staff members comfortable discussing medical transition goals with students?			
3. Are regular in-service trainings offered to medical health providers regarding the needs of transgender students?			
4. Are providers trained in the most recent WPATH standards of care (these provide clinical guidance for working with transgender patients)?			

Documentation	Yes	No	Maybe
1. Can students request being called a different name and pronoun from those in their records?			
2. Are there policies in place to make sure that the student's identity remains confidential?			
3. Are there procedures in place for making sure that the student is called by their preferred name and pronoun?			
4. Are there procedures in place for making sure that insurance billing, prescriptions, etc., are consistent with legal documentation (but that the preferred name and pronouns are used in the office)?			

→

Health Insurance	Yes	No	Maybe
1. Are hormones and related services covered under student health insurance?			
2. Are surgery and related services covered under student health insurance?			
3. Are there are policies in place for billing insurance companies for services related to medical transition that protect students from denial of coverage, discrimination, or being red-flagged?			
4. Are staff members trained to help students understand the ramifications of submitting transgender-related procedures to their health insurance carrier (e.g., parental notification)?			

Processes, Policies, Procedures	Yes	No	Maybe
1. Do the intake forms provide an option for students to self-disclose their gender identity as being different from their assigned sex?			
2. Does the medical software provide an option for alerting providers to a transgender students' preferred (chosen) name and pronouns? If not, is there an alternate plan in place?			
3. Are there policies and procedures in place for students who need physical examinations (for sports or otherwise) to ensure the student's confidentiality?			
4. Does the health center have an up-to-date list of community referrals for transgender-inclusive mental health and medical providers?			
5. Are regular in-service trainings offered to help medical health providers understand the implications of the campus's physical health, mental health, and sexual/reproductive health services, the campus pharmacy, peer health programs, health promotion services, etc.?			
6. Are there established policies and procedures that determine whether or not transgender students will be required to have a letter from a mental health provider in order to access medical transition?			
7. Are there established connections with mental health providers (on and off campus) who are transgender affirming?			

Affirmation	Yes	No	Maybe
Does the Health Center have the means in place to provide affirming support for transgender students who:			
1. Lack the support of family, friends or peers?			
2. Cannot come out to their parents due to the safety reasons?			
3. Fear for their physical safety on campus?			
4. Consider seeking hormones outside of a healthcare setting?			
5. Engage in unsafe or unmonitored use of hormones?			
6. Inject free-form silicone as a method of expediting transition?			
7. Need to take a medical leave of absence to focus on medical transition (or to deal with the psychological consequences of not being able to medically transition)?			
8. Have other mental health issues, not directly related to their identity?			
9. Avoid routine or necessary health monitoring or concerns for other existing health conditions because they fear stigma, discrimination, lack of confidentiality (re: institution, parents, peers)?			
10. Have difficulty in accessing medical care in general?			
11. Wish to study abroad and need support regarding documentation, hormones, access to care, etc., while traveling?			

MEDICAL & MENTAL *Health Providers*

Recognizing Our Common Humanity

By Jennifer Hastings, MD
Director of the Transgender Health Care Program,
Planned Parenthood Mar Monte

• • •

A medical visit can be frustrating. As patients, we want to be seen and understood, and hope for an intimacy that helps us address whatever ailment befalls us, but sometimes we feel scared, ashamed, or vulnerable, there is no "connection" with our provider, and we can leave dissatisfied. For a transgender or gender non-conforming person, the experience of seeking care is all too often traumatic and not necessarily just from the provider. It can start at the front office reception with a furrowing of eyebrows or shifting eyes. A core aspect of identity is not understood or respected, and without this understanding and respect, it is impossible for a client to feel comfortable, and for healing to take place. In 2011, the National Transgender Discrimination Survey of health experiences published by the National Center for Transgender Equality showed us what we have known for years: the medical community does not know how to provide health care for transgender people. For a transgender person, the shocking statistics from this study are a daily reality. Over 19 percent of transgender patients were refused care because of their transgender identity, and 28 percent of respondents were harassed during their medical visit. Because of discrimination and the frequency of abuse, a majority of transgender individuals do not seek medical care.

Using the lessons and materials in this chapter, as a facilitator you will help participants to learn about the challenges transgender individuals face when trying to access medical care, and what they can do to create a safe and welcoming setting. As front office staff, medical assistants, medical and mental health providers and billers, they will gain knowledge, skills and compassion to transform the health care experience from traumatic to positive. Medical and mental health providers have much to learn from the courageous and remarkable journeys of gender outside the normative definitions of sex assigned at birth. Learning about how to provide culturally compassionate and affirming care invites a personal exploration of gender that may challenge participants to view the world differently.

As you embark on facilitating these lessons, it is important to remember that in order for a didactic method to be effective, to actually change behavior, we must engage our participant's minds and hearts. To this goal, a fundamental concept within these lessons is that cisgender and transgender people are in fact more alike than we may imagine, and by recognizing our common humanity, we can greatly improve medical and mental health services for transgender and gender non-conforming people. As a facilitator, when you help participants to open their hearts and minds to the experiences of people who are different than themselves, you will take them on a journey to be a better provider for all patients.

WHAT TO DO WHEN THE PHONE RINGS:
Welcoming Transgender Clients

By Maureen Kelly

• • •

Overview & Rationale

This lesson provides healthcare providers—frontline staff, nurses, practitioners, mental health providers, billing staff—an opportunity to talk through the various aspects of a clinical visit with a transgender client and explore how paperwork, language, and clinical and administrative procedures may require important new steps or adaptations to existing systems to provide exceptional and affirming healthcare experiences for transgender clients. During this lesson, participants will have the opportunity to brainstorm various aspects of a clinic visit for a transgender client with a focus on what can be done to create such experiences.

Audience

This lesson is designed for healthcare providers, including frontline staff, nurses, practitioners, mental health providers, and billing staff. This activity works best with 10–30 participants.

Objectives

By the end of this lesson, participants will be able to:
- Describe 2 ways in which staff can be affirming to transgender patients on the phone.
- Explain 2 ways in which check-in and medical in-take procedures can be updated to include transgender patients.
- Identify 2 resources to turn to for additional tips to provide exceptional care to transgender people.

Background Knowledge for Facilitators

It will be useful for facilitators to understand the common barriers that transgender people face when they are trying to access medical care or other social services—particularly when interacting with non-medical staff.

Time

- Preparation: 10 minutes
- Implementation: 60 minutes

Materials

- Large easel paper
- Tape
- Markers
- Copies of *Useful Words and Phrases* handout (1 per participant)
- Copies of *Strategies for Better Serving Transgender Patients* from Lesson 24 on page 206 (1 per participant)

Preparation

- Make copies of the handouts
- Create posters with **PHONE CALLS, CHECK-IN/IN-TAKE, THE VISIT,** and **CHECK-OUT/BILLING** labeled in large print on the top so that each sheet has a different phrase. Hang the sheets of paper around the room. You may wish to have an additional blank sheet for each phrase in case the participants run out of room on the original sheets.

www.TeachingTransgender.com • THE TEACHING TRANSGENDER TOOLKIT • 193

Procedure

1. Break participants into 4 small groups by having them count off by 4's. Direct the participants to stand in front of the paper on the wall that matches the number they were assigned. Pass out 1-2 markers to each group.

2. Tell the group there will be 2 rounds. Explain that this is a brainstorming process, so getting everyone's thoughts and ideas out is important. Direct participants to assume that they are or will be interacting with someone who is transgender.

3. **First round:** Instruct each group that they will have 4 minutes at each poster to list as many possible challenges, worries, concerns, and "how would I . . ." questions about potential interactions with transgender patients as they can. So, for example, for the **PHONE CALLS** poster, what concerns do you have about interacting with transgender patients by phone?

4. Time each group, and after 4 minutes, instruct them to move clockwise to the next poster, at which they will again write as many possible challenges, worries, concerns, and "how would I . . ." questions as they can. Continue this until each group has had 4 minutes at each poster.

5. **Second round:** Instruct each group that will now have 5 minutes at each poster to write out as many possible solutions, fixes, workarounds, suggestions, and examples of best practices related to providing potential affirming services for transgender patients as they can.

6. Time each group and, after 5 minutes, instruct them to move clockwise to the next poster, at which they will again write as many possible solutions, fixes, workarounds, suggestions, and examples of best practices related to the part of the clinical visit written on their paper as they can in 5 minutes. Continue this until each group has had 5 minutes at each poster.

7. Once all of the groups have completed the circuit, instruct the groups to mingle and read the content on each of the posters.

8. Discussion:
Lead the group in reflective discussion about what they find on the posters using some or all of the questions below:

Discussion Questions
- What are your initial reactions to this activity?
- Were their specific topics that were harder or easier to discuss?
- Did you notice any consistent barriers among topics?
- Were there any specific best practices that you want to call out and talk about?
- What are the possible effects of how these systems work on a transgender patient's experience and willingness to seek care?

Talking Points
- Words: Pronouns matter. Names matter. Use what patients ask you to use.
- Paperwork: Whenever possible, add a blank space for the patient to fill in their identity. If that's not an option, explain why it is not an option and honor the patient's self-identification in every other way possible.
- Conversations: Be kind and take your patient's lead.

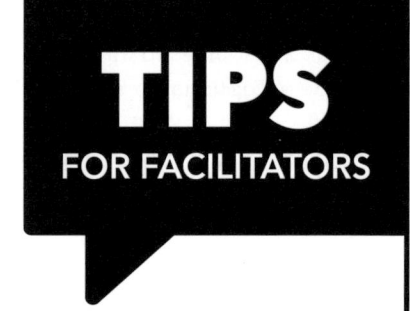

TIPS FOR FACILITATORS

Participants may exhibit frustration or resistance to the topics being presented, particularly if they have a hard time acknowledging that their actions may cause harm—even when it is not intended. It is important to stress the difference between impact and intent, and help participants to see that their actions can have significant ramifications that are not intended.

• • •

Participants may also exhibit frustration or resistance because they feel unsupported or overburdened in their professional roles, and do not wish to add to their workload. It can be useful to validate that this is a challenging process.

9. If using as a standalone lesson, conclude by distributing the *Strategies for Better Serving Transgender Patients* handout (from Lesson 24) and explain that this resource was created by transgender people to help communicate what they would like medical providers to remember when working with them. Also distribute the *Useful Words and Phrases* handout and explain that this will help serve as a reminder of what was covered today.

10. *Optional:* If technology is available in your training setting, guide participants through 2 websites to highlight training modules and continuing education opportunities related to providing transgender care. If technology is not easily accessible, provide the URLs and a verbal description of the resources that are available for continuing education.
    - Center of Excellence for Transgender Health: transhealth.ucsf.edu
    - The National LGBT Health Education Center: fenwayhealth.org

Evaluation Questions

✔ What are 2 ways to be affirming of transgender people when answering the phone?

✔ What are 2 ways check-in and medical in-take procedures can be updated to include transgender patients?

✔ What are 2 resources to turn to for additional tips to provide exceptional care to transgender people?

Talking Points for Each Assigned Area
FACILITATOR RESOURCE

The following are some sample responses for the brainstorming activity that you may hear or wish to add if they do not come up.

PHONE CALLS

CHALLENGE	TIP FOR ADDRESSING
I'm afraid to mis-gender them because it's hard to tell if it's a male or female voice.	Don't use pronouns or gendered language until you ask for what pronoun the patient wishes to be used.
I get worried saying the word "transgender" sometimes.	It's really important to say the word "transgender" as that is the specific kind of service the transgender patient is seeking from you.

CHECK-IN/IN-TAKE

CHALLENGE	TIP FOR ADDRESSING
I don't know what form to give them at check in.	Consider having ONE form with information for both men and women to fill out and the patient can fill in the information that pertains to them. If you cannot combine these into one form, you can hand them all forms for all genders and ask them to fill out the pertinent forms.
I don't want to assume they're here for transgender services if they aren't.	Always ask the patient why they are visiting and provide them with care that pertains to their needs.

THE VISIT

CHALLENGE	TIP FOR ADDRESSING
What name should I use when I call them back for their appointment? What pronouns? I don't know and I don't want to do it wrong?!	Have a procedure in place to ask the patient about this when they call to make the appointment.
I don't want to offend them if I slip up and use the wrong name or pronoun	Quickly recognize your mistake, apologize, and correct yourself.

CHECK-OUT/BILLING

CHALLENGE	TIP FOR ADDRESSING
What if the insurance is registered in a different name or gender from the ones we use during the visit?	Ask the patient under what name and gender they are insured. If it is under a different name or gender let them know that in order to bill insurance the name and gender need to match; this is an administrative procedure and simply letting the patient know—patients are often well aware of this mismatch of names and gender already—that you need to submit insurance claims under the name designated on the insurance card.

PARTICIPANT HANDOUT

Useful Phrases and Words

Two things that can make it difficult for staff to communicate easily with transgender or gender non-conforming patients are confusion about what to do, and fear about saying the wrong thing. Here is some guidance about how to navigate such common concerns.

- When a patient calls to make an appointment and comes out as transgender on the call, consider saying "Okay, great. Is the name you have given me the one you'd like us to call you when you are at your appointment?" You can also follow up and ask specifically: "What pronouns would you like us to use?"

- When a patient is checking in and you are unsure of the name or pronouns consider a simple "How would you like me to address you?" There will be mistakes with names and pronouns. Acknowledging a mistake and offering a sincere, simple, and brief correction and apology is key. If this occurs consider saying, "I just used the wrong name, I'm sorry," and correct yourself.

- Be aware that some patients may wish to be addressed differently in a public space versus a private space, preferring one name when being addressed in a public waiting room or when you are leaving them a voicemail but another name within a private and confidential setting. You can simply ask, "Is that the name you would like to have used throughout for visit?" and "Are there any times or places that you would like me not to use this name or pronoun?"

- Review your paperwork and intake forms and procedures to identify where patients are asked to select a gender marker. Consider whether this is a required inclusion and, if not, consider removing it. There are times when a gender marker may be required (such as insurance billing, official reports, grant reporting, ordering lab work or making referrals). Make sure that there is ample space for a person to indicate how they would like to be addressed, so that assumptions are not made based on the required marker. Consider providing a blank line for preferred name and pronouns for the patient to self-identify rather than check boxes.

- Let transgender patients know if and when you are required to use their legal name. This may be a requirement for insurance billing or other official paperwork; inform the patient by saying, "I wanted to let you know we will need to use your legal name to submit this paperwork, but we will continue to use the name that is most affirming for you in all of our other interactions."

- Remember that being "outed" as transgender can be a major safety risk for that individual. It is essential to consider if/how this information will be recorded, with whom it will be shared and what the potential consequences of disclosure might be. Let the client know who will have access to the information, under what circumstances and why, so that they can create a safety plan as needed. Avoid referring to the client as "the transgender client" or having conversations in spaces where this information might be overheard.

23

THE VIEW FROM HERE:
Accessing Medical Care from a Transgender Perspective

By Eli R. Green, PhD & Courtney Weaver, PhD

• • •

Overview & Rationale

This lesson helps healthcare providers increase their cultural competency and sensitivity when working with transgender patients by raising awareness of the discrimination that transgender people experience when accessing medical care. Through the use of video clips and case examples, this session provides a starting point from which providers can begin to understand—as a core piece of cultural competency—some of the reservations transgender people may have about accessing medical facility. This lesson is designed to be paired with **Lesson 24: It's Not Always About Transition** on page 206.

Audience

This lesson works well with medical students, and current medical/health care practitioners. This activity works best with groups 10-30.

Objectives

By the end of this lesson, participants will be able to:
- Describe 3 major barriers that currently inhibit transgender people from accessing culturally competent medical care
- Identify 2 strategies for being more culturally competent when working with transgender patients

Background Knowledge for Facilitators

Facilitators will benefit from understanding the common narratives of transgender people's experiences with medical care—particularly stories of negative experiences. Familiarity with the *Injustice at Every Turn: A Report of the National Transgender Discrimination Survey* results related to medical discrimination will be helpful in managing resistance. While an in-depth understanding of the specifics of medical transition is not necessary to facilitate this lesson, some understanding of how transition works and the available options will be useful.

Time

- Preparation: 15 minutes, plus 75 minutes to watch documentaries
- Implementation: 60-75 minutes

Materials
- Index Cards
- Documentary film "Southern Comfort"
- Computer with Internet access, projector and speakers
- Copies of the *Transgender People Accessing Care Case Examples* handout (1 per participant)

Preparation
- Make copies of the handouts.
- Watch the entire *Southern Comfort* documentary to become familiar with Robert's life and story. Watch the video of Jay and become familiar with his case: *www.huffingtonpost.com/2015/06/15/transgender-health-care_n_7587506.html*
- Read through all of the vignettes and be familiar with the talking points corresponding to each one.
- Prepare all appropriate audio/visual equipment so that it is ready to play. Cue the film at 13:14, press "pause" and black out the screen, so that the documentary will not require other preparation (other than turning on the screen and pressing play) during the presentation.

Procedure
1. Explain: You will be exploring some of the challenges that transgender people face when they are trying to access medical care. The lesson will begin with a clip from a documentary called *Southern Comfort,* which records the last year of Robert Eads's life. Robert was a transgender man who was diagnosed with ovarian cancer, and was refused treatment by over two-dozen medical providers. It took him over a year to find a provider to treat him, but by that point the cancer had metastasized and was too far advanced to prevent his death. Robert died in 1999. The clip that we are going to watch briefly addresses Robert's struggle with trying to find medical care.

2. Cue film at: 13:14 and play it until: 15:53. Lead participants in a group discussion based on the *Southern Comfort: Facilitator's Guide.* The length of the discussion will vary based on the amount of time available and participant engagement.

3. Explain that for the next portion of the lesson you will be using some case examples to explore the common barriers and challenges that transgender people face when accessing medical care.

4. Divide the class into small groups of 3-5 people. Assign each group a number (1-5) and explain that this number corresponds to the case example that their group will read and discuss. If there are more groups than case examples available, then assign the same case example to 2 groups.

5. Instruct participants to read their assigned case example and then, as a small group, answer the questions at the end. Explain to the participants that they will be coming together at the end of this activity to share their answers/reactions with the rest of the group.

6. Allow participants 10 minutes for group reading/discussion/processing. (Note: participants may not be able to get through all the questions in the time allotted, depending on the depth of their conversation). During small-group discussion, the facilitator should rotate around the room, stopping to listen to each group and making sure the group is on task. Following group discussion, the facilitator should direct attention back to the front of the space and then go around to each group to discuss their case example.

7. In turn, ask each group to briefly summarize the contents of the case example and have one representative from each small group share what the group learned, based on the questions that were asked at the end of the case examples. Use the *Transgender People Accessing Care Case Examples: Facilitator's Guide* to guide the discussion and cover key talking points.

Evaluation Questions

✔ What are 3 major barriers that currently inhibit transgender people from accessing culturally sensitive medical care?

✔ What are 2 strategies that you can use to make your services more affirming for transgender people?

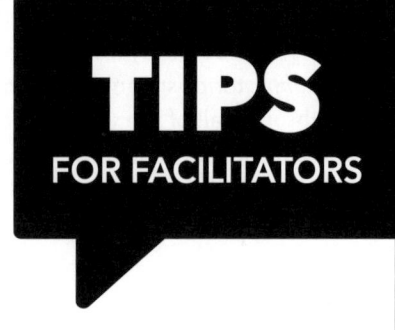

TIPS FOR FACILITATORS

One common source of pushback on this lesson is that participants assume that what happened to Robert doesn't happen today, or that it doesn't happen in a particular location or community. It is important to help participants understand that this is not true, and that these situations do still happen frequently everywhere.

• • •

It is also important to note that because the transgender communities are small, experiences such as Robert's will be shared widely within an individual's transgender community, which may discourage people from seeking care. This may result in the expectation of poor treatment when accessing medical care, which will increase anxiety about receiving treatment. As a result, many transgender people report postponing or delaying medical care until a condition has become urgent or is an emergency.

• • •

Participants may resist the idea that medical providers are harming transgender patients and will often make excuses to explain why a provider might have denied a person care or why a transgender person may have misread a situation. It can be useful to help providers see that, regardless of the cause or intention, the end result is still that transgender people do not feel safe in most healthcare settings and are not receiving needed medical care.

• • •

Be prepared to explain that much of the discrimination that transgender people experience comes in the form of microaggressions, such as mis-gendering, using the wrong name or non-affirming pronouns, or cultural insensitivity, such as announcing someone's transgender identity in a public space, referring to someone as a transgender patient, or asking inappropriate questions that are not relevant to the person's presenting concerns.

REFERENCE:
Davis, K. (Ed.). (2012). *Southern Comfort*. Films Transit International.

Southern Comfort:
FACILITATOR'S GUIDE

Discussion Questions and Talking Points

1. First, before we talk about your reactions to this clip, does anyone have any questions about what you just saw?

2. What are your reactions to this clip?

3. Robert died in 1999. What do you think has changed about the medical care that transgender people receive today? Do you think that cases like Robert's still happen?
   - *Talking Point: Explain that similar cases do still happen today, such as the case of Jay Kallio, a transgender man whose doctor refused to tell him that he had breast cancer because he was transgender (Buxton, 2015).*
   - *Optional: Show video of Jay talking about his story and his diagnosis: www.huffingtonpost.com/2015/06/15/transgender-health-care_n_7587506.html*

4. As the title suggests, this occurred in the Deep South. Do you think this type of treatment is isolated to conservative and rural settings? Why or why not?
   - *Talking Point: Jay Kallio's case happened in New York City (Buxton, 2015). Prejudice and discrimination happen across medical settings, whether urban or rural. Nearly 20% of transgender people are outright denied medical care because of being transgender (Grant et al., 2011), and 1 out of 4 transgender people who have already medically transitioned are denied non-transition-related medical care. Many transgender people try to avoid sharing that they are transgender in medical settings (when not medically necessary) to avoid the higher rates of discrimination that occur in conjunction with disclosure.*

5. In the clip several doctors said that Robert's presence would make their other patients uncomfortable. What are some other reasons that 26 doctors and hospitals refused to treat him?
   - *Possible reasons: Their own discomfort, lack of knowledge about transgender people, believing that being transgender requires someone to be seen by a provider who is a specialist in medical transition, concerns about backlash from other patients, staff discomfort.*

6. What effects do you think Robert's being turned down by so many people have had on his emotional and physical health?
   - *Possible effects: Increased depression, fear, anxiety, distrust of other doctors, and ultimately death.*

Transgender People Accessing Care Case Examples:
FACILITATOR'S GUIDE

Vignette 1

- *Positives* – The doctor asked what James likes to be called and then used that name. The doctor explained the effects of testosterone on the body, but also ordered a pregnancy test to ease James's mind.
- *Negatives* – Asked impertinent and impolite questions about James's body.

TALKING POINTS:

- Even if the doctor was just trying to make a joke or had otherwise benign intentions, it does not mean the patient will interpret it the same way. Transgender people are often nervous with new medical providers, and have reasonable expectations that they will face discrimination or prejudice. Research has shown this is particularly true for transgender men, who report higher levels of prejudice and discrimination from medical providers.
- Transgender people engage in a range of sex acts based on their desires, partners, and comfort with their bodies. It is important not to make assumptions about the gender of partners, the type of sex acts being engaged in, or a person's degree of comfort with their bodies.

Vignette 2

- *Positives* – The secretary was very helpful, pointing out a place on her form where Pam could write her gender choice.
- *Negatives* – The doctor asked probing questions, urged Pam to undergo a physical examination even though Pam may or may not be comfortable doing that just yet, refused to use the affirming pronouns, and diagnosed her with a mental disorder and suggested a psychiatrist without first knowing Pam's medical history.

TALKING POINTS:

- The secretary's actions clearly indicate a level of cultural competency, and respectful behavior. When accessing care, transgender people have to engage with many people. It is essential that security, front desk staff, intake staff and other frontline staff have transgender-related cultural competency training.
- Medical transition is an appropriate medical treatment for transgender people, and should not be considered a sign of mental illness. Likewise, it is important to remember that all transgender people need access to non-transition-related medical care as well.

Vignette 3

- *Positives* – Kelly informed the exam room nurse of the secretary and the other nurse's inappropriate behavior. The same nurse informed the doctor, who issued a verbal warning to the secretary and male nurse. The doctor asked Kelly to help him make his office more transgender friendly.
- *Negatives* – The secretary made a big deal out of the gender issue, and decided to mock the patient as opposed to helping her, humiliating Kelly by making her stand up in front of all the other patients in the waiting room while they laugh at her. Refused to answer any of Kelly's questions.

TALKING POINTS:

- Not all people who are gender non-conforming are transgender. It is important not to make assumptions about gender identity.
- Not all gender non-conforming or transgender people wish to serve in an advocacy or educational role. There are people who are professional facilitators who are able to help provide training and education. A patient should never be required to educate their provider about their identity.

Vignette 4

- *Positives* – Politely approached the presenter and asked for scientific references. The doctor realized that some of those sources are extremely biased. The doctor also gave the presenter more LGBT-friendly resources that might be more useful.

- *Negatives* – Presentation is riddled with falsehoods and stereotypes that are old and ingrained, which also hints at reparative therapy. Sources that presenter used were full of bias, which the doctor presenting didn't check on. Presenter was stubborn and told LGBT-friendly doctor to shove off.

TALKING POINTS:
- This vignette highlights negative attitudes and beliefs about transgender people. The person is clearly very anti-transgender– although much prejudice against transgender people comes from well-intentioned people who mean no harm.

- This is an excellent opportunity for an ally to speak up and intervene in a situation marked by prejudice or discrimination.

Vignette 5

- *Positives* – The ER staff treated the victim with the necessary care despite any apparent gender disparity. The EMS staff was confronted about its incompetency and reported to a higher authority. The doctor clearly is an ally of the transgender population, and made it known.

- *Negatives* – The victim arrived untreated to the ER even though her injuries were life-threatening. The EMS team stood around and gawked, as though the victim was an act in a side show. When the doctor complained about their negligence, they muttered something derogatory under their breath, assuming that since the doctor is an ally he/she is one of "them."

TALKING POINTS:
- While this vignette seems implausible, this scenario is based on real cases. It is a strong indicator of the amount of work that needs to be done with all medical professionals to ensure that transgender people receive full medical care, particularly in emergency situations when they are unable to advocate for themselves.

For more information on the factual portions of Vignette 5, please see the following articles:

Shaun Smith (2013): Available online at: http://bit.ly/1EF1um8
Tyra Hunter (1995): Available online at: http://bit.ly/1AxTJh2

PARTICIPANT HANDOUT

Case Examples

TRANSGENDER PEOPLE ACCESSING CARE

1. James comes into your office. Biologically, he was born a female, but identifies as a man and expresses his gender in a masculine way. He has had a bilateral mastectomy, but has not had a hysterectomy or oophorectomy, and is on a regimen of testosterone. He has recently had a one-night stand with another man. During intercourse, the condom broke, and the man ejaculated into James' vagina. James is now worried that he is pregnant. The doctor enters the exam room. The first thing she does is ask what name he likes to be called. James tells her, and the doctor replies with, "So I guess you're not just an uber-butch lesbian then?" James politely responds with "No, I am not" and then proceeds to tell the doctor what the problem is. The doctor explains that it is rare for someone to become pregnant while on a consistent regimen of testosterone, but recommends that they run a quick pregnancy test, just to make sure.

   - Can you identify some positive aspects of this situation?
   - Can you identify some negative aspects of this situation?
   - How do you think James felt during this appointment?

2. Pam is a first-year college student and identifies as a transgender woman. She goes into her campus health center for the first time during her first week of class. When entering the outer office, Pam has to fill out some new forms. She does this to the best of her ability, asking the secretary questions about what to put for the "gender" part of the form. The secretary points out that there is a third box on the form that can be checked if one does not identify as either male or female. Pam thanks her, finishes the form, and is ushered into an exam room. When the doctor enters the room, Pam begins to tell her about her required hormone regimen, as she has marked that she is a male-to-female transsexual. The doctor begins to ask Pam very probing and personal questions ("Oh, do you have a history of sexual abuse?"; "So you intend to cut off your penis?"), suggests that Pam undergo a complete and thorough physical examination, refuses to use female pronouns, and then recommends that Pam see a psychiatrist for Dissociative Identity Disorder. Pam leaves the health center, literally shaking with emotion.

   - Can you identify the positive aspects of this situation?
   - Can you identify the negative aspects of this situation?
   - How would you react, if you were in Pam's situation?

3. Kelly identifies as female, uses female pronouns, and dresses androgynously. When out in public, Kelly is often identified by strangers as male. This is especially likely when she begins to talk due to her rather deep voice. She goes in to her new physician's office. In the waiting room, she is asked by the secretary to fill out some new patient forms. When she returns them to the secretary, the secretary looks them over and asks Kelly to remain where she is standing. The secretary picks up her phone and requests that a nurse be called out front. When the nurse appears, the secretary takes Kelly's form over to him, and they begin to talk in low voices. Kelly keeps asking them what the issue is, but they refuse to answer and actually begin to laugh. When Kelly is finally allowed into an exam room to see her new doctor, she is ashamed but angry, and relates what happened to another nurse who is taking her vitals. This nurse is also outraged and informs the doctor, who serves a verbal warning to the secretary and male nurse involved. The doctor then speaks with Kelly about how he can train his office staff to be more transgender friendly, even asking if Kelly can help him.

   - Can you identify the positive aspects of this situation?
   - Can you identify the negative aspects of this situation?
   - How can Kelly help the doctor train his staff? Should it be Kelly's responsibility?

4. At an annual medical conference, a presentation on LGBT health care and concerns is given, so you attend. The presentation is riddled with falsehoods, such as that all homosexuals will try to recruit you, all transgender-identified individuals suffer from psychosis, etc., and that you as their doctor can teach them how to repress their urges to express themselves. You, being an LGBT-friendly provider, are outraged. You approach the presenter following the presentation, and ask him where he found the research to back up some of the claims that he made. You are vaguely familiar with the resources he gives you, but you know that they are extremely biased, based more on religion than anything else. Not wanting to insult him, you gently suggest some more LGBT-friendly resources that he can use, at which point he tells you to stuff it and walks off.

   - Can you identify the positive steps that were taken by the LGBT-friendly provider?
   - Can you identify the negative aspects of this situation?
   - As a medical professional, would you have reacted differently? Why or why not?

5. You are a physician in the ER. One night, a traffic accident occurs and the victim is rushed to your hospital. When the victim arrives, the doors of the ambulance are opened and the entire EMS team is standing around the gurney, staring at the victim. Apparently, when the team had arrived on the scene, they had thought that the victim was female, as that was how she presented, but when cutting off the victim's clothes to assess injuries, they found that she had a penis. Stunned and repulsed, the EMS team ceases all activity, and she arrives at the ER untreated. You and your staff have to work in double time in order to save the victim's life, while the EMS team hangs around and gawks. When the patient has reached a stable condition, you scold the EMS team, asking "What's the matter with you?" They try to explain why they demonstrated such incompetence while you listen calmly. When they have finished you inform them that you will be reporting them for negligence, and that if they ever try something like that again, they'll have a lot more to answer to. As they walk out, you hear one of them mutter something derogatory under their breath.

   - Can you identify the positive aspects of this situation?
   - Can you identify the negative aspects of this situation?
   - How would you have reacted if you were the doctor in this situation? Would you have handled things differently? Why or why not?

24
IT'S NOT ALWAYS ABOUT
Transition...

Overview & Rationale

This lesson helps healthcare providers increase their cultural competency and sensitivity when working with transgender patients by exploring the impact of the discrimination that transgender people experience when accessing medical care. Through the use of case examples and analysis of best practices, this session increases awareness of the specific challenges that transgender people face when accessing medical care as well as ways in which providers can convey support to transgender patients and encourage proactive work to create affirming spaces. This lesson is designed to be paired with **Lesson 23: The View from Here: Accessing Medical Care from a Transgender Perspective** on page 198.

Audience

This lesson works well with providers who are relatively new to learning about transgender people and for more advanced participants who have a strong knowledge base but will benefit from increased understanding of the challenges of non-affirming medical care. This lesson works best with groups of 20 or less.

Objectives

By the end of this lesson, participants will be able to:
- List 3 barriers that transgender patients face when they are accessing medical services.
- Name 1 way in which these barriers affect how transgender people make decisions regarding accessing medical care.
- Provide 1 strategy that can be used to help create a more affirming space for transgender patients.

Background Knowledge for Facilitators

It will be particularly useful for facilitators to have background knowledge of the challenges that transgender people face when accessing general (non-transgender-specific) medical services, such as preventative health screenings, specialized medical treatment, and emergency care.

Time

- Preparation: 10 minutes
- Implementation: 60 minutes

Materials

- *Stories of Transgender Patient Experiences* (1 per participant)
- *Strategies for Better Serving Transgender Patients* (1 per participant)
- Easel paper & markers
- Masking tape
- Good/Meh/Bad signs and activity cards

Preparation

- Make copies of the handouts.
- Print off the Good/Meh/Bad signs and activity cards from: www.teachingtransgender.com/printables (PW: TTTprep15). Alternatively, prepare large index cards or posters with each of the items from the Good/Meh/Bad facilitator's resource on page 212, so that each of the statements is on a separate card or poster. Keep the statements separated into piles by row.
- Create and hang Good, Meh, and Bad signs on the wall with enough distance between each so that the participants can tape the activity cards underneath.

Procedure

1. Ask participants to take a few minutes and create a list of the top 5 reasons that patients seek their medical services. (For example: annual physical, the flu, medication refills, etc.). Once everyone has created their list, ask participants to share 1 item from the list (without repeating a prior response). Record their responses on the easel paper so that you have a list of at least 10 common reasons that people access medical care.

2. Explain that transgender people have the same medical concerns as people who are not transgender, but often have significant challenges when they are trying to access medical care. National research has indicated the following talking points:
   - Of the 6,456 respondents to the *National Transgender Discrimination Survey,* 19% reported that they were refused medical care because of their identity, with 28% reporting that they were harassed by medical providers, and 2% reporting that they were victims of violence in medical settings (Grant et al., 2011).
   - Many transgender people do not disclose their transgender status unless they deem it medically necessary (Grant et al., 2011). Those who do so face higher rates of discrimination. Transgender people who have undergone some form of medical transition are at higher risk for discrimination in medical settings, with 1 out of 4 people reporting that they were denied medical treatment. (The denial of service was not specific to accessing medical transition and includes access to general medical care and emergency services.)
   - Transgender People of Color are disproportionately impacted (Grant et al., 2011), as 34% of Black, 36% of Latino/a, and 47% of Asian & Pacific Islander (API) transgender people actively postpone medical care out of fear of discrimination. Moreoever, 21% of Black and 23% of Latino/a transgender people were denied medical care because they were transgender.

3. Break the participants into 5 small groups, and pass out the **Stories of Transgender Patients** handout. Assign each of the groups one of the stories, ask them to read it and briefly discuss the 3 questions on the back. Ask the participants to share their discussion points. Use the *Stories of Transgender Patient Experiences: Facilitator's Guide* to guide the discussion and correct/add information as needed.

4. Keeping the participants in their small groups, explain that the next part of the lesson will involve a brief activity that will help participants better understand how providers can be proactive in creating safer and more affirming services for transgender people. Give each of the groups one of the stacks of three cards, and ask them to figure out what indicates BEST/MEH/BAD, and tape their responses to the wall in the appropriate place.

5. Compare each of the responses with the answers on the *Best/Meh/Bad Facilitator Resource* and make any necessary corrections. Ask the participants to explain their rationale for placing the cards where they did (particularly for any that were incorrectly placed). Provide additional information and clarification as needed.

TIPS FOR FACILITATORS

Medical providers often have the reputation of preferring didactic PowerPoint lectures to interactive learning. This is generally exacerbated by short training times and conflicting demands during that time. Don't be discouraged by this reputation. Many medical providers genuinely appreciate the opportunity to engage with materials in a more involved and in-depth manner. It can be helpful to explain up front that you will not be using a traditional format for your presentation.

• • •

For the Good/Meh/Bad activity, participants may push back against the particular placement of each of the cards in a given category. Provided that their explanation is affirming, it is more important that participants base their reasoning on transgender-affirming concepts than it is to come to a "correct" response.

Discussion Questions:
- How did you determine what was a best practice versus one that was "meh" or bad?
- Which practices do you think occur most commonly? Why?
- How does seeing providers who are not transgender inclusive or affirming affect a patient's willingness to seek out medical services?
- Which of these best practices can you commit to incorporating into your own patient care?

6. Ask participants to reflect on where their own medical practices or locations fall on this spectrum, and identify areas where they might advocate for improvement. Distribute the *Strategies for Better Serving Transgender Patients* handout, and ask participants to identify 1 strategy that they feel they would be able to implement after this training.

Evaluation Questions

✔ Based on what we have discussed today, what are 3 barriers that transgender patients face when they are accessing medical services?

✔ What is 1 way in which these barriers affect how transgender people make decisions regarding if and when they will access medical care?

✔ What is 1 strategy that can be used to help create a more affirming space for transgender patients?

Stories of Transgender Patient Experiences:
FACILITATOR'S GUIDE

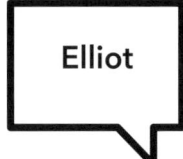 Elliot

1. **What were the patient's presenting medical concerns?**
   - Seeking a skin check, due to family history of skin cancer

2. **How did Elliot's being transgender impact the experience of accessing care?**
   - The insurance card's incongruent gender marker caused mis-gendering and additional questions
   - The staff used non-affirming pronouns
   - Having to come out to all of the medical students and staff caused discomfort
   - Genitals are exposed

3. **How did their prior experiences inform/affect the patient's decisions about accessing care?**
   - Postponed screenings to avoid dealing with the stress, which increases risk

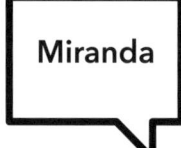 Miranda

1. **What were the patient's presenting medical concerns?**
   - Pelvic discomfort, pain while urinating
   - Sharp stabbing pains

2. **How did Miranda's being transgender impact the experience accessing care?**
   - The staff asked inappropriate questions, used non-affirming language
   - The person inserting the catheter was rough and looked revolted
   - Cannot afford insurance, possibly due to employment discrimination

3. **How did Miranda's prior experiences inform/affect decisions about accessing care?**
   - Having been treated poorly before resulted in her putting off getting treated, in turn resulting in a medically urgent situation

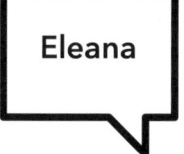 Eleana

1. **What were the patient's presenting medical concerns?**
   - Has a long-term chronic illness

2. **How did Eleana's being transgender impact the experience accessing care?**
   - Having to decide whether to disclose and deal with the impact of disclosing
   - Not having the option to find transgender-affirming specialists
   - Managing doctors' assumptions that chronic illness is related to medical transition

3. **How did Eleana's prior experiences inform/affect decisions about accessing care?**
   - The stress of navigating non-affirming providers had a negative impact on health

PARTICIPANT HANDOUT

Stories of...

TRANSGENDER PATIENT EXPERIENCES

Elliott's Story

I have a history of skin cancer in my family, and so I have to go to the dermatologist a few times a year to make sure that I don't have any emerging problems. Every time I go in for a screening, I have to navigate several additional barriers because I am transgender. First, my insurance card reflects the sex I was assigned at birth, to ensure that I can access related coverage if needed. But rather than having my affirming gender recognized at check-in, the front desk always tells me that they made a mistake with my record and had incorrectly recorded my gender. I then have to explain and ask them to leave the marker alone. Then, when I am called to the back, the person always calls my name using pronouns based on the sex assigned in my records. This usually happens in front of a full waiting room, and the front desk publically outs me to all the people who are there. Then, when I get to the back, I have to see the screening nurse and two medical students before I can see my doctor. I have to come out to each of them; otherwise there is a lot of confusion and discomfort for all of us. Then when my doctor comes in and conducts the exam (in front of the medical students), she requires me to pull down my underwear so that she can examine my skin, which means that my genitals are exposed. I have never had anyone say anything negative during these visits, and everything has been handled professionally, but the stress of having to navigate being outed and having to come out makes me postpone appointments—which, given my history of melanoma, poses a significant risk for early detection.

(Read and respond to the discussion questions on the back of this sheet).

Miranda's Story

I hate going to the doctor because there are always issues related to my being visibly transgender. Someone either says something rude, asks me inappropriate questions, or is just generally unpleasant. It's not always the medical staff; often it is the other people who are accessing services there—security or front desk staff. I can honestly say that I have never had a positive experience at the doctor. Even with Obamacare, I can't afford insurance, so routine care is totally unavailable to me. Last year, I was experiencing some pelvic discomfort and trouble urinating. I figured that it wasn't a really big deal and decided to try drinking extra water and some cranberry supplements. I ignored it for as long as I could, but in the middle of the night I started having sharp, stabbing pains in my side. I got really scared that my appendix was going to burst or something, so I went to the ER. As usual, I was treated rudely, pointed at, laughed at, and I overheard the nursing assistants talking about the "tranny" in Room # 4. If I hadn't been in so much pain, I would have gotten up and walked out. It turned out that I had kidney stones, and had to have a catheter. Because I have not been able to afford genital surgery, it was a particularly grueling process—the person who was inserting it looked visibly revolted by me, and was not particularly gentle about it. I can't stand being treated like I am less than everyone else. It just makes an already bad situation worse.

(Read and respond to the discussion questions on the back of this sheet).

> **Eleana's Story**
>
> I have been battling a long-term chronic illness for several years, and I have had to see a significant number of specialists to try to figure out what is wrong. Every time I see one of these doctors, I have to decide whether or not I am going to come out as transgender. I don't want to hide information that might have an impact on figuring out what is wrong with me, but it is also really uncomfortable to have to tell them that I was assigned a different sex at birth. I have never been denied treatment, but I have had to consistently manage the doctors' reactions to the information, and often I have to answer extra questions about what it means to be transgender (that are not related to my illness or treatment). There was one time when a neurologist said "Oh, okay" but started visibly shaking and accidentally knocked papers off of his desk. At other times, doctors have insinuated that I am chronically ill because I medically transitioned—even though my illness did not emerge until many years after that—which clearly indicates a lack of knowledge about medical transition. I did find a doctor who was supportive and sought out additional information on her own, but I did not want the office staff to know, so we had to figure out what to put into the notes in my medical record so that it would not catch their attention. These experiences don't even include all of the other types of medical staff that I have to interact with when getting various tests or treatments. Because I am chronically ill, my body can't handle extra stress, and having to navigate this contributes to my physical exhaustion. It's hard enough to be sick without having to come out all the time.

DISCUSSION QUESTIONS:

1. What were the patients' presenting medical concerns?

___

2. How did their being transgender affect their experience accessing care?

___

3. How did their prior experiences inform/affect their decisions about accessing care?

___

BEST/MEH/BAD
FACILITATOR RESOURCE

DIRECTIONS: Distribute copies of the cards to participants and ask them to determine the appropriate classification. Once they have decided, ask them to tape the cards under the appropriate heading. Use this as an answer key.

Good	Meh	Bad
(1) Medical provider asks for affirming pronouns from the patient and uses them.	(1) Medical provider avoids using pronouns and gendered language for the patient.	(1) Medical provider assumes pronouns and does not check with the patient.
(2) Medical provider uses transgender-inclusive sex history questions with all patients.	(2) Medical provider identifies possible need for transgender-inclusive sex history questions and creates them on the fly.	(2) Medical provider does not use or have access to transgender-inclusive sex history questions.
(3) Medical providers include transgender-identity options on all their patient forms, including information on insurance handling. Staff is trained to handle these transgender-inclusive forms with sensitivity.	(3) Medical providers include transgender-identity options on some of their forms, but do not ask about insurance handling, or train the staff on proper use.	(3) Medical providers do not have transgender-inclusive options on their patient forms.
(4) Medical care facility has single-stall, gender-neutral restrooms.	(4) Medical care facility has multi-stall gender-neutral restrooms.	(4) Medical care facility does not have gender-neutral or single-stall restrooms.
(5) Medical provider is knowledgeable and sensitive to transgender issues, and feels comfortable discussing related client needs.	(5) Medical provider has limited knowledge, but is empathetic to transgender issues, and asks a lot of questions to ascertain information about these issues.	(5) Medical provider has no knowledge of transgender issues, uses insensitive language, or body language that shows distaste for/discomfort with transgender people.

PARTICIPANT HANDOUT

Strategies for...

BETTER SERVING TRANSGENDER PATIENTS*

- **Transgender people are a lot more like cisgender people ("those whose self-identity conforms with the gender that corresponds to their biological sex") than unlike them.** Get to know transgender people as *people*.

- **Focus on the client's specific needs, rather than on their gender identity** (unless the client's issue is specifically gender related). You don't have to be an endocrinologist or gender specialist to help transgender patients, and they probably will not expect this of you. Transgender people need routine preventative care in a safe and welcoming environment, just like everyone. In the words of transgender educator Rebecca Kling: *"I often joke that I don't go to the trans-dentist to get my trans-teeth trans-cleaned. That's a healthcare situation where my trans identity is irrelevant."*

- **Don't rely solely on your clients to educate you.** Do your own homework as well. Check out the resources on the following page as a great place to start! Also accept that there are things you don't/won't know or understand, and *be willing to be humble and listen*.

- **Offer sex and gender blanks on the intake forms, rather than male/female check boxes.** Ask ALL clients about preferred names and pronouns, including those who "appear" cisgender. This questions assumptions based on appearances, and offers a teachable moment for cisgender patients to understand why these issues matter. Also respect that not all transgender patients may feel comfortable disclosing this information to you.

- **Understand the power you have as a provider when navigating insurance and other bureaucratic challenges.** Help your clients determine what services their insurance (if they have it) will cover, offer support with obtaining insurance (if needed), and work with your billing department to determine the best way to code services to maximize coverage.

- **Understand the importance of intersectionality.** Transgender people who are People of Color, disabled, female-identified, or a member of another oppressed group may struggle with discrimination on multiple levels. Be sensitive as to how intersectionality may affect the healthcare experiences of your clients.

- **Involve transgender people in your practice.** Hire transgender-identified health educators and advocates to educate you and your staff about inclusivity. Invite transgender people to apply for open positions in your practice or organization. Promote your practice or organization as a transgender-affirming space.

- **Network with transgender-affirming clinicians and organizations in your field.** They may be able to offer additional models and strategies for creating more transgender-affirming environments, and can serve as referrals for clients when needed.

---

* Crowdsourced from transgender and gender non-conforming people and those who serve them; compiled by Bianca Jarvis, MPH. Used with permission.

Educational Resources:

Understanding Health Disparities in Transgender Populations www.indiana.edu/~isitjust/

The National Transgender Discrimination Survey Report www.endtransdiscrimination.org/report.html

Transgender Health Learning Center (UCSF) www.transhealth.ucsf.edu/trans?page=lib-00-00

American Medical Student Association: Transgender Health
www.amsa.org/advocacy/action-committees/gender-sexuality/transgender-health/

Resources for Transgender People and Their Friends and Families (pamphlets)
www.kinseyconfidential.org/resources-transgender-people-friends-families

Organizations:

UCSF Center of Excellence for Transgender Health (SF) www.transhealth.ucsf.edu

Tom Waddell Transgender Clinic (SF) www.sfdph.org/dph/comupg/oservices/medSvs/hlthCtrs/TransgenderHlthCtr.asp

Howard Brown Health Center (Chicago) www.howardbrown.org/

Chicago Women's Health Center (Chicago) www.chicagowomenshealthcenter.org/services-page/trans-health-services

Lurie Children's Hospital Gender & Sex Development Program (Chicago)
www.luriechildrens.org/en-us/care-services/specialties-services/gender-program/Pages/index.aspx

Callen Lorde Transgender Health Services (NYC)
www.callen-lorde.org/our-services/sexual-health-clinic/transgender-health-services/

Fenway Institute National LGBT Health Education Center (Boston) www.lgbthealtheducation.org

25

PROVIDING TRANSGENDER-AFFIRMING THERAPY
Applying Pre-Existing Clinical Strengths

...

Overview & Rationale

The lesson gives participants the opportunity to increase awareness and empathy for the challenges related to having a transgender identity, with a specific focus on how this may affect a person's access to and engagement in therapeutic settings. The lesson allows participants to consider and explore themes common to the experience of many transgender people, through the lens of the therapeutic process and setting. Vignettes provide the opportunity to assist participants in making connections between informational content and lived experiences. Through this process, participants will develop a better understanding of themes that many transgender people face, common issues and barriers for transgender people in therapeutic settings, and will be better prepared to act as informed allies to or advocates for transgender clients.

Audience

This lesson is designed for mental health counselors, therapists and other clinicians. This activity works best with groups of 10–30.

Objectives

By the end of this lesson, participants will be able to:
- Describe 2 reasons transgender people seek out therapeutic and mental health services.
- Identify 3 commonalities between the mental health needs of transgender and cisgender clients.

Background Knowledge for Facilitators

It will be useful for facilitators to understand mental health and therapeutic settings, related clinical skills, and common barriers that transgender people face when accessing these services. It will also be helpful for facilitators to understand the WPATH Standards of Care, letter-writing requirements that support medical transition, local legal requirements for changing a person's name or gender marker on identity documents, and local affirming referral options for people who wish to transition medically.

Time

- Preparation: 10 minutes
- Implementation: 75 minutes

Materials

- Copies of *Clinical Vignettes & Discussion Questions* handout (1 per participant)

Preparation

- Make copies of the handouts.
- Research local and online resources that can provide additional information, continuing education, or referrals on transgender topics for counselors and therapists.

Procedure

1. Ask participants to break into small groups of 4, 5 or 6 people (depending on the size of the group). Once participants have settled into their groups, distribute the vignettes handout.

2. Assign each group 2-3 of the vignettes to work on. (Depending on the number of groups, there may be multiple groups working on the same vignette). Instruct participants to read their assigned vignettes and then answer the questions in their small groups. Explain that they will have 30 minutes to discuss the vignettes and the questions, and that they will be reporting back to the large group. During this time, rotate through the small groups and provide assistance as needed.

3. After 30 minutes, ask everyone to return to the large group and have each group take turns reporting. Have someone from each group read the vignettes their group discussed aloud to the large group. Ask the groups who worked on each vignette to share some of their answers to the discussion questions as well as any common themes that arose.

4. Once all or a majority of the vignettes have been discussed, use the following discussion questions to lead a large-group discussion.

   Discussion Questions:
   1. What themes were found in all of the vignettes?
   2. What were some common feelings the people in the vignettes expressed or manifested?
   3. How can you as a therapist support transgender people?
   4. In what ways are transgender and cisgender clients similar?
   5. If using this as a standalone lesson, conclude the activity by inviting participants to share 1 thing they learned during the session and 1 thing they will do in their clinical work as a result of today's session. This can be done as a whip (where each person shares in turn) or by simply having participants share as they feel ready.

Evaluation Questions

✔ What are 2 reasons transgender people seek out therapeutic and mental health services?

✔ What are 3 commonalities between transgender and cisgender clients when they are seeking support?

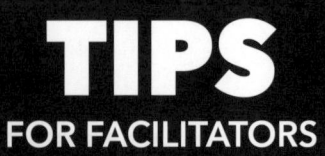

TIPS FOR FACILITATORS

Clarify that not all transgender-related therapy is about transition; much is often about coming out to family/friends/partners, venting fears, navigating challenges, and determining aspects of self. It is important to remember that not all transgender people wish to transition medically. It may be irrelevant to their current therapeutic work.

•••

It is important to remember that participants may become fixated on the medical aspects of transgender experience. Help facilitate participants' questions, acknowledging how medical and legal issues may be fascinating or complicated, while assisting them in assigning these an appropriate but not undue degree of significance.

•••

Providers may be particularly concerned about the vignettes that involve writing letters to support medical transition because it potentially involves medical and legal systems with which they may not be familiar. Additional resources and support for this are available via the WPATH website: www.wpath.org.

PARTICIPANT HANDOUT

Clinical Vignettes

AND DISCUSSION QUESTIONS

1. Nafeesa's partner has recently disclosed to her that they identify as transgender and Nafeesa is accessing therapy so that she can have a safe space to work through the complexities of her feelings.

2. Ronni is struggling with sexual orientation and gender identity, and is not sure who they are, or what labels they should use. They are coming to you seeking a safe space in which to work through their identity-related thoughts and feelings.

3. Stefanie's 7-year-old son has recently been saying that they wish they had been born as a girl, and is upset that God made a mistake. She is unsure of how to support her child, and needs a safe space to manage her feelings and concerns.

4. Taja is a 35-year-old transgender woman who is considering using hormones, but is having a lot of anxiety about how she will manage the increased public scrutiny, particularly around violence and harassment. She needs a safe space to talk through her anxiety and figure out how she will manage these situations.

5. Ben is a 45-year-old transgender man who has been managing chronic health challenges and is considering having genital surgery, but is concerned about how surgery will affect his ongoing health issues. He is seeking a safe space in which to determine the potential costs and benefits of having surgery.

6. Jessica is a 20-year-old transgender woman who is coming to you because her doctor has requested a therapist's letter to meet the WPATH Standards of Care requirements before she is able to go on hormones. She is coming to you as a formality to meet the requirements, and is resistant to engaging in a non-superficial way.

7. Jorge is an 18-year-old transgender man who is coming to you because his doctor has requested a therapist's letter to meet the WPATH Standards of Care requirements before he can have top surgery. He is coming to you as a formality to meet the requirements, and is resistant to engaging in a non-superficial way.

8. Leslie is a 17-year-old person who identifies as genderqueer and wants to come out to their parents, but is unsure of how the information will be received.

9. Pat is a 55-year-old person who has recently lost their parents and who has been waiting to transition medically. Pat is now experiencing intense feelings of sadness about not having given their parents the chance to know them in their true gender, and is experiencing a lot of guilt for using the money left from the sale of the parents' house to pay for surgery.

10. Ty is a 30-year-old whose parents disowned them 10 years ago after they came out as transgender and medically transitioned. They have recently learned that their mother has cancer, and needs a safe place to work through whether or not to contact her.

11. Lamia is a transgender woman who is trying to figure out how to come out to her elderly grandparents. Her parents would prefer that she not disclose her identity, but it is important to her that her grandparents be included in her coming-out process.

12. Bianca is a young transgender woman who needs to go home for a family function, but is very nervous about how her extended family will receive her now that she has transitioned. She is unsure who knows what. A few cousins have friended her on Facebook and follow her on Twitter/Tumblr, but she has not had any conversations with them, or with anyone else beyond her immediate family.

Small-Group Discussion Questions:

1. How would you react initially to the client and presenting issues?

2. What would you say to the client during your first meeting?

3. What challenges might the client face?

4. What would you consider doing to be supportive of the client and assist them in realizing their treatment goals?

5. Are there resources that your or your colleagues can access to develop or strengthen your skills in working with transgender clients?

6. Are there any policies or processes to which you can turn, if your work is in an agency or organizational setting?

7. How do you handle your personal feelings when clients recount that others use inappropriate or offensive language, or engage in microaggressions toward them?

8. Therapists may find the actions of others towards their clients upsetting. In addition, if a therapist or colleague has strong gender-conforming beliefs, they may find these vignettes troubling as well. Resources may be available, in your community as well as online, to assist you and your colleagues with processing your feelings and supporting your clients. Can you identify a few of these resources to which you can turn?

SERVICE PROVIDING & NON-PROFIT Settings

Creating Transgender Affirming Services & Organizations

By Rhodes Perry, MPA
Director, Office of LGBTQ Policy & Practice, NYC Administration for Children's Services

• • •

Human services offered by government and non-profit organizations exist to serve as life-saving social safety nets for the most vulnerable people in our communities. Such services exist to mitigate the significant trauma of family rejection, homelessness, school bullying, unemployment, and physical or mental health crises. Unfortunately, these services are not immune from implicit bias and discrimination toward transgender and gender non-conforming (TGNC) people. In fact, a majority of TGNC people report that they have experienced poor treatment or discrimination when attempting to access social services like mental health care, substance abuse treatment, domestic violence shelters, and rape crisis centers; a disproportionate number of TGNC people reporting this type of discrimination were People of Color (Whitfield, Kattari, & Langenderfer-Magruder, 2014). Tragically, human services designed to respond to the needs of the most vulnerable continue to exacerbate severe and pervasive rejection, discrimination, and violence experienced by TGNC people.

Such harsh realities should be a call to action for leadership to work in alliance with all levels of staff to build sustainable TGNC-affirming human service organizations. Managing such organizational change requires hiring experts, dedicating program resources, implementing policy changes, and mandating training for staff at all levels—especially those staff working directly with clients. These staff members wield enormous power that influences a client's overall experience with the organization. Experience tells us that it takes all staff—receptionists, security guards, intake workers, HIV counselors, therapists, truancy officers, service coordinators, hotline volunteers and others—to create a TGNC-affirming organization, but only one staff member to create a hostile environment.

Training and coaching that provides best practices regarding how to respectfully interact with TGNC clients will dramatically improve how safe, respected, and affirmed the clients feel at an organization, and will often improve overall service engagement. Staff members and volunteers who are proactively trained in respectfully interacting with TGNC clients are best equipped to meet these clients at times of greatest need. Training is the essential starting point to open an ongoing dialogue encouraging staff members to recognize and unpack their personal, cultural, or religious biases toward TGNC people. Committing staff time and resources to training and coaching is a critical investment for transforming an organizational culture into one that affirms, respects, and supports TGNC people.

I am proud to be a national leader in such efforts thanks to my role as the Director of the Office of LGBTQ Policy and Practice at New York City's Administration for Children's Services. My responsibilities include leading the implementation of one of the nation's strongest LGBTQ policies that includes language requiring all staff to respect, affirm, and meet the specific needs of TGNC young people involved in the City's foster care and juvenile justice systems. To expand our policy expectations as we seek to create a more TGNC-affirming agency, my office developed Safe & Respected, the nation's first-ever TGNC Best Practices guide, published by a child welfare and juvenile justice government agency. As we were rolling out this guide, it became very clear that even with strong policy and written guidance, staff were struggling profoundly with how best to support TGNC young people in their care. To support our staff, we successfully launched our LGBTQ & TGNC training initiatives, which have provided cultural competency trainings for thousands of administrators, direct service practitioners, foster parents, and volunteers providing services for LGBQ and TGNC youth. As a result of these trainings, staff and volunteers are reporting increased confidence in their abilities to provide affirming services to TGNC young people. These training efforts have significantly contributed to our success in shifting people's attitudes, transforming organizational culture, and equipping direct service staff with the best practices and skills necessary to provide TGNC-affirming services.

When combined with the content of the Transgender 101 and Addressing Anti-Transgender Prejudice sections of this Toolkit, the lessons presented in this section are specifically designed to help direct service staff to expand their professional skills, examine their practices and identify action steps within their organizations. Whether you are training ten people or ten thousand, you have the opportunity and power to help ensure that TGNC people are treated with respect and compassion at the times that they need it the most. Consider this your opportunity to help create the change you wish to see!

Whitfield, D., Kattari, S. K., & Langenderfer-Magruder, L. (October 26, 2014) Differential Treatment Of Transgender People In Social Services: A Social Work Response. Presented at Council on Social Work Education Annual Meeting, 2014.

26
CONTEXT IS EVERYTHING:
The Journey to Accessing Services

...

Overview & Rationale

This lesson gives participants an opportunity to explore some of the barriers that transgender people experience when they are trying to access supportive services from the client perspective. Using a detailed case example and related discussion, participants will develop a better understanding of why transgender people may be hesitant to access social services, identify common areas of challenge, and consider how transgender people are affected by non-affirming services. This lesson works particularly well when implemented with **Lesson 27: How Inclusive and Affirming Are We?** on page XX.

Audience

This lesson is designed for people who are working in service-providing organizations, including support staff, direct service, administration and leadership. This lesson works best with groups of 10-30, and with careful facilitation can work with larger audiences.

Objectives

By the end of this lesson, participants will be able to:
- Identify 3 common barriers transgender people face when trying to access social services.
- Name 2 strategies that they can personally implement in their work to help reduce or remove these barriers.

Background Knowledge for Facilitators

It will be useful for facilitators to understand social service settings and common barriers that transgender people face when accessing these services. It will also be helpful to have a list of other local services that work with transgender people.

Time

- Preparation: 10 minutes
- Implementation: 45 minutes

Materials

- Copies of *The Client's Journey to Accessing Services* handout (1 per participant)
- Tips for Providing Transgender Affirming Services (1 per participant)

Preparation

- Make copies of the handout.
- In advance of the session, research local and online resources that can serve as additional referrals or potential community partners.

Procedure

1. Explain: To understand how to make social services more affirming for transgender clients, it is critical to examine such services from a transgender client's perspective, and this activity will help us consider that perspective.

2. Break participants into groups of 4-5 people per group. Distribute the handout, and direct participants to read through Amari's story and then work together to discuss the questions. Allow about 15-20 minutes for this activity. As groups are working on the discussion questions, rotate through the groups and provide support as needed.

3. Using the discussion questions and talking points provided in *Discussing Amari's Journey: Facilitator's Guide*, lead the group in a discussion about Amari's experiences in the scenario. After discussing Amari's experience in the organization, direct participants to imagine that Amari has now appeared at their organization, and discuss how Amari's experiences would be similar or different from those depicted in the scenario.

4. Pass out the *Tips for Providing Affirming Services* handout and review the tips with the group.

5. If using this as a standalone lesson, conclude by asking participants to take 5 minutes to write down 5 things that they or their organization could do to make their organization more welcoming for transgender clients. Have each participant report 1 action item, without repeating any of the ones that have already been named.

Evaluation Questions

✔ What are 3 common barriers transgender people face when trying to access social services?

✔ Describe 2 strategies that you can personally implement in your work to help reduce these barriers.

TIPS FOR FACILITATORS

Participants may experience worry, anger, frustration, or hopelessness if they feel they have no control over aspects of how affirming their organization is. In these situations, the facilitator may refocus the discussion on the impact that very small changes can make, or on strategies for working toward organizational policy or process change that in turn can move the environment toward greater inclusivity.

•••

It is important to be vigilant about participants' potentially blaming Amari for getting into the situation depicted in the scenario. People who work with clients directly may be more comfortable viewing the situation from the perspective of Amari's decisions and circumstances, rather than focusing on how the organization failed. Redirecting the conversation back to the organizational perspective will help participants stay focused.

Discussing Amari's Journey:
FACILITATOR'S GUIDE

Report Back on Small-Group Discussions

1. Why was Amari seeking services?

    Possible responses:
    Individual factors: Due to a court requirement, counseling and mental health support, housing resources, schooling resources, help to improve overall life circumstances

    Systematic factors: Family rejection, employment discrimination, violence and prejudice toward transgender people

2. What are Amari's options in this situation?

    Possible responses: Continue to live on the street, try to access other organizations, try to find other people/ strangers to provide support, attempt to return home

3. What were Amari's challenges?

    Possible responses: Being in a city with limited resources, lacking a support network, facing threats of physical and sexual violence, lacking housing and food security, being treated poorly/turned away by the social service organization, being 19 years old, sleeping in the park, coping with extensive stress and insecurity.

4. What were Amari's strengths and resiliencies?

    Possible responses: Left a home situation that was not affirming, being willing to seek out supportive services, wishing to continue education and get a stable job

5. What services would Amari benefit most from?

    Possible responses: Crisis services for housing and food security, ongoing case management and supportive services, mental health counseling, educational services, legal support for navigating arrest and probation, transgender-specific supportive services, creative outlets, positive peer networks

Large-Group Discussion:

- If Amari were asked to name their two or three most important needs, what do you think Amari might say?

- What are Amari's potential avenues for obtaining this support? (Or, where is Amari most likely to be able to access services?)

- What might be the ongoing impact of the microaggressions Amari faced? The impact of the overt prejudice and discrimination? How will these affect Amari's access to services?

- How might this scenario have been different if Amari were not visibly transgender? We do not know what sex Amari was assigned at birth. How would this scenario have changed if Amari were born male? Born female?

- How might intersecting oppressions affect Amari's journey, reception in care, or services offered/provided?

Applications to Current Organization

Direct participants to consider that Amari has now appeared at their organization, which is the second organization on the referral list.

- What is Amari's frame of mind likely to be when entering your organization?

- How will the prior instance at the other organization affect how Amari navigates your organization?

- How will Amari's experience be different at your organization? Why? How do you know?

- What are the potential impacts/outcomes if Amari is not able to access services, transgender-affirming or otherwise?

- If Amari were to go to an organization that was completely transgender affirming, what would be different about Amari's experience? How would that affect the outcomes?

Talking Points:

- Amari's situation is very common. The combination of systematic, organizational and individual prejudices can effectively bar transgender people from accessing social services. It is the rare organization that is affirming, which leaves transgender people very vulnerable.

- Amari's scenario told us little about how Amari interacted with people, but it is common that transgender people enter a space assuming that it will not be affirming and are defensive from the start (and reasonably so, given that most places are not affirming). Also, even if the provider at the end of the line is affirming, the non-affirming interactions prior to reaching that person will negatively affect that person's experience.

- Even in situations in which the receptionist or caseworker intends to be affirming but is having a bad day, their actions are likely to be perceived by the client as a result of hostility toward transgender people.

PARTICIPANT HANDOUT

The Client's Journey
To Accessing Services

The following scenario outlines the challenges that transgender clients may face when they are trying to access services in non-profit and community-based settings. While everyone's experience of transgender identity varies based on their individual identity, gender expression, race/ethnicity, socioeconomic status, support network, and communities—there are common themes. This scenario helps us explore some of these challenges.

Amari is a 19-year-old who is originally from Smithville, a small rural town. Life at home was challenging. Amari's family members were loving in their own way, but Amari's interests were very different from theirs, and at times this made Amari feel misunderstood. They didn't understand why Amari didn't dress or act like everyone else, and while they acted like it didn't bother them in front of Amari, they were often embarrassed when people couldn't tell if Amari was male or female, particularly because Amari dressed rather androgynously. When the family went out, others would often mis-gender Amari, and Amari's family would make it a point to correct them. As Amari matured, this become more and more uncomfortable, and it gradually became clear that the family would not support Amari's transitioning. The family started disengaging. Amari no longer felt welcome at home and so stayed with friends whenever possible.

While the family relationship was deteriorating, Amari was also facing more verbal and physical harassment for being transgender. After a particularly scary incident involving harassment by some people from a neighboring town, Amari and a gay friend (Magik) packed up and left for the city. Once they arrived in the city, Amari and Magik stayed with Magik's cousin, and tried to find jobs. Magik got a retail job, but Amari was never called by any of the places to which they applied, presumably for being transgender. Amari mainly hung around the cousin's apartment while Magik was at work because of not feeling safe going out alone, and after a few weeks it was clear that the cousin was becoming annoyed because Amari was always around and not contributing to paying the household expenses.

Amari decided to look into medical assistant programs after hearing that it was possible to finish the training in a year and then land stable job with good pay. Upon looking into the programs, Amari realized that applicants needed to have taken a few college courses in advance. Amari went to the local community college to talk about enrolling in classes, but the financial aid office personnel were very mean and pretty much refused to help with the paperwork.

All of the stress was taking a toll on Amari; having not really been accepted by family, being socially isolated from peers in middle and high school, targeted for verbal and physical harassment—in both the hometown and now the new city, not being sure how much longer Magik's cousin would allow them to continue to stay, not being able to find even a crappy job, not being able to enroll in school or a job program . . . . To cope with this Amari began smoking pot regularly with some new acquaintances from the park. One Friday evening a police officer approached them in the park while Amari was holding a joint, and arrested Amari. The arresting officers said nasty things about Amari being transgender and were physically rough while conducting the arrest. Amari was placed in custody based on sex assigned at birth, and even though Amari requested being placed in the other part of the facility, the request was ignored. The other detainees made sexual and physical threats and

Amari was really concerned about being sexually assaulted, but the officers refused to change placements. At the hearing on Monday, the judge released Amari on probation and a requirement of connecting with a local non-profit agency to take a required drug intervention course.

Upon being released, Magik made it clear that Amari could no longer stay at his cousin's place. Amari slept in the park that night. In the morning Amari decided to go to one of the places on the drug intervention course referral sheet to see about getting some services. On the way to the organization, some guys on the bus started making a lot remarks about Amari's androgynous appearance and demanding to know whether or not Amari is male or female. It seemed as though they might have tried to touch Amari's crotch to find out. Amari was shaken and got off the bus to walk the rest of the way.

Upon arriving at the organization, the security guard made some disparaging remarks about Amari being transgender. The receptionist was not much better and was very rude and abruptly handed Amari a clipboard with the intake forms on it that to fill out. Amari looked at the intake paperwork and decided to leave the gender marker question blank. When Amari returned the paperwork to the receptionist, the receptionist saw that the question was blank and said: "Well, which are you? You can't leave this blank. We can't enter you into our computer system without it." Amari said "Pick whatever, I don't care." The receptionist sneered and said that a worker would be out sometime soon.

After 15 minutes, no one had come to ask for Amari. About a half hour later, the caseworker appeared, immediately mis-gendering Amari. The intake session was not particularly helpful—it was mainly questions about types and duration of drug use, why returning home wasn't an option, and a few questions about whether Amari had been doing sex work. The case worker told Amari that they didn't have services for transgender people, and while they could probably work something out, Amari would be better off going to the LGBTQ Community Center, since they know about transgender people. Amari left with the impression that they didn't really want to help, returning to the park to figure out the next steps.

1. Why was Amari seeking services?
   _____
   _____

2. What are Amari's options in this situation?
   _____
   _____

3. What were Amari's challenges?
   _____
   _____

4. What were Amari's strengths and resiliencies?
   _____
   _____

5. What services would Amari benefit most from?
   _____
   _____

PARTICIPANT HANDOUT

Tips for Providing Transgender-Affirming Services

Use Affirming Name & Pronouns

Always use the name and pronouns that are most affirming to a person. This is one of the most fundamental signs of respect. If you accidentally use the wrong name or pronoun, apologize, correct yourself and move on. Acknowledging the mistake and offering a sincere, simple, and brief correction and apology is key. Don't make excuses or give explanations as it often shifts the burden onto the transgender person to have to make you feel better about your mistake. Be aware that some clients may wish to be addressed differently in different spaces. For example, some clients may wish to use one name when being addressed in a public waiting room but use a more affirming name when they are in a one-on-one setting.

Review Intake Forms & Procedures

Review all of your clients' paperwork and note where clients are asked to identify their gender. Remove any instances where this information is not required. In case the gender marker is needed for official reasons (insurance billing, grant reporting, government databases), consider including a blank line for affirming name and pronouns. Let transgender patients know if and when you are required to use their legal name. Inform the patient by saying, "I wanted to let you know we will need to use your legal name to submit this paperwork, but we will continue to use the name that is most affirming for you in all of our other interactions."

Consider Confidentiality

Being "outed" as transgender can be a major safety risk for that individual. It is essential to consider if/how this information will be recorded, with whom it will be shared and what the potential consequences of disclosure might be. Let the client know who will have access to the information, under what circumstances and why, so that they can create a safety plan as needed. Avoid referring to the client as "the transgender client" or having conversations in spaces where this information might be overheard.

Staff Training

Make sure that all staff—including security personnel, hotline workers, front desk staff, maintenance employees—attend at least a Trans 101 training. This will help ensure that all staff, particularly those who see clients first, have basic cultural competency skills and can contribute to creating an affirming space and organization. From a client perspective, even one negative interaction reflects upon the organization as a whole.

Resources & Referrals

Do some proactive work to figure out which other organizations also provide transgender-affirming services so that you know where you can make referrals when needed. Call and ask in advance to inquire about policies and procedures for working with transgender clients, and inquire if there is a particular staff member for whom someone should ask. Create a referral list and update it periodically.

27

HOW INCLUSIVE & AFFIRMING ARE WE?

Overview & Rationale

This lesson gives participants an opportunity to consider all the direct and indirect messages their agency, organization, or office projects about gender identity through the physical environment, materials, handouts, and images present in their space and programs. This will help participants understand changes they may need to make to their physical environment to make it more visibly affirming for transgender people and their loved ones.

Audience

This lesson is designed for people working at community-based and non-profit organizations. This activity works best with 10–30 participants.

Objectives

By the end of this lesson, participants will be able to:
- Demonstrate an understanding of the purpose of an inclusion audit and of how it can help their organization or agency become more welcoming to transgender people.
- Identify 2 of the messages projected by images or materials in their physical or programmatic space regarding gender identity and expression.
- Identify 2 things that they can do in the physical space of their environment to make their agency or organization more welcoming to transgender people and their families.

Background Knowledge for Facilitators

It will be useful for facilitators to understand issues and barriers that transgender people commonly face when they are accessing services, and to be familiar with first-person narratives about how these barriers have affected transgender clients. It will also be useful to have examples for each of the stages of the *Transgender Inclusion Scale*.

Time

- Preparation: 15 minutes
- Implementation: 90 minutes

Materials

- *Guided Imagery Notes* handouts (1 per participant)
- Index cards (1 per participant)
- *Transgender Inclusion Audit* handouts (1 per participant)
- *Transgender Inclusion Scale* handouts (1 per participant)
- Easel paper and markers (or computer, projector & PowerPoint)

Preparation

- Make copies of the handouts
- Practice reading the *Guided Imagery* out loud
- Review the *Transgender Inclusion Scale* and become familiar with each of the stages
- Write the discussion questions from Procedure step 4 on the easel paper (or download the PowerPoint slides from www.teachingtransgender.com/printables PW: TTTprep15).

Procedure

1. Explain: This lesson guides participants through an exercise called an Inclusion Audit. This is a process used to examine the direct and indirect messages an agency, organization, or office projects about gender, gender identity and the inclusion of transgender and gender non-conforming people. For counselors, doctors, or nurses, this might include taking a new look at the waiting room. For facilitators, case managers or outreach workers, it might include looking at forms, handouts, and pamphlets, and typical interactions while out in the community.

2. Ask participants to break into small groups. Once participants have settled into their groups, distribute the *Guided Imagery Notes* handout to each participant.

3. Explain that since they are not presently in their workspaces, you will be using a guided imagery exercise to help them evaluate their workplace and the messages it may send intentionally or unintentionally to clients or patients who use their services. Read the imagery from the *Guided Imagery: Facilitator Guide*. Be sure to take your time, and read slowly.

4. After you finish reading the guided imagery content, ask the small groups to discuss the following questions for 15 minutes, using their experiences from the imagery as well as the notes they wrote on their handouts. Rotate among the small groups and provide support as needed.

   Discussion Questions:
   - What are some of the challenging aspects of seeking services at your organization as a transgender person, based on the environment? What intentional and unintentional messages are projected by the physical environment?
   - What are some of the positive aspects of seeking services at your organization for transgender people, regarding these intentional and unintentional messages?
   - What are some things that you might be able to do to better support transgender people seeking the services of your organization, after completing this survey of your workplace and the messages it projects about gender identity and expression?

5. After 15 minutes, have the small groups redirect their attention to the large group, and invite each small group to share a few of the things they discussed.

6. Remind participants that the purpose of an inclusion audit is to consider all the direct and indirect messages their agency, organization, or office projects about gender identity and expression, through the physical environment. These include materials, handouts, and images present in their space and programs.

7. Ask participants to consider the impact of non-affirming spaces on potential transgender clients, and invite them to share a few of their thoughts.

8. Explain that, due to systematic marginalization, many transgender people are in need of supportive services to assist with survival and basic needs, and that many transgender people are especially marginalized due to having to navigate multiple oppressions related to intersecting identities. When potential transgender clients access services that are non-affirming, this further increases the stigma that they experience and makes it even harder to access the services they most need. This is why it is essential that service-providing organizations take on the work to become affirming.

9. Distribute the *Transgender Inclusion Scale* handout to the participants and explain that this handout provides information on what a truly affirming organization looks like. Give participants about 10 minutes to review the handout. Guide them in thinking about how their organization rates as they read through each of the stages.

10. Once everyone has had a chance to read through the handout, call out of each of the stages and ask the participants to raise a hand (or stand) to indicate which stage best represents their organization. For each of the stages, ask for volunteers to share a few of the reasons that they believe that their organization falls into this stage.

11. Through discussion, help participants understand that there are two key factors to figuring out an organization's placement on the scale: 1) An organization is only as strong as its least-affirming staff member and 2) transgender and gender non-conforming clients are the ones who ultimately decide how affirming a space is. Transgender clients rarely report this; they just don't return.

12. Distribute an index card to each participant and ask them to write down 2 things that they can do (or continue to do) in the physical space of their environment to make their agency or organization more visibly welcoming to transgender people and their loved ones. Once the participants have completed their responses, collect the index cards, shuffle them and return them to participants, so that each person has a new card (not their own card). Have each participant read off the responses written on their cards in turn until everyone's cards are read aloud.

13. To conclude the lesson, distribute the *Transgender Inclusion Audit* handout, and ask that participants take this back to their workplaces and fill it out while moving through their workplace. Explain that having staff, clients or patients, youth, or anyone who interacts with their agency can also be encouraged to fill out the handout. Involving many people in the inclusion audit process can often yield valuable information that supports creating and maintaining an environment that is safe, welcoming, and inclusive.

Evaluation Questions

✔ What did the inclusion audit reveal about your organization and what steps need to be taken to make your organization more transgender affirming?

✔ What are 2 messages projected by images or materials in your physical or programmatic space regarding gender identity and expression?

✔ What are 2 things that you can do in the physical space of your work environment to make your agency or organization more welcoming to transgender people and their families?

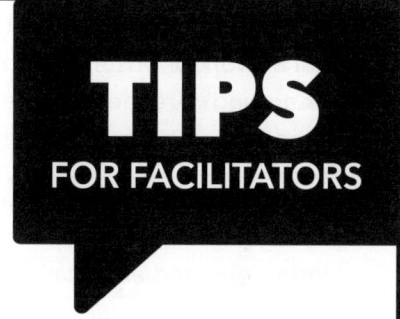

TIPS FOR FACILITATORS

Participants may experience worry, anger, frustration, or hopelessness if they feel they have no control over aspects of their physical work environments or changes that must be implemented by organizational leadership. In these situations, the facilitator may refocus the discussion on the impact that very small changes can make or on strategies for working toward organizational policy or process change that in turn can move the environment toward greater inclusivity.

• • •

If using this lesson in partnership with **Lesson 26: Context Is Everything: The Journey to Accessing Care** it can be useful to make Amari's experience the focal point of the discussion if participants are getting stuck. For example: Imagine that Amari walks into your organization's waiting room—what transgender-affirming messages would Amari see in the waiting room? Or, what might Amari look for to gauge if this organization is going to be any more welcoming than the last?

SOURCES

Kelly, M, & Maurer, L. (Mar-Apr 1999). The Inclusion Audit: Evaluating Your Camp's Efforts To Include Diverse Populations. Camping Magazine, v72 n2 p39-40,42.

Kelly, M, & Maurer, L. (2008). Out for Health's LGBT Inclusion Audit. Retrieved February 22, 2015, from www.outforhealth.org/lgbt-inclusion-audit.html

The Transgender Inclusion Scale is adapted from: "Stages and Levels of Cultural Competency Development" originally created by *Addressing Health Disparities Through Cultural Competency Initiatives – The Migrant Experience*. Available online at: http://bit.ly/1JxJvVd

Guided Imagery:
FACILITATOR'S GUIDE

Read the following script aloud. Italicized items are instructions for facilitators and do not need to be read out loud.

1. We'll be taking a journey through your workplace. Sit back, relax and, if you wish, close your eyes as you listen. Imagine with me an average day at your workplace. Although you may have been working at the same place for months or even years, imagine you are visiting your workplace or usual work surroundings for the very first time. *(Pause)*

2. Imagine that you have arrived at your workplace. Imagine going up to the building where you work, whether it's an office, clinic, hospital, or some other place. Take a look at the sign or signs on the door outside. What do they say? Open the door, and walk in. As you take in the indoor space, what do you see? What artwork or posters do you see as you look around? Are there a variety of types of individuals, couples, and families represented? *(Pause)*

3. Do the images show people who challenge gender roles and expectations? Will the people looking at your walls see themselves represented in the images here? Will they recognize the artists of any artwork as those who share dimensions of diversity with themselves? *(Pause)*

4. Now please open your eyes, and write down a few bullet points for prompts 1-3 of your Guided Imagery Notes handout that reflect what you observed.

(Allow 3-4 minutes for completion.)

5. Now we'll be continuing with the imagery, and I invite you to close your eyes again, if you wish.

6. Is there music playing? Do you recognize the artists or composers? If there are lyrics, are they about conventionally gendered people, people whose gender differs from what society might expect, or both? Is there a television? Do you recognize the program or channel? Is the program in a language you speak and understand? *(Pause)*

7. Now please open your eyes, and write down a few bullet points on prompt 4 of your Guided Imagery Notes handout that reflect what you observed.

(Allow 2-3 minutes for completion.)

Now we'll be continuing with the imagery, and I invite you to close your eyes again, if you wish.

8. Look around some more. Are there magazines on the table for you to read as you wait? Are their pamphlets or other written materials displayed? Promotional materials for the agency or organization? Do these include words or images that represent gender diversity? Are there any magazines or pamphlets that are specifically about, or for, transgender people? *(Pause)*

9. Now please open your eyes, and write down a few bullet points on prompt 5 of your Guided Imagery Notes handout that reflect what you observed.

(Allow 2-3 minutes for completion.)

10. Now we'll be continuing with the imagery, and I invite you to close your eyes again, if you wish.

11. If there is a receptionist or front desk, imagine approaching it. What do you see? Are there signs or directions that you see? Is there a non-discrimination statement displayed? And if so, does it include "gender identity and expression"? Are there other signs or symbols posted that indicate this is a transgender-friendly office? And, are there forms to be filled out? Is the information and the choices on the forms inclusive of transgender people? Where are the restrooms located? Are they male and female? Or for all genders? *(Pause)*

12. Now please open your eyess and write down a few bullet points on prompts 6-7 of your *Guided Imagery Notes* that reflect what you observed.

(Allow 2-3 minutes for completion.)

13. Now we'll be completing the imagery with one more aspect of the workplace. Please feel free to relax and close your eyes, if you wish.

14. If you go out into the field to do your work, in what ways do images, sounds, forms, handouts, lesson plans, and other surroundings and themes reflect the diversity of people's gender identity and expression? Over which of these might you have control? Are there some over which you have no control? If so, what can you do about that? (Pause)

15. Now please open your eyes, and write down a few bullet points on prompt 8 of your *Guided Imagery Notes* that reflect what you observed.

(Allow 2-3 minutes for completion.)

16. Reflect on the space as a whole. Ask yourself: Is what I am seeing, hearing, reading and experiencing in my workplace setting congruent with messages of acknowledging diversity regarding gender identity and presentation, and respect for transgender people and their families and allies? (Pause)

17. Now please open your eyes, and write down a few bullet points on prompts 9-10 of your *Guided Imagery Notes* that reflect what you observed.

(Allow 2-3 minutes for completion.)

PARTICIPANT HANDOUT

Guided Imagery Notes

INSTRUCTIONS: Note your mental observations for each of the components below.

1. Approaching the Building _____
   _____
   _____

2. Entering the Building & Opening the Door _____
   _____
   _____

3. Walls of the Waiting Room (or equivalent space) _____
   _____
   _____

4. Sounds of the Waiting Room (or equivalent space) _____
   _____
   _____

5. Materials in the Waiting Room (or equivalent space) _____
   _____
   _____

6. Approaching & Interacting with Reception (or equivalent) _____
   _____
   _____

7. The Bathrooms _____
   _____
   _____

8. Out In the Field _____
   _____
   _____

9. Overall Impressions of Transgender Inclusion _____
   _____
   _____

10. Areas Needing Improvement _____
    _____
    _____

PARTICIPANT HANDOUT

Transgender Inclusion Audit

This handout will help you monitor your workplace to answer the question: Do the messages and images that people see, hear, and experience match our commitment to making transgender people, and their families and allies, feel welcome and respected?

Anyone can fill out this form—staff, clients or patients, youth, others who interact with your agency or organization. Involve as many people as possible to collect information on what is working well and where there may be room for updates or changes.

Take this sheet with a pen or pencil and move around your workplace. Look at the walls, forms, magazines, pamphlet racks, promotional items and publications, and other materials, and take note of what you experience and what you think. Then, take action to create or maintain a more inclusive environment.

Which will you keep? Replace? Find more of? Which are okay but you could keep looking for better?

Magazines:

Posters and artwork:

Music, sounds, and television:

Pamphlets and brochures:

Other materials, handouts, and forms:

Adapted from the work of Kelly & Maurer 1999, 2008

PARTICIPANT HANDOUT

Transgender Inclusivity Scale

FOR NON-PROFIT & SERVICE PROVIDING ORGANIZATIONS

Review the following 6 stages of transgender inclusion and determine into which stage you believe that your organization falls.

1. **Actively Discriminatory** - An organization that is "Actively Discriminatory":
   - Has policies and procedures that ban/inhibit transgender people from accessing the space or services.
   - Operates under the idea that transgender people are mentally ill.
   - Has staff people who view transgender people as freaks, or deviants.
   - Assumes that there are only two sexes and genders, and that gender must be or should be congruent with the sex assigned at birth.
   - Has no desire to learn about or provide services for transgender people.
   - Actively discriminates against transgender people, has actively enforced policies of transgender exclusion.

2. **Overtly Prejudiced** - An organization that is "Overtly Prejudiced":
   - Has only a vague awareness of the existence of transgender people
   - Does not welcome transgender people or only specific staff members welcome transgender people.
   - Does not acknowledge or address microaggressions (such as rudeness, funny looks or derogatory remarks) made by staff about transgender people.
   - May look down on transgender people as people who are always in a lot of emotional pain.
   - Believes that "there are no transgender clients" within their client base or community.
   - Unintentionally ignores the specific needs of transgender people due to ignorance about related identities and challenges.
   - Frequently discriminates against transgender people, has policies of transgender exclusion that are enforced on a case-by-case basis.

3. **Aware** - An organization that is "Aware":
   - Has a staff that acknowledges that there may transgender clients, and that the organization may not be meeting their needs
   - Has organizational leadership that may not acknowledge the importance of being proactive about transgender issues and minimizes the differences between LGB and Transgender clients.
   - Lacks the desire or action to increase understanding of transgender identities and issues.
   - Has staff that are nervous or unsure in their work with transgender people.
   - May feel that because transgender people are statistically infrequent, that it is not a wise use of time or money to serve transgender clients.
   - Has staff that believes strongly that transgender people are victims of their identities and will face a lifetime of pain because of their transgender identity and experience.

→

4. **Active** – An organization that is "Active":
   - Acknowledges its weaknesses in serving transgender clients, with an understanding that there is room for improvement (may not understand what or how to improve).
   - Has a preliminary understanding of intersectionality and how it affects transgender clients.
   - Has some staff working to create organizational changes to make it safer for transgender clients.
   - Begins to assess how the organization can meet the needs of transgender clients.
   - Hires transgender people to help diversify the staff.
   - Works to create inclusive spaces by modifying the forms and physical space (e.g., gender-neutral bathrooms or a safe alternative, intake forms, client records, etc.)
   - Attempts to meet the needs of transgender clients, but perhaps with only marginal success.
   - Has transgender-inclusive human resources policies (legal name protections, etc.).

5. **Friendly** – An organization that is "Friendly":
   - Is accepting and respecting of differences between LGB and Transgender clients.
   - Has a solid understanding of intersectionality and how that affects transgender clients.
   - Routinely seeks out transgender voices to find ways to improve services.
   - Implements training to increase awareness of transgender identities and issues; seeks out areas of ignorance and addressing them.
   - Tokenizes transgender people, staff or clients, and expects them to take on a primary role in making the organization more fully transgender inclusive because they are transgender.
   - Does not address the negative behaviors of clients who are transphobic or provide education for clients who are ignorant about transgender issues.

6. **Fully Inclusive & Affirming** – An organization that is "Fully Inclusive & Affirming":
   - Truly respects and values transgender people
   - Has staff all of whom make transgender inclusivity a priority, and work together to achieve the goal of full inclusion.
   - Provides transgender-inclusive health care, and transition-related medical leave.
   - Requires that new staff be knowledgeable about transgender identities, and/or requires training to become so as a condition of hire.
   - Continues to explore and build knowledge about transgender identities and issues, and pro-actively seeks out ways to improve.
   - Takes actions to address intersecting oppressions, particularly as it relates to advocacy work to include transgender people in other social justice movements, and includes intersectional approaches in work with transgender clients and communities.
   - Advocates for the inclusion of transgender people in partner organizations and communities.
   - Proactively discusses transgender inclusion with funders and encourages funders to prioritize the needs of transgender clients and communities.
   - Has staff members all of whom role-model transgender-sensitivity for clients and address transphobia between clients.
   - Publically speaks out against anti-transgender prejudice and discrimination.
   - Mandates that transgender people serve in leadership roles within the organization and actively seeks to overcome social barriers to transgender people serving in leadership roles.

MAKING MEANING: *Closing Activities*

While it can be tempting to cut closing activities due to lack of time or energy, well-planned closing activities are an essential component of an effectively facilitated training. The end of the training is your opportunity to help your participants make sense of what they have learned during the session, start thinking about how they will apply the information moving forward, and evaluate their experience. It also provides the facilitator with valuable information about whether any needs for clarifying information remain, or whether follow-up might be necessary with the group. This closure process will also help you as a facilitator assess what your participants have gained during the session and transition back to non-facilitator mode. Each of the closing activities that we have provided is designed to provide all of these benefits.

We have included three types of concluding activities here:

1 Impact & Reflection Circle: A group activity for sessions in which there are groups with strong cohesion and ample time for participants to speak openly. This activity can bring out strong emotions in participants and in the group dynamics, which is often a positive experience that speaks to participants' level of interest and engagement.

2 Navigating Next Steps: A group activity in which participants work together to strategize how the session's contents can be applied to their work as individuals and overall as an organization. This activity works best when people either all work in the same organization or there are enough people from each organization to create small groups.

3 Reflections Sheets: An individual activity for sessions where there are participants from a variety of settings (instead of a session that is specific to one location), or time is limited.

28

IMPACT & REFLECTION CIRCLE

...

Overview & Rationale

In this closing activity, participants will briefly share their reflections about what they have learned during the session. This activity serves to help participants contextualize the information presented in the training, and re-focus on specific strategies that can be applied to their personal and professional lives. It also provides closure for the group as well as the facilitator.

Audience

Can be used with all audiences. Works best with 30 participants or fewer.

Objectives

By the end of this lesson, participants will be able to:
- Identify 2-3 pieces of information gained during the session.
- Name 1 concrete way that this information can personally or professionally applied.

Background Knowledge for Facilitators

None needed.

Time

- Implementation: 10 minutes

Materials

- Koosh ball, foam ball, ball of yarn, or other small, soft item that can easily be tossed from person to person

Preparation

- Obtain ball.

Procedure

1. Tell the group that we'll be playing a game with the koosh ball as a fun closing exercise after having completed the main lesson.

2. Ask the group to form a circle in the center of the room. (Participants may stand or sit as needed).

3. Explain the directions for this activity before beginning:
   - The facilitator will introduce a question, and then toss the koosh ball to someone else in the circle. When another person catches it, it is their turn to quickly answer the question using only a few words or a brief phrase. After answering, they then throw it to another person in the group. When that person catches it, it is their turn to answer the question in the same manner. Anyone may elect to "pass" and answer the question later or not at all.

- The goal is for each person to have a turn, and for the question to be answered quickly by everyone in the group when it is their turn (when they catch the koosh ball). After everyone has had a turn, the last participant to have a turn will toss the ball back to the facilitator, and the facilitator will introduce a new question and the process begins again.

- During the activity, others are instructed to listen to everyone's responses. Only one person may speak at a time—the person holding the koosh ball. After all of the questions have been answered by everyone, discuss any insights gained during the activity.

Discussion:

1. What is 1 thing that stood out for you after having participated in the lesson?
2. What is 1 thing that you will take forward in your work, after having participated in the lesson?

The facilitator leads the group in this activity, introducing one question at a time. The activity concludes when everyone has answered both questions. Thank the participants for their hard work during the training and congratulate them on their success.

Evaluation Questions

✔ What are 2 pieces of information you learned during today's session?

✔ What is 1 concrete way that you can apply this information personally or professionally?

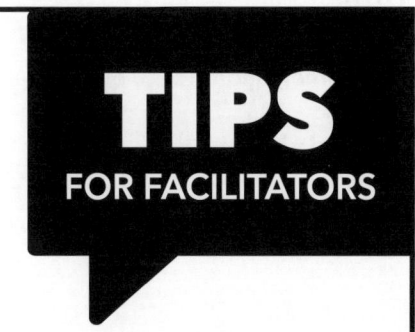

Depending on the group or the intensity of the training experience, a circle may be too intense for some participants. If there have been a lot of emotions present during a training, it may be best to have participants stay in their seats.

• • •

Some participants may feel pressured or put on the spot when they are called on by another peer. It may be helpful to use a "popcorn" style response wherein participants volunteer when they are ready to speak.

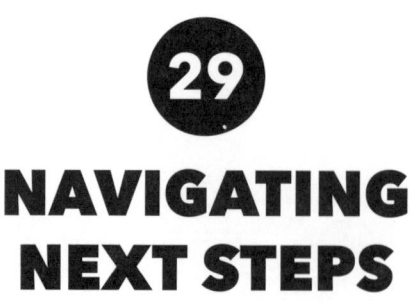

29
NAVIGATING NEXT STEPS

Overview & Rationale

In this closing activity, participants are asked to work together to identify next steps they can commit to moving forward with after the training. It also provides closure for the group and the facilitator.

Audience

Can be used with all audiences. Works best with 30 participants or less.

Objectives

By the end of this lesson, participants will be able to:
- Identify 2 individual next steps for applications outside this training.
- Identify 2 organizational next steps for applications outside of the training.

Background Knowledge for Facilitators

It will be useful for facilitators to be familiar with a variety of strategies individuals and organizations can use to be allies to transgender people.

Time

- Preparation: 2 minutes
- Implementation: 15–20 minutes

Materials

- Easel paper and markers

Preparation

- Label 2 sheets of easel paper so that one reads "Individual" and the second reads "Organizational." Hang these where both can be seen and written on.

Procedure

1. Explain to the group that for a closing activity everyone will be working together to brainstorm next steps that they can take personally and professionally to be better transgender allies.

   Examples include:

   - *Individual:* Reading additional literature and materials about transgender people
   - *Individual:* Making an extra effort to be friendly with visibly transgender people and gender non-conforming people when in public by doing things such as holding the door open or smiling (to help counteract microaggressions)
   - *Organizational:* Checking the outreach materials to make sure they are transgender-inclusive
   - *Organizational:* Evaluating agency forms to ensure that they provide options for transgender people to accurately reflect their identity.

2. Using your method of choice, break participants into small groups of 3-4 people. Instruct each small group to create two lists—1 list of individual actions and 1 list of organizational actions—that can be taken after leaving the training. Explain that they will have 5 minutes to create their list and that these lists will be shared with the large group. During the small-group session, rotate among the small groups and offer support as needed.

3. After 5 minutes, bring the small groups back to the large group. Ask each small group in turn to share a few of their strategies with the large group and then write them on the appropriate piece of easel paper so that all participants can see the resulting list.

4. At the end of the brainstorming and sharing session, congratulate the participants on their success in the training and creating the lists, and thank them for their efforts toward being better allies for transgender people.

5. Optional: You may wish to type participants' responses to these questions and send them out to the group after the training as a follow-up piece to help remind them of their commitment.

Evaluation Questions

✔ What are 2 next steps you can take as an individual for applications outside of this training?

✔ What are 2 next steps you help your organization take for applications outside of the training?

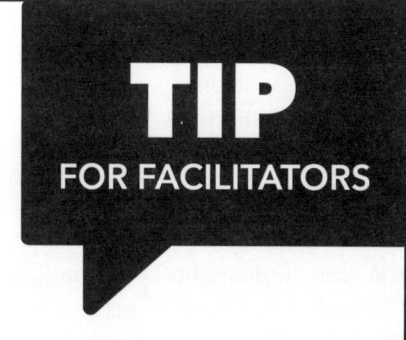

At times, a participant—or many participants—may be highly motivated but feel "stuck" that they don't have the power to make organizational changes. Help refocus the conversation—perhaps many people speaking up can bring about change at an organization that moves slowly or is not particularly embracing of change. There may also be participants in the room who have witnessed the impact that one person can have, even in systems that are slow to change, who would like to share their story or their strategies.

30

REFLECTION SHEET

Overview & Rationale

In this closing activity, participants will briefly share their reflections on what they are taking away from the sessions. In doing so, the participants will have a chance to synthesize what they have learned, and the facilitator will be able to better assess the success of the training and make decisions about future trainings.

Audience

Can be used with all audiences, provided that participants are comfortable with and are able to write. There is no limit on the number of participants and works well with large groups.

Objectives

By the end of this lesson, participants will be able to:
- Identify 2 pieces of information they have learned during the session.
- Describe 2 next steps for personal and professional application outside of the training.

Background Knowledge for Facilitators

None required.

Time

- Preparation: None
- Implementation: 10–15 minutes

Materials

- *Training Reflection Sheet* handout (1 per participant)
- Writing implements (1 per participant)

Preparation

- Make copies of the handout.

Procedure

1. Explain to the group that for a closing activity each participant will be completing a brief reflection sheet to help them summarize their experiences.

2. Distribute the handouts and explain that the participants will need to hand in their sheet before they depart the training, indicating where the participants should leave them on their way out. Thank the participants for their hard work during the training and congratulate them on their success.

3. Plan for the participants to spend 10-15 minutes completing their sheets.

4. Optional: Reflection sheets may be handed out earlier in the session so that participants can record their responses throughout the training.

Evaluation Questions

✔ What are 2 pieces of information you've learned during this session?

✔ What are 2 next steps you can take to apply what you've learned, personally or professionally?

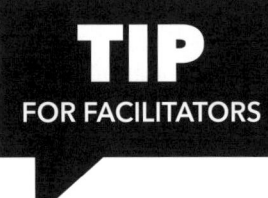

TIP FOR FACILITATORS

It will be helpful to build time into the schedule for this activity and notify participants earlier in the training that there will be a short written closing activity prior to ending the session. Explain to participants that this is a valuable tool for you as a trainer and encourage them to take the time to fill it out carefully and in detail (rather than rushing).

TRAINING REFLECTION
WORKSHEET

NAME_____ DATE_____

Based on your experiences in today's training, please answer the following questions.
If you run out of space, please use the back of this worksheet.

One thing I learned today:
_____
_____
_____

One thing that surprised me today:
_____
_____
_____

One thing that I will apply to my work/life is:
_____
_____
_____

One way that I will act differently moving forward is:
_____
_____
_____

One thing that I am still wondering about is:
_____
_____
_____

One thing that was particularly helpful for me today was:
_____
_____
_____

WORKS CITED

Addis, S., Davies, M., Greene, G., MacBride-Stewart, S., & Shepherd, M. (2009). The health, social care, housing needs of lesbian, gay, bisexual and transgender older people. *Health and Social Care in the Community, 17*(6), 647–658.

Addressing Health Disparities Through Cultural Competency Initiatives - The Migrant Experience (n.d.) Stages and levels of cultural competency development. Retrieved from: http://bit.ly/1JxJvVd

Alcorn L. (December 28, 2014). Untitled. Originally posted on: http://lazerprincess.tumblr.com/ Retrieved from: http://www.dailymail.co.uk/news/article-2891267/Transgender-teenager-leaves-heartbreaking-suicide-note-blaming-Christian-parents-walking-tractor-trailer-highway.html

American Medical Association. 2014. AMA Policies on GLBT Issues. Available online at: http://www.ama-assn.org/ama/pub/about-ama/our-people/member-groups-sections/glbt-advisory-committee/ama-policy-regarding-sexual-orientation.page?

American Psychological Association. 2014. Answers to your questions about transgender people, gender identity and gender expression. Available online at: http://www.apa.org/topics/lgbt/transgender.aspx

Annika. (September 13, 2012). Disowned: When Coming Out Doesn't Go As Planned. Retrieved from: http://www.autostraddle.com/disowned-when-coming-out-doesnt-go-as-planned-145663/

Anon. (May 6, 2011). My Mom's first post-transition visit. Retrieved from: http://faggotboi.wordpress.com/2011/05/06/my-moms-first-post-transition-visit/

Beam, C. (2007). *Transparent: Love, Family and Living the T with Transgender Teenagers*. Orlando, FL: Harcourt Books.

Beemyn, B. G. (2005). Making campuses more inclusive of transgender students. *Journal of Gay & Lesbian Issues in Education*, 3(1), 77–87

Bellino, D. (July 2, 2014). Exclusive: Drea Kelly on Her Transgender Son, Her Pending Divorce and Life After the Show. VH1. Retrieved from: http://m.vh1.com/blog/2014-07-02/drea-kelly-on-transgender-son-pending-divorce/

Bettcher, T. M. (2007). Evil deceivers and make-believers: On transphobic violence and the politics of illusion. *Hypatia: A Journal of Feminist Philosophy*, 22(3), 43–65.

Bloom, B. S., & Krathwohl, D. R. (1956). *Taxonomy of educational objectives: The classification of educational goals.* Handbook I: Cognitive domain. Longmans: McKay.

California School Success and Opportunity Act. 2013. AB 1266.

Center of Excellence for Transgender Health. (2015) Fertility Issues. Retrieved from http://transhealth.ucsf.edu/trans?page=protocol-fertility

De Vries, A. L., Steensma, T. D., Doreleijers, T. A., & Cohen-Kettenis, P. T. (2011). Puberty suppression in adolescents with gender identity disorder: A prospective follow-up study. *The Journal of Sexual Medicine*, 8(8), 2276–2283.

De Vries, A. L., McGuire, J. K., Steensma, T. D., Wagenaar, E. C., Doreleijers, T. A., & Cohen-Kettenis, P. T. (2014). Young adult psychological outcome after puberty suppression and gender reassignment. *Pediatrics, 134*(4), 696–704.

Gates GJ. *How Many People Are Lesbian, Gay, Bisexual and Transgender? Los Angeles, CA: UCLA-Williams Institute; 2011.*

GLAAD. (2014). GLAAD Media Reference Guide, 9th Edition. Retrieved from http://www.glaad.org/reference/

GLAAD. (2015). Tips for Allies of Transgender People. Retrieved from http://www.glaad.org/transgender/allies

GLSEN & Harris Interactive (2008). *The principal's perspective: School safety, bullying and harassment, a survey of public school principals.* New York: GLSEN.

GLSEN & Harris Interactive. (2012). *Playgrounds & prejudice: Elementary school climate in the United States.* New York: Gay, Lesbian & Straight Education Network.

Grant, J., Mottet, L., Tanis, J., Harrison, J., Herman, J., & Keisling, M. (2011). Injustice at every turn: A report of the National Transgender Discrimination Survey. Retrieved from http://endtransdiscrimination.org/PDFs/NTDS_Report.pdf

Green, E. R. (2010). Shifting paradigms: Moving beyond "Trans 101" in sexuality education. *American Journal of Sexuality Education*, 5(1). 1–16.

Green, E. R. (2013). The SIEO Model of Gender & Orientation. Retrieved from: http://www.elirgreenphd.com

Green, E. R. (2014). Does Teaching Transgender Content Effectively Reduce Anti-Transgender Prejudice? The Assessment Findings from a National Study. (Unpublished doctoral dissertation). Widener University, Chester, PA.

Green, E. R. & Perry, J. R. (2014). Safe & Respected: Providing Culturally Competent Services for Transgender and Gender Non-Conforming Youth in ACS Care (Training Curriculum). New York City, NY: New York City's Administration for Children's Services.

Greytak, E. A., Kosciw, J. G., & Boesen, M. J. (2013). Putting the "T" in "resource": The benefits of LGBT-related school resources for transgender youth. *Journal of LGBT Youth*, 10(1-2), 45-63.

Greytak, E. A., Kosciw, J. G., and Diaz, E. M. (2009). *Harsh Realities: The Experiences of Transgender Youth in Our Nation's Schools*. New York: GLSEN.

Hall, D. M. (2009). *Allies at Work: Creating a Lesbian, Gay, Bisexual and Transgender Inclusive Work Environment*. San Francisco, CA: Out and Equal Workplace Advocates.

Harrison, J., Grant, J., & Herman, J. L. (2012). A gender not listed here: Genderqueers, gender rebels, and otherwise in the National Transgender Discrimination Survey. *LGBTQ Public Policy Journal at the Harvard Kennedy School*, *2*(1).

Herman, J. L., Haas, A. P., & Rodgers, P. L. (2014). Suicide attempts among transgender and gender non-conforming adults. American Foundation for Suicide Prevention & Williams Institute: UCLA School of Law.

Intersex Society of North America. (2008). What's the difference between being transgender or transsexual and having an intersex condition? Retrieved from http://www.isna.org/faq/transgender

Kellaway, M. (July 8, 2015). Two Black Trans Boys, Two NY Families and Boundless Love. *The Advocate*. Available at: https://www.advocate.com/families/2015/07/08/two-black-trans-boys-two-ny-families-and-boundless-love

Kelly, M, & Maurer, L. (Mar-Apr 1999). The Inclusion Audit: Evaluating Your Camp's Efforts To Include Diverse Populations. *Camping Magazine*, *72*(2), p39–40, 42.

Kelly, M, & Maurer, L. (2008). Out for Health's LGBT Inclusion Audit. Retrieved February 22, 2015, from http://www.outforhealth.org/lgbt-inclusion-audit.html

Keyishian, A. (September 15, 2011). Cher defends transgender son, Chaz Bono, on 'Ellen.' *The Stir*. Retrieved from: http://thestir.cafemom.com/entertainment/126049/cher_defends_transgender_son_chaz

Kosciw, J., Greytak, E. A., Palmer, N. A., & Boesen, M. J. (2014). *The 2013 National School Climate Survey: The experiences of lesbian, gay, bisexual, and transgender youth in our nation's schools*. New York: GLSEN.

Kull, R. (2014). Preparing school counselors, psychologists, and social workers to support lesbian, gay, bisexual, and transgender students: The role of pre-service education and training. American Education Research Association Annual Meeting. Philadelphia, PA.

Lambda Legal. (n.d.) FAQ About Identity Documents. Retrieved from http://www.lambdalegal.org/know-your-rights/transgender/identity-document-faq

Lambda Legal. (n.d.) FAQ About Transgender People and Marriage Law. Retrieved from http://www.lambdalegal.org/know-your-rights/transgender/trans-marriage-law-faq#basics

Lambda Legal. (n.d.) FAQ on Access to Transition-Related Care. Retrieved from http://www.lambdalegal.org/know-your-rights/transgender/transition-related-care-faq#q7

Marriage Equality and Transgender People. (July 1, 2015). Retrieved from http://marriageequalityfacts.org/trans/

McClouskey, M. (2014). Trans women are not drag queens. *Everyday Feminism*. Retrieved from: http://everydayfeminism.com/2014/04/trans-women-not-drag-queens/

McGuire, J. K., Anderson, C. R., Toomey, R. B. & Russell, S. T. (2010). School climate for transgender youth: A mixed method investigation of student experiences and school responses. *Journal of Youth and Adolescence, 39*(10), 1175-1188.

McNaught, B. (2011). Guided Imagery. Anyone Can Be An Ally. SunShower Learning.

Media Matters, http://mediamatters.org/research/2015/06/03/17-school-districts-debunk-right-wing-lies-abou/203867 accessed 6/24/2015

Mezirow, J. (1991). *Transformative dimensions of adult learning*. San Franciso, CA: Jossey-Bass.

Mitchell, K. J., Ybarra, M. L., & Korchmaros, J. D. (2014). Sexual harassment among adolescents of different sexual orientations and gender identities. Child Abuse & Neglect, 38(2), 280-295.

Movement Advancement Project. (July 1, 2015). Non Discrimination Laws. Retrieved from http://www.lgbtmap.org/equality-maps/non_discrimination_laws

Nadal, K. L. (2013). That's so gay! Microaggressions and the lesbian, gay, bisexual, and transgender community. American Psychological Association.

National Center for Transgender Equality. (2012.) Injustice at Every Turn: A Look at Latino/a Respondents in the National Transgender Discrimination Survey; Injustice at Every Turn: A Look at Asian American, South Asian, Southeast Asian and Pacific Islander (API) Respondents in the National Transgender Discrimination Survey; Injustice at Every Turn: A Look at Black Respondents in the National Transgender Discrimination Survey. Retrieved from www.endtransdiscrimination.org.

Nelson, J. B. (1978). *An approach to sexuality and Christian Theology*. Minneapolis: Augsburg Publishing House.

Oh, Inae. (June 29, 2015). John Oliver: Quit Asking Transgender People About Their Genitals. *Mother Jones*. Retrieved from http://www.motherjones.com/mixed-media/2015/06/john-oliver-transgender-rights

Perrson, D. (2009). Unique challenges of transgender aging: Implications from the literature. *Journal of Gerontological Social Work, 52*, 633-646.

Center of Excellence for Transgender Health. (April 2011). *Primary Care Protocol for Transgender Patient Care*. University of California, San Francisco, Department of Family and Community Medicine.

Rankin, S. (2007). Campus climate for sexual minority students: Challenges and best practices. In J. Jackson & M. Terrell (Eds.), *Toward administrative reawakening: Creating and maintaining safe college campuses*. Herndon, VA: Stylus Publications.

Reisner, S. L., Bradford, J., Hopwood, R., Gonzalez, A., Makadon, H., Todisco, D., Cavanaugh, T., VanDerwarker, R., Grasso, C., Zaslow, S., Boswell., S., & Mayer, K. (2015). Comprehensive Transgender Healthcare: The Gender Affirming Clinical and Public Health Model of Fenway Health. *Journal of Urban Health*, 1-9.

Reisner, S. L., Greytak, E. A., Parsons, J. T., & Ybarra, M. L. (2014). Gender minority social stress in adolescence: Disparities in adolescent bullying and substance use by gender identity. *The Journal of Sex Research. 52*(3), 243-256.

Robison, M. (1998). The residence hall: A home away from home. In R. Sanlo (Ed.), *Working with lesbian, gay, bisexual and transgender college students: A handbook for faculty and administrators* (5366). Westport, CT: Greenwood Press.

Rolling Stone. (July 1, 2015). Kim Kardashian gets real: 11 revelations from the new cover story. Retrieved from: http://www.rollingstone.com/culture/news/kim-kardashian-gets-real-11-revelations-from-the-new-cover-story-20150701

San Francisco Human Rights Commission, 2002.

Satterly, B. A., & Dyson, D. A. (2010). Social work practice with gay, lesbian, bisexual, and transgender persons. In J. Poulin (Ed.), *Collaborative social work: Strengths-based generalist practice (3rd ed.)*. Belmont, CA: Wadsworth.

Scarleteen. (April 22, 2014). With Pleasure: A View of Whole Sexual Anatomy for Every Body. Retrieved from http://www.scarleteen.com/article/bodies/with_pleasure_a_view_of_whole_sexual_anatomy_for_every_body

Smith Y., Van Goozen S., Kuiper A., Cohen-Kettenis P. (2005). Sex reassignment: outcomes and predictors of treatment for adolescent and adult transsexuals. *Psychological Medicine*; 35(1): 89-99.

Spack, N. P., Edwards-Leeper, L., Feldman, H. A., Leibowitz, S., Mandel, F., Diamond, D. A., & Vance, S. R. (2012). Children and adolescents with gender identity disorder referred to a pediatric medical center. *Pediatrics*, *129*(3), 418-425.

Stotzer, R. (2009). Violence against transgender people: A review of United States data. *Aggression and Violent Behavior*, 170-179.

Title IX of the Education Amendments of 1972, 20 U.S.C.A. §§ 1681-1688 (West Supp. 2014).

Valenti, J. (June 20, 2014). Transgender people want to exist without having to prove they are 'real'. Retrieved from http://www.theguardian.com/commentisfree/2014/jun/20/transgender-janet-mock-passing-realness

Veale J., Saewyc E., Frohard-Dourlent H., Dobson S., Clark B. & the Canadian Trans Youth Health Survey Research Group (2015). *Being Safe, Being Me: Results of the Canadian Trans Youth Health Survey*. Vancouver, BC: Stigma and Resilience Among Vulnerable Youth Centre, School of Nursing, University of British Columbia.

Whitfield, D., Kattari, S. K., & Langenderfer-Magruder, L. (2014) Differential Treatment of Transgender People In Social Services: A Social Work Response. Presentation at Council on Social Work Education Annual Meeting, October 26, 2014.

World Professional Association for Transgender Health. (2012). Standards of Care, v7. Retrieved from: http://www.wpath.org/site_page.cfm?pk_association_webpage_menu=1351&pk_association_webpage=3926

RESOURCES & RECOMMENDED READING

There are more transgender-related books, films, websites, research, organizations and resources than ever before, and titles continue to be added. This list provides some suggestions as a starting point, and is not intended to be an exhaustive list. Use the Internet and local libraries to learn more about the many books on this topic to find those that best suit your needs. Also be sure to check **www.TeachingTransgender.com** for updates and additions.

BOOKS

General/Transgender 101

Doing Gender Diversity: Readings in Theory and Real World Experience. Rebecca F. Plante and Luca Maurer (eds.). 2009. Westview Press.

Gender Outlaw: On Men, Women & the Rest of Us. Kate Bornstein. 1994. Vintage Books.

My New Gender Workbook. Kate Bornstein. 2013. Routledge.

Trans Bodies, Trans Selves: A Resource for the Transgender Community. Laura Erickson-Scroth (ed.). 2014. Oxford University Press.

Transgender History

The Gender Frontier. Marriette Pathy Allen. 2003. Kehrer.

How Sex Changed: A History of Transsexuality in the United States. Joanne Meyerowitz. 2002. Harvard University Press.

Transgender History. Susan Stryker. 2008. Seal Press.

Transgender Warriors: Making History from Joan of Arc to Dennis Rodman. Leslie Feinberg. 1996. Beacon Press.

Raising Transgender & Gender Non-Conforming Children

Angels & Allies: A Memoir of Our Family's Transition. Terri Cook and Vince Cook. 2013. Hallowed Birch Publishing.

Beyond Magenta: Transgender Teens Speak Out. Susan Kuklin. 2014. Candlewick Press.

Gender Born, Gender Made: Raising Healthy Gender Non-Conforming Children. Diana Ehrensaft, PhD. 2011. The Experiment Press.

Now What? A Handbook for Families With Transgender Children. (2015). Rex Butt, PhD. Transgress Press.

Raising My Rainbow: Adventures in Raising a Fabulous, Gender Creative Son. Lori Duron. 2012. Broadway Books.

Trans Forming Families: Real Stories About Transgender Loved Ones. Mary Boenke (editor). 2008. PFLAG Transgender Network.

The Transgender Child: A Handbook for Families & Professionals. Stephanie Brill and Rachel Pepper. 2008. Cleis Press.

Transitions of the Heart: Stories of Love, Struggle and Acceptance by Mothers of Transgender and Gender Variant Children. Rachel Pepper (editor). 2012. Cleis Press.

Trans-Kin: A Guide for Family and Friends of Transgender People. Eleanor Hubbard and Cameron Whitley (editors). 2012. Bolder Press.

Transparent: Love, Family & Living the T with Transgender Teenagers. Cris Beam, PhD. 2007. Harcourt Press.

Personal Narratives (Non-Fiction)

A Queer & Pleasant Danger: A Memoir. Kate Bornstein. 2012. Beacon Press.

Becoming a Visible Man. Jamison Green. 2004. Vanderbilt University Press.

Body Alchemy: Transsexual Portraits. Loren Cameron. 1996. Cleis Press.

Dress Codes: Of Three Girlhoods – My Mother's, My Father's, and Mine. Noelle Howey. 2003. Picador.

Finding the Real Me: True Tales of Sex and Gender Diversity. Tracie O'Keefe and Katrina Fox (eds.). 2003. Wiley and Sons.

From the Inside Out: Radical Gender Transformation FTM and Beyond. Morty Diamond. 2004. Manic D Press.

Gender Outlaws: The Next Generation. Kate Bornstein and S. Bear Bergman (eds.). 2010. Seal Press.

Genderqueer: Voices From Beyond the Sexual Binary. Joan Nestle, Clare Howell and Riki Wilchins (eds.) 2002. Alyson Books.

The Last Time I Wore a Dress: A Memoir. Dylan Scholinski. 1997. Riverhead Books.

Man Alive: A True Story of Violence, Forgiveness, and Becoming A Man. Thomas Page McBee. 2014. City Lights Publishers.

Mark 947: A Life Shaped by God, Gender, and Force of Will. Calpernia Addams. 2002. iUniverse.

My Husband Betty: Love, Sex and Life with a Crossdresser. Helen Boyd. 2003. Thunders Mouth Press.

Nobody Passes: Rejecting the Rules of Gender and Conformity. Mattilda AKA Matt Bernstein Sycamore (editor). 2006. Seal Press.

Out of the Ordinary: Essays on Growing Up With Gay, Lesbian and Transgender Parents. 2010. Stonewall Inn Editions.

Real Man Adventures. T. Cooper. McSweeney's. 2012.

Redefining Realness: My Path to Womanhood, Love & So Much More. Janet Mock. 2014. Atria Books.

Sexual Metamorphosis: An Anthology of Transsexual Memoirs. Jonathan Ames (editor). 2005. Vintage Books.

She's Not the Man I Married. Helen Boyd. 2007. Seal Press.

She's Not There: A Life in Two Genders. Jennifer Finney Boylan. 2013. Broadway Books.

Stuck In The Middle With You: A Memoir of Parenting in Three Genders. Jennifer Finney Boylan. 2014. Broadway Books.

The Testosterone Files: My Hormonal and Social Transformation from Female to Male. Max Wolf Valerio. 2006. Seal Press.

Through the Door of Life: A Jewish Journey Between Genders. Joy Ladin. 2013. University of Wisconsin Press.

Whipping Girl: A Transsexual Woman on Sexism and the Scapegoating of Femininity. Julia Serrano. 2007. Seal Press.

Relationships:

Love, Always: Partners of Trans People on Intimacy, Challenge & Resilience. Becky Garrison & Jordan Johnson (eds). 2015. Transgress Press.

My Husband Betty: Love, Sex and Life with a Crossdresser. Helen Boyd. 2003. Thunders Mouth Press.

She's Not the Man I Married: My Life with a Transgender Husband. Helen Boyd. 2007. Seal Press.

Transition:

Freeing Ourselves: A Guide to Health and Self Love for Brown Bois. 2011. The Brown Boi Project.

Hung Jury: Testimonies of Genital Surgery by Transsexual Men. Trystan T Cotton (editor). 2013. Transgress Press.

Letters for My Sisters: Transitional Wisdom in Retrospect. Andrea James & Deanne Thornton (eds). 2014. Transgress Press.

Manning Up: Transsexual Men on Finding Brotherhood, Family & Themselves. Zander Keig & Mitch Kellaway. 2014. Transgress Press.

REAL TALK for TEENS: Jump Start Guide to Gender Transitioning and Beyond. 2015. Seth Jamison Rainess. Transgress Press.

CHILDREN'S BOOKS

10,000 Dresses. Marcus Ewert. 2008. Seven Stories.

About Chris. Nina Benedetto. 2015. CreateSpace.

All I Want to Be Is Me. Phyllis Rothblatt. 2011. CreateSpace.

Be Who You Are. Jennifer Carr. 2012. Author House Press.

Call Me Tree/LLamame Arbol. Maya Christina Gonzalez. 2014. Children's Press.

George. Alex Gino. 2015. Scholastic Press.

I am Jazz. Jessica Herthel, Jazz Jennings, and Shelagh McNicholas. 2014. Dial Press.

Jacob's New Dress. Sarah Hoffman and Ian Hoffman. 2014. Albert Whitman and Company.

My Favorite Color is Pink. Nina Benedetto. 2015. CreateSpace.

My New Daddy. Lilly Mossiano. 2013. CreateSpace.

My New Mommy. Lilly Mossiano. 2012. CreateSpace.

My Princess Boy: A Mom's Story About a Young Boy Who Loves to Dress Up. Cheryl Kilodavis. 2009. Simon and Schuster Press.

Nonnie Talks About Gender. Mary Jo Podgurski, PhD. 2014. CreateSpace Independent Publishing.

Roland Humphrey Is Wearing a WHAT? Eileen Kiernan-Johnson. 2013. Huntley Rahara Press

What Makes a Baby. Cory Silverberg. 2012. Seven Stories.

When Kayla was Kyle. Amy Fabrikant. 2013. Avid Readers Publishing Group.

When Leonard Lost His Spots: A Trans Parent Tail. Monique Costa. 2012. DodiPress.

YOUNG ADULT

Adam. Ariel Schrag. 2014. Mariner Books.

Alex As Well. Alyssa Brugman. 2015. Henry Holt and Company.

Almost Perfect. Brian Katcher. 2010. Delacorte Books for Young Readers

Beautiful Music For Ugly Children. Kirstin Cronn-Mills. 2012. Flux.

Gracefully Grayson. Ami Polonsky. 2014. Disney-Hyperion.

Hello, Cruel World: 101 Alternatives to Suicide for Teens, Freaks, and Other Outlaws. Bornstein, Kate. 2006. Seven Stories Press.

I Am J. Chris Beam. 2011. Little, Brown Books for Young Readers

Lost Boi. Sassafras Lowrey. 2015. Arsenal Pulp Press.

Luna. Julie Anne Peters. 2006. Little Brown Books.

Parrotfish. Ellen Wittlinger. 2011. Simon and Schuster Books for Young Readers.

Rethinking Normal: A Memoir In Transition. Katie Rain Hill. 2014. Simon and Schuster Books for Young Readers.

Roving Pack. Sassafras Lowrey. PoMo Freakshow. 2012.

Some Assembly Required: The Not-So-Secret Life of a Transgender Teen. Arin Andrews. 2014. Simon & Schuster Books for Young Readers.

DOCUMENTARIES

This is a selection of documentaries about transgender people and related themes. Many more can be found online. These are suggested starting points for facilitators using this book, both for use in trainings (see **Guidance on Transgender Documentaries** on page 38) and for personal knowledge development.

100% Woman: www.100percentwoman.com

The Aggressives: www.7thart.com/films/The-Aggressives

Austin Unbound: www.austinunbound.org

Becoming Me – In The Life: www.youtube.com/watch?v=IxzKlPVceWg

Becoming Me – The Gender Within: digital.films.com/play/RHFWJ7

The Believers: cart.frameline.org/ProductDetails.asp?ProductCode=T642

Boy I Am: www.wmm.com/filmcatalog/pages/c696.shtml

Call Me Malcolm: www.callmemalcom.com

Cruel & Unusual: www.outcast-films.com/films/cu/

Diagnosing Difference: www.diagnosingdifference.com

Ethical is Not Just: Transgender Populations and Health Care: https://www.youtube.com/watch?v=XKUG6-saDio

Everyone Matters: www.glad.org/work/everyone-matters

FREE CeCe: www.freececedocumentary.net

Girl Inside: www.wmm.com/filmcatalog/pages/c708.shtml

Georgie Girl: www.pbs.org/pov/georgiegirl

Growing Up Trans PBS Frontline: www.pbs.org/wgbh/pages/frontline/growing-up-trans/

How Do I Look: www.howdoilooknyc.org

I Am: Transgender People Speak (Series): www.transpeoplespeak.org

I'm Just Anneke: www.newdaydigital.com/I-m-Just-Anneke.html

I am Jazz: A Family In Transition: www.transkidspurplerainbow.org/featured/i-am-jazz-a-family-in-transition

I am Jazz (Series): www.tlc.com/tv-shows/i-am-jazz/

In The Turn: www.intheturn.com

I Stand Corrected: www.istandcorrectedmovie.com

Just Call Me Kade: cart.frameline.org/ProductDetails.asp?ProductCode=T526

Kumu Hina: www.kumuhina.com

Lady Valor: www.ladyvalorfilm.com/

Mala Mala: www.facebook.com/malamalathemovie

No Dumb Questions & No Dumb Questions 5 Years Later: www.nodumbquestions.com

On The Male Side of Middle: www.calvinneufeld.com/2011/07/on-male-side-of-middle.html

Paris Is Burning: www.miramax.com/movie/paris-is-burning/

Passing Ellenville: www.facebook.com/passingellenville

Pay It No Mind: The Life & Times of Marsha P Johnson: www.frameline.org/now-showing/frameline-voices/pay-it-no-mind-marsha-p-johnson

Prison Industrial Complex: Trans Views: www.youtube.com/watch?v=S5qw2kViAaM

Prodigal Sons: www.prodigalsonsfilm.com

Queer and Pleasant Danger: www.katebornsteinthemovie.com

Red Without Blue: www.redwithoutblue.com

Riot Acts: Flaunting Gender Deviance in Music Performance: www.riotactsfilm.com

The Same Difference: thesamedifferencedocumentary.tumblr.com/

Screaming Queens: The Riot at Compton's Cafeteria: http://cart.frameline.org/ProductDetails.asp?ProductCode=T636

She's a Boy I Knew: outcast-films.com/shes-a-boy-i-knew/

Southern Comfort: www.nextwavefilms.com/southern/

Still Black: Portrait of Black Transmen: www.stillblackfilm.org

Straightboy Lessons: cart.frameline.org/ProductDetails.asp?ProductCode=T527

Straightlaced: How Gender's Got Us All Tied Up: http://groundspark.org/our-films-and-campaigns/straightlaced

Switch: A Community in Transition: http://www.boxxo.org/id2.html

Three to Infinity: Beyond Two Genders: www.threetoinfinity.com

Thy Will Be Done: www.newday.com/film/thy-will-be-done-transsexual-womans-journey-through-family-and-faith

TRANS The Movie: www.transthemovie.com

Transforming Families: vimeo.com/44406099

Transforming Gender: www.cbc.ca/doczone/episodes/transforming-gender

TRANSforming Healthcare: Transgender Cultural Competency for Medical Providers: http://cart.frameline.org/ProductDetails.asp?ProductCode=T810

Transforming Justice: Ending the Criminalization & Imprisonment of Transgender & Gender Non-Conforming People: https://vimeo.com/16952110

Transgeneration Series: www.docurama.com/docurama/transgeneration

TransMormon: vimeo.com/82104871

Transparent (Documentary): www.julesrosskam.com/transparent/

Two Spirits: www.twospirits.org

Working Together to Protect Our Transgender Community (Law Enforcement): http://www.sunandmoonvision.org/working_together.html

Zanderology: http://auralstories.blogspot.com/p/zanderology.html

ORGANIZATIONS

This is a selection of organizations that provide resources about, by, or for transgender people and communities and those that serve them. Many more can be found online. These are suggested starting points for facilitators using this book. We encourage you to find out more about the many organizations doing this important work, and the roles they can play in supporting your efforts.

Black & Pink: www.blackandpink.org
　An open family of LGBTQ prisoners and "free world" allies who support each other via the LGBTQ Pen Pals program that works toward the abolition of the prison industrial complex, rooted in the experiences of currently and formerly incarcerated people.

Brown Boi Project: www.brownboiproject.org
　Works to build leadership, economic self-sufficiency, and health of young masculine of center womyn, trans men, and queer/straight men of color—pipelining them into the social justice movement.

Campus Pride: www.campuspride.org
　Serves LGBTQ and ally college student leaders and campus organizations in leadership development, supports programs and services to create safer, more inclusive LGBTQ-friendly colleges and universities. Includes a Trans Policy Clearinghouse, LGBTQ-friendly college ratings, resources and research, national LGBTQ student college fairs, and tools for ongoing measurement to improve *campus* LGBTQ policies, programs, and practices.

Center of Excellence for Transgender Health: transhealth.ucsf.edu
　Works to increase access to comprehensive, effective, and affirming healthcare services for trans and gender-variant communities. Serves as a central hub for a wide variety of medical information including a learning center with online trainings, guides, reports, and fact sheets for health care professionals.

CLAGS: The Center for LGBTQ Studies www.clags.org
　CLAGS provides a platform for intellectual leadership in addressing issues that affect LGBTQ individuals and other sexual and gender minorities.

FORGE: www.forge-forward.org
　An organization dedicated to raising awareness about the ways in which violence affects the lives of transgender people and their loved ones, particularly as it relates to training providers around the provision of culturally competent services related to sexual violence, intimate partner violence, and hate-related violence.

Gender Spectrum: www.genderspectrum.org
　Seeks to create gender-sensitive and inclusive environments for all children and teens. Resources for parents and families who have transgender children in many topic areas including education, medical, faith, legal, social services, parenting and family.

GLAAD: www.glaad.org
　Works with print, broadcast and online news sources, and responds to and advocates for fairness and accuracy in media. Provides many transgender resources including FAQ and terminology guides, Transgender Day of Remembrance and Transgender Awareness Week resources, media reference guides, and more.

GLSEN: www.glsen.org
　Wants every K–12 student in every school to be valued and treated with respect, regardless of their sexual orientation, gender identity or gender expression; and believes that all students deserve a safe and affirming school environment. Provides resources for educators and professional development, and also conducts research and evaluation on LGBT issues in K–12 education. A wide-range of national reports and briefs detailing experiences of LGBT students are available.

Keshet: www.keshetonline.org
　A religious organization working for the full equality of LGBT Jews in Jewish Life. Keshet advocates to cultivate the spirit and practice of inclusion in all parts of the Jewish community.

Lambda Legal: www.lambdalegal.org
　National legal organization whose mission is to achieve full recognition of the civil rights of lesbians, gay men, bisexuals, transgender people and those with HIV through impact litigation, education and public policy work. Provides resources and referral, and a selection of resources on the rights of transgender people.

Many Voices: www.manyvoices.org
: A Black church movement for gay and transgender justice that envisions and works towards a community that embraces the diversity of human faith and ensures that all are treated with love, compassion and justice.

Movement Advancement Project: www.lgbtmap.org
: Provides research, insight and analysis to speed equality for lesbian, gay, bisexual and transgender (LGBT) people. Provides issues maps with information about transgender rights in each state, as well as policy and issues reports.

National Black Justice Coalition: www.nbjc.org
: A civil rights organization dedicated to empowering Black lesbian, gay, bisexual and transgender people.

National Center for Transgender Equality: www.transequality.org
: Comprehensive information on topics including aging, anti-violence, employment, families, health, HIV, housing, homelessness, identity documents, privacy, immigration, international transgender issues, military and veterans issues, non-discrimination laws, police and prisons, racial and economic justice, research and data, travel, voting rights, youth and student needs.

National Center for Lesbian Rights: www.nclr.org
: Advances the civil and human rights of lesbian, gay, bisexual, and transgender people and their families through litigation, legislation, policy, and public education. Provides resources on transgender law, and the needs and issues of transgender parents and transgender youth.

National LGBTQ Task Force: www.thetaskforce.org
: Advances freedom and justice for LGBTQ people. Fact sheets, infographics, reports and studies on topics impacting transgender people.

Out for Health: www.outforhealth.org
: Planned Parenthood of the Southern Finger Lakes LGBT Health and Wellness Project provides outreach, education, and information to LGBT people, their healthcare providers and the community at large about the importance of inclusive, welcoming, respectful care.

PFLAG: www.pflag.org
: Parents, Families, Friends, and Allies United with LGBTQ people to move equality forward. Support for transgender and LGBQ people and their families. Resources include pamphlets on supporting transgender family members, and being an ally to transgender people.

Religious Institute: www.religiousinstitute.org
: A multi-faith organization dedicated to advocating for sexual health, education and justice, including LGBTQ rights, in faith communities and society.

Straight for Equality: www.straightforequality.org
: An education and outreach project of PFLAG National to help empower straight allies in supporting and advocating for LGBTQ people.

Sylvia Rivera Law Project: www.srlp.org
: Works to guarantee that all people are free to self-determine gender identity and expression, regardless of income or race, and without facing harassment, discrimination, or violence. Provides legal assistance, prisoner advocacy, policy advocacy, tips for communicating with transgender clients in prisoners' rights cases, tips for transgender people when interacting with the police and jails, and more.

Trans* Athlete: www.transathlete.com
: A resource project for students, athletes, coaches and administrators to learn about transgender inclusion at various levels of play, including example policies.

Transgender Law Center: www.transgenderlawcenter.org
: A civil rights organization advocating for *transgender* communities. Provides legal information, attorney resources, and publications on issues impacting transgender people.

Transgender Law & Policy Institute: www.transgenderlaw.org
: An advocacy organization that brings together experts and advocates to work on law and policy initiatives that advance transgender equality.

Trans Lifeline: www.translifeline.org
: A U.S. and Canadian hotline run by transgender people for transgender people who are in crisis and in need of support.

Trans People of Color Coalition: www.transpoc.org
   The national social justice organization that promotes the interest of transgender people of color.

Trans Youth Family Advocates: www.imatyfa.org
   Empowers children and families by partnering with educators, service providers and communities, to develop supportive environments in which gender may be expressed and respected. Provides a wide variety of resources for parents youth, and educators.

The Trevor Project: www.thetrevorproject.org
   Provides resources, including a 24-hour hotline, for LGBTQ youth who are considering suicide.

Williams Institute: williamsinstitute.law.ucla.edu
   Conducts rigorous, independent research on sexual orientation and gender identity law and public policy.

World Professional Association for Transgender Health: www.wpath.org
   An international multidisciplinary professional association that promotes evidence-based care, education, research, advocacy, public policy and respect in transgender health.

ADDITIONAL ONLINE RESOURCES

There are many websites that provide information, support, resources and referral. This list includes some of the most commonly sought topics, along with a few suggested sources for each. Please note that Internet URL addresses, and the locations at which various reports are available online, can change periodically. Searching using the title of a resource or organization can frequently locate the desired information quickly and easily. If the topic in which you're interested does not appear below, consider searching for it using the search bar on several of the organizations' websites listed below, or under the *Organizations* heading in this section. This can help narrow results to those that are credible and of use to professionals.

Being an Ally

Guide To Being A Trans Ally. PFLAG. www.straightforequality.org/TransMaterials

Tips For Allies of Transgender People. GLAAD. www.glaad.org/transgender/allies

Trans* Ally Workbook: Getting Pronouns Right and What It Teaches Us About Gender. Think Again Training and Consultation. thinkagaintraining.com/resources/publications/trans-ally-workbook/

Discrimination

Injustice at Every Turn: A Report of the National Transgender Discrimination Survey by the National Center for Transgender Equality and The National Gay and Lesbian Task Force. 2011. www.endtransdiscrimination.org and www.ustranssurvey.org

Transgender Day of Remembrance. www.tdor.info

Family

Our Trans Loved Ones: Questions and Answers for Parents, Families, and Friends of People Who Are Transgender And Gender Expansive. 2015. PFLAG. www.pflag.org

If You Are Concerned About Your Child's Gender Behaviors: A Guide for Parents. Children's National Medical Center. childrensnational.org/~/media/cnhs-site/files/departments/gender-and-sexuality-development-program/gvparentbrochure.ashx?la=en

Health

How I Help Transgender Teens Become Who They Want To Be: Dr. Norman Spack. www.ted.com/speakers/norman_spack

Primary Care Protocol for Transgender Patient Care – A practical reference for clinicians caring for transgender patients. Center of Excellence for Transgender Health. transhealth.ucsf.edu

Providing Transgender-Inclusive Healthcare Services. Out for Health. www.plannedparenthood.org/files/4414/0606/9716/PPSFL_Providing_Transgender_Inclusive_Healthcare_Handbook.pdf

Trans Health Fact Sheets (Bilingual English and Spanish). Center of Excellence for Transgender Health and California Family Health Council. transhealth.ucsf.edu

WPATH Standards of Care, 7th Version by the World Professional Association for Transgender Health (WPATH). Available at wpath.org

Therapy

American Psychological Association. (2015). *Guidelines for Psychological Practice with Transgender and Gender Nonconforming People.* www.apa.org/practice/guidelines/transgender.pdf

Identity Documents & Legal Rights

Choose Your Issue Equality Maps. Movement Advancement Project. www.lgbtmap.org/transgender-americans

Identity Documents Center. National Center for Transgender Equality. www.transequality.org

Know Your Rights (Series). National Center for Transgender Equality. www.transequality.org

Lambda Legal Transgender Rights Toolkit. Lambda Legal. www.lambdalegal.org

Understanding Issues Facing Transgender Americans. 2015. By The Movement Advancement Project, National Center for Transgender Equality, and Transgender Law Center, in partnership with GLAAD. www.lgbtmap.org/file/understanding-issues-facing-transgender-americans.pdf

Personal Narratives

I AM: Trans People Speak – a collection of videos in which transgender people share their experiences www.transpeoplespeak.org

Transgender Lives: Your Stories – a collection of personal stories of transgender people www.nytimes.com/interactive/projects/storywall/transgender-today

Religion

A Jewish Guide for Marking Transgender Day of Remembrance. Keshet. www.keshetonline.org/2013/11/tools-to-observe-transgender-day-of-awareness/

Made In God's Image and *All God's Children.* Many Voices. www.manyvoices.org/get-involved/shop/

K-12 Schools

Bending the Mold: An Action Kit for Transgender Students, Lambda Legal and National Youth Advocacy Coalition. 2008. www.lamdalegal.org

Harsh Realities: The Experiences of Transgender Youth in Our Nation's Schools, GLSEN. 2009. www.glsen.org

Model District Policy on Transgender and Gender Nonconforming Students: Model Language, Commentary, and Resources, GLSEN and National Center for Transgender Equality. 2014. www.glsen.org

Ready! Set! Respect! GLSEN's Elementary Toolkit. Developed in partnership with National Association for Education of Young Children (NAEYC) and the National Association of Elementary School Principals (NAESP). 2012. www.glsen.org

Title IX Resource Guide US Department of Education Office for Civil Rights. April 2015. www.ed.gov

Social Service Inclusion Guides

A Place of Respect: A Guide for Group Care Facilities Serving Transgender & Gender Non-Conforming Youth by The National Center for Lesbian Rights & The Sylvia Rivera Law Project. 2011. www.nclrights.org/legal-help-resources/resource/a-place-of-respect-a-guide-for-group-care-facilities-serving-transgender-and-gender-non-conforming-youth/

Hidden Injustice: LGBT Youth in Juvenile Courts by Legal Services for Children, National Juvenile Defender Center, & National Center for Lesbian Rights. 2009. www.equityproject.org/pdfs/hidden_injustice.pdf

Know Your Rights: A Guide for Transgender and Gender Non-Conforming Students by American Civil Liberties Union (ACLU) and Gay, Lesbian, Straight Education Network (GLSEN). 2012.
www.aclu.org/files/assets/transstudent_kyr_20120508.pdf

Safe & Respected: Policy, Best Practices & Guidance for Serving Transgender & Gender Non-Conforming Children & Youth Involved in the Child Welfare, Detention & Juvenile Justice Systems by NYC Administration for Children's Services, LGBTQ Policy & Practice Office. 2014.
www.nyc.gov/html/acs/downloads/pdf/lgbtq/FINAL_06_23_2014_WEB.pdf

Sexuality & Relationships

Brazen: Trans Women Safer Sex Guide:
www.springtideresources.org/sites/all/files/Trans%20Women%20Safer%20Sex%20Guide.pdf

Fucking Trans Women zine, Issue #0.
fuckingtranswomen.tumblr.com

Let's Get Real: A Question & Answer Guide for Dating Trans Folks
www.rainbowresourcecentre.org/

Primed: The Back Pocket Guide for Transmen & The Men Who Dig Them.
www.optionsforsexualhealth.org/sites/optionsforsexualhealth.org/files/primed.pdf

Queer Tips
www.queertips.org

Sports

Guidelines for Creating Policies for Transgender Children in Recreational Sports, Transgender Law and Policy Institute. 2009. www.transgenderlaw.org

NCAA Inclusion of Transgender Student-Athletes, NCAA Office of Inclusion. 2011.
www.ncaa.org/sites/default/files/Transgender_Handbook_2011_Final.pdf

On the Team: Equal Opportunities for Transgender Student Athletes, by Pat Griffin and Helen Carroll. 2010.
www.nclrights.org

Workplace

Everyone Matters: Dignity and Safety for Transgender and Transsexual People, a movie focusing on workplace issues, by Gay and Lesbian Advocates & Defenders (GLAD) www.glad.org

Model Transgender Employment Policy: Negotiating for Inclusive Workplaces, by the Transgender Law Center. 2013.
www.transgenderlawcenter.org

RESEARCH STUDIES

A Gender Not Listed Here: Genderqueers, Gender Rebels, and OtherWise in the National Transgender Discrimination Survey. Harrison, Jack; Grant, Jaime; Herman, Jody L. LGBTQ Policy Journal; 2011-2012, 2, 13. williamsinstitute.law.ucla.edu/wp-content/uploads/Harrison-Herman-Grant-AGender-Apr-2012.pdf

Gender Identity and Sexual Orientation in People with Developmental Disabilities. Bedard, Zhang & Zucker, Sexuality and Disability, September 2010, 28(3), 165–175.

Harsh Realities: The Experiences of Transgender Youth in Our Nation's Schools. GLSEN. 2009. glsen.org/learn/research/national/report-harsh-realities

Injustice at Every Turn: A Report of the National Transgender Discrimination Survey. The National Center for Transgender Equality and The National Gay and Lesbian Task Force. 2011. endtransdiscrimination.org/report.html

Suicide Attempts Among Transgender and Gender Non-Conforming Adults: Findings of the National Discrimination Survey. Ann Hass, PhD, Phillip Rodgers, PhD, and Jody Herman, PhD. The American Foundation for Suicide Prevention and The Williams Institute. 2014. williamsinstitute.law.ucla.edu/wp-content/uploads/AFSP-Williams-Suicide-Report-Final.pdf

The 2013 National School Climate Survey: The experiences of lesbian, gay, bisexual and transgender youth in our nation's schools. Kosciw, J. G., Greytak, E. A., Palmer, N. A., & Boesen, M. J. New York: GLSEN. 2014.

The School Discipline Consensus Report: Strategies from the Field to Keep Students Engaged in School and Out of the Juvenile Justice System. **School Discipline Consensus Project. 2014.** csgjusticecenter.org/wp-content/uploads/2014/06/The_School_Discipline_Consensus_Report.pdf

When Health Care Isn't Caring: Lambda Legal's Survey of Discrimination Against LGBT People and People with HIV. Lambda Legal. 2010. lambdalegal.org/health-care-report

CONTRIBUTOR BIOS

Jennifer Finney Boylan, the author of thirteen books, is the inaugural Anna Quindlen Writer in Residence at Barnard College of Columbia University. She also serves as the national co-chair of the Board of Directors of GLAAD, the media advocacy group for LGBT people worldwide. She has been a contributor to the op/ed page of the *New York Times* since 2007; in 2013 she became Contributing Opinion Writer for the page. Jenny also serves on the Board of Trustees of the Kinsey Institute for Research on Sex, Gender, and Reproduction. Her 2003 memoir, *She's Not There: a Life in Two Genders* (Broadway/Doubleday/Random House) was the first bestselling work by a transgender American. A novelist, memoirist, and short story writer, she is also a nationally known advocate for civil rights. Jenny has appeared on the *Oprah Winfrey Show* on four occasions; *Live with Larry King* twice; the *Today Show*, the *Barbara Walters Special*, *NPR's Marketplace* and *Talk of the Nation*; she has also been the subject of documentaries on *CBS News' 48 Hours* and *The History Channel*. She lives in New York City, and in Belgrade Lakes, Maine, with her wife, Deedie, and her two sons, Zach and Sean. Check out the Twitter feed @JennyBoylan; or follow Jennifer Finney Boylan on facebook.

Jaymie Campbell, MEd has been working in health promotion, social services, HIV research, and education since 2007. After obtaining a Bachelor of Arts in Feminist Studies from the University of California, Santa Cruz, Jaymie took great interest in working with trans* populations in San Francisco. While conducting HIV tests and volunteering at the safe syringe exchange, he became enthralled with the wisdom of the harm-reduction model and decided to continue his academic career by achieving a Master's in Counseling Psychology, with emphasis in Community Mental Health, from the California Institute of Integral Studies. He focused his clinical practice on working with homeless and marginally housed queer and trans* youth as well as African American adults living with or at risk for HIV. Currently, Jaymie is the Ally Safe Schools Program Coordinator for Mazzoni Center in Philadelphia, PA. He works with lesbian, gay, bisexual, queer, and/or trans* (LGBQ/T+) youth establishing, and building capacity for, Gay/Queer Straight Alliances (GSA/QSA) in Pennsylvania middle and high schools. Jaymie also conducts professional development trainings for adults and is most passionate about the topic of racial microaggressions within education. He has created and developed workshops on race, gender, and sexuality microaggressions and has facilitated in both non-profit and academic settings for community members, educators, and providers. A third-year doctoral student in the Human Sexuality Studies PhD program at Widener University, Jaymie plans to focus his dissertation on strategies for recognizing racial microaggressions in sexuality education and non-violent strategies for response.

Emily A. Greytak, PhD, is the Director of Research for GLSEN (the Gay, Lesbian & Straight Education Network), a non-profit organization dedicated to furthering LGBT issues in K–12 education. She has particular expertise in transgender and gender non-conforming youth and authored the only national study on the school experiences of transgender adolescents. Her research is regularly cited by the media, including *USA Today, Education Week, The Advocate, Huffington Post,* and *People Magazine*. She is published in both practitioner and scholarly outlets such as *Transgender Studies Quarterly, Journal of LGBT Youth, Teaching Education, Journal of School Violence,* and the *Prevention Researcher*. Prior to her research career, Emily worked as a prevention-educator and professional trainer on child welfare and anti-bias issues for a variety of organizations including the Anti-Defamation League and the Pennsylvania Coalition Against Rape. She currently serves on the GenIUSS (Gender Identity in United States Surveillance) Group convened by UCLA's Williams Institute and the SAMHSA (U.S. Substance Abuse and Mental Health Services Administration) National Workgroup to Address the Needs of LGBT Youth. Emily holds a Bachelor's Degree in Psychology with a minor in Feminist and Gender Studies from Haverford College, and a Master's of Science in Education and a Doctorate of Philosophy in Education Policy from the University of Pennsylvania.

Jennifer Hastings, MD, was an art teacher and painter before medical school at UCSF, and is grateful for varied life experiences before medicine. As Assistant Clinical Professor, UCSF, Department of Family and Community Medicine, Jen is a family practice physician who started and is Director of the Transgender Health Care Program at Planned Parenthood Mar Monte Santa Cruz and has been actively involved in supporting Transgender Health Care Services around the country. Jen teaches abortion care through the UCSF TEACH program. Jen works closely with the Santa Cruz Transgender Therapist Team, and is involved in the integration of Behavioral Health and Primary Care for Safety Net Clinics and with Mindfulness and Medicine. Jen is a member of the Medical Advisory Board of the UCSF Center of Excellence for Transgender Health and intimately involved with Medical Conference Programming for Gender Spectrum. Jen works to increase medical access and understanding about the gender journey.

Calvin J. Kasulke is a writer and has been the Social Media Manager for upstate New York's Planned Parenthood of the Southern Finger Lakes LGBT Health and Wellness Program, Out for Health, since 2012. He was formerly a BuzzFeed editorial fellow and has recently been selected as a Wurlitzer Foundation Playwright in Residence in Taos, New Mexico. He is a graduate of Ithaca College where he was inducted into the ICTV Hall of Fame and is a recipient of the Harvey Milk Award for outstanding efforts to increase awareness and visibility of LGBT issues at Ithaca College.

Maureen Kelly, Vice President for Programming and Communications at Planned Parenthood of the Southern Finger Lakes, has trained locally, nationally and internationally for over 20 years. Her published work includes her book "My Body, My Rules," and a variety of articles in print and on the web for the SIECUS Report, American Journal of Sexuality Education, Advocates for Youth, Camping Magazine, the National Council on Family Relations, and chapters in "Trans Forming Families: Real Stories About Transgendered Loved Ones," "Sexual Lives: Theories and Realities of Human Sexualities," and a chapter in the *Encyclopedia of Africa and the Americas*. Kelly's media work includes a documentary film and a TV commercial that have won five international honors, including a Telly Award. Kelly is a Robert Wood Johnson Foundation Fellow and is designated as a Certified Family Life Educator, a Certified Sexuality Educator, and a Certified Sexuality Counselor. She is also the founder of Planned Parenthood's LGBT Health and Wellness Program, Out for Health.

Rhodes Perry, MPA, is a nationally recognized expert on LGBTQ and anti-poverty public policy matters, with nearly two decades of leadership experience innovating policy and program solutions for nonprofit organizations and government agencies. As Director of the Office of LGBTQ Policy and Practice at New York City's Administration for Children's Services (ACS), Rhodes leads a team of principal consultants informing the implementation of system-wide policy and practice changes. With his leadership, the Agency has developed a national LGBTQ policy implementation model, resulting in critical service delivery improvements for LGBTQ children, young adults and their families. During his time at ACS, Rhodes crafted one of the nation's most progressive child welfare and juvenile justice LGBTQ policies, designed a model training curriculum for thousands of staff and provider agencies, implemented a reporting and monitoring system, chartered a LGBTQ youth advisory council, and authored resources to equip staff with the necessary skills to address the specific needs of LGBTQ populations. Prior to joining Children's Services, Rhodes served as Director of Policy for PFLAG National where he led the policy strategy and advocacy efforts for the organization's 350 chapters located throughout the U.S. Prior to this, he served as a Program Examiner at the White House Office of Management & Budget, where he developed policy recommendations to improve the efficacy of federal benefit programs that provide assistance to low-income communities. Rhodes earned a Bachelor of Arts in Economics and Gender Studies from the University of Notre Dame, and obtained a Master's of Public Administration in Public and Non-Profit Management from New York University.

Elizabeth Schroeder, Ed.D., M.S.W., is an internationally recognized educator, trainer, and consultant specializing in sexuality education pedagogy, LGBTQ issues and working with adolescent boys. She has provided consultation to and direct education and training for schools, parent groups and youth-serving organizations in countries around the world for more than 20 years. The former executive director of Answer, a national sexuality education organization serving young people and the adults who teach them, Dr. Schroeder played a leadership role in the development of the *National Sexuality Education Standards: Core Content and Skills, Grades K–12* and the *National Teacher Preparation Standards for Sexuality Education*. She was a co-founding editor of the *American Journal of Sexuality Education,* and has authored or edited numerous publications. She is a frequently sought-out spokesperson and guest blogger in the news media on issues related to sexual health education and youth development and provides national and international conference keynotes on sexuality and adolescent development. Dr. Schroeder has received numerous honors throughout her career, including the Healthy Teen Network Carol Mendez Cassell Award for excellence in leadership in sexuality education, the American Association of Sexuality Educators, Counselors and Therapists' Schiller Prize for her approaches to teaching Internet safety to youth, Widener University's William R. Stayton Award in recognition of outstanding contributions to the field of human sexuality, and the Planned Parenthood Mary Lee Tatum Award. She has an MSW from New York University and a doctorate in Human Sexuality Education from Widener University. Her website is www.drschroe.com.

Nancy Jean Tubbs has directed the University of California, Riverside's LGBT Resource Center since 2000. She holds a Master's degree in Educational Administration from Texas A&M University, and has published articles on allies development and transgender-inclusive campus policies. Working closely with center staff, colleagues, and students, she has taken the lead in developing best practices and policies related to gender identity and expression. In 2005, UCR was the first public institution in the nation to offer a gender-inclusive housing option to all students. In 2009, after several years of advocacy work, UCR became one of the first campuses to offer trans-inclusive student health insurance. In 2012, Nancy Jean helped develop the nation's first intercampus retreat for Trans* and gender-questioning college students, T*Camp. She is currently working with students to host the inaugural Asterisk Trans* Conference in 2015. Nancy Jean is a radical bureaucrat who enjoys improving policies, spending budgets, writing reports, questioning gender, dialoguing sexuality, challenging systems of oppression, and wearing comfortable shoes.

Courtney Weaver, PhD, is currently the Assistant Director of Owls Care Health Promotion at Florida Atlantic University in Boca Raton, Florida. She earned both her Masters of Education and her Ph.D. in Human Sexuality Education at Widener University, where her dissertation examined implicit power motivation and risky sexual behavior. Throughout her time in graduate school, Courtney enjoyed designing curricula, particularly that which served medical students. Currently, in her full-time position, she educates college-aged individuals, but she also continues to work with medical students, and remains passionate about educating the next generation of healthcare professionals. She also serves as an adjunct professor at Florida Atlantic University, where she trains peer sexuality educators.

EDITORIAL & EXPERT REVIEW BOARD

Elizabeth Amaya-Fernandez, MPH, Senior Program Coordinator of Community Outreach; Center for Alcohol Studies, Rutgers University

Sarah Axelson, MSW, Instructor, Milken Institute School of Public Health, George Washington University

Jaymie Campbell, MA Professional Development Manager, Mazzoni Center

Stephanie Chando, MEd, MSW, LSW, Palliative Care Social Worker, Pennsylvania Hospital, University of Pennsylvania Health System

Melanie Davis, PhD, CSE, Our Whole Lives Program Associate, Unitarian Universalist Association

Laura Erickson-Schroth, MD, MA, Public Psychiatry/LGBT Health Fellow, Columbia University Medical Center; Editor, Trans Bodies, Trans Selves

Eva S. Goldfarb, PhD, MA, Professor of Public Health, Montclair State University

Emily A. Greytak, PhD, Director of Research, GLSEN (Gay, Lesbian & Straight Education Network)

David M. Hall, PhD President of David M Hall Associates, Teacher at North Penn School District, Lansdale, PA & Author of *Allies at Work: Creating a Lesbian, Gay, Bisexual, and Transgender Inclusive Work Environment*

Liam Heerten-Rodriguez, MSW, CSE, Instructor, Grace Abbott School of Social Work, University of Nebraska - Omaha

Maureen Kelly, VP for Programming and Communications, Planned Parenthood of the Southern Finger Lakes

Melissa Keyes DiGioia, CSE, Co-Founder & Director of Education, Finding Your Individuality (FYI), LLC

Michael McGee, PhD, Assistant Professor in Health Education, Borough of Manhattan Community College

Mary Jo Podgurski, RNC, EdD, President, Academy for Adolescent Health

Karen Rayne, PhD, Founder, Unhushed

Monica Rodriguez, MS, President and CEO, Sexuality Information and Education Council of the United States (SIECUS)

Jen Mainville, Project TEACH Facilitator, Philadelphia FIGHT

Konnie McCaffree, PhD, CFLE, CSE, CSES, Sexuality Education Consultant

Ryan W. McKee, MS, MEd, Adjunct Instructor, Center for Human Sexuality Studies, Widener University

Susan Milstein, PhD, MCHES, CSE, Professor, Montgomery College

Marcia Quakenbush, MS, MFT, MCHES, Senior Editor and Health Education Specialist, ETR

Michelle C. Scarpulla, MPH, MCHES, Assistant Professor of Public Health, Temple University

Elizabeth Schroeder, EdD, MSW, Sexuality Education & Training Expert

Lisa Schulze, MEd, CSE, Training and Education Coordinator, The Adolescent Health Project, Women's Fund of Omaha

Avery B. Tompkins, PhD Assistant Professor and Bingham Diversity Scholar, Transylvania University

Roey Thorpe, Director of Advocacy Programs, Equality Federation

Al Vernacchio, MSEd, Sexuality Educator, Friends' Central School; Author of *For Goodness Sex: Changing the Way We Talk to Kids About Sexuality, Values, and Health*

ACKNOWLEDGEMENTS

We wish to personally thank the following people for their contributions and assistance in creating this book:

The generous and learned experts who wrote introductory selections to help frame the content of each section: Elizabeth Schroeder, Jennifer Finney Boylan, Emily Greytak, Jaymie Campbell, Nancy Jean Tubbs, Jennifer Hastings, and Rhodes Perry.

Our amazing Editorial & Expert Review Board, who devoted countless hours to this project; and Liam Heerten-Rodriguez, who wrangled all their input as our fantastic Review Editor.

Our publisher, Planned Parenthood of the Southern Finger Lakes' LGBT Health and Wellness Program Out for Health, which believed in us and brought our dream to life and to the printed page.

Our copyeditor, William E. Barnett, PhD, WordCraft Editing & Writing Services, Ithaca, New York.

Book layout graphic designer Torri Bennington of West Hill Graphics, Ithaca, New York.

Artist Ketch Wehr, who created the cover design and other graphics.

Our legal sage, Gabrielle Sellei.

And all those who provided other help in specific topic areas and resources, especially Matt Dankanich, Calvin Kasulke, David Hall, Sue Milstein, and Bianca Jarvis. In particular, we thank Maureen Kelly and Elizabeth Schroeder for their generosity of time, energy and spirit in helping us make this work the best it could be, and providing ongoing support throughout the project.

We also wish to thank our countless dear colleagues, friends, and families who provided encouragement, good company, moral support, perspective, diversion and, occasionally, comestibles and libations, which were savored and greatly appreciated. We couldn't have done this without the gracious and persistent support of those who believed in us, our mission, and our work.

And above all, we hold in memory those members of our community that we have lost along the way and we honor the activists, advocates, teachers, and mentors who came before us and on whose shoulders we stand. We are privileged to continue the life work of creating a world in which transgender equality was a battle fought and won.